BIOLOGY AND MANAGEMENT OF MULTIPLE MYELOMA

CURRENT CLINICAL ONCOLOGY

Maurie Markman, MD, SERIES EDITOR

Biology and Management of Multiple Myeloma

Edited by

James R. Berenson, MD

Institute for Myeloma and Bone Cancer Research,
Los Angeles, CA

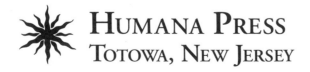

Humana Press
Totowa, New Jersey

© 2004 Humana Press Inc.
999 Riverview Drive, Suite 208
Totowa, New Jersey 07512
www.humanapress.com

For additional copies, pricing for bulk purchases, and/or information about other Humana titles, contact Humana at the above address or at any of the following numbers: Tel.: 973-256-1699; Fax: 973-256-8341, E-mail: humana@humanapr.com; or visit our Website: humanapress.com

Production Editor: Robin B. Weisberg.

Cover Illustration: From Fig. 2, Chapter 14, "Renal Diseases Associated With Multiple Myeloma and Related Plasma Cell Dyscrasias," by Alan Solomon, Deborah T. Weiss, and Guillemo A. Herrera.

Cover design by Patricia F. Cleary.

This publication is printed on acid-free paper. ∞
ANSI Z39.48-1984 (American National Standards Institute) Permanence of Paper for Printed Library Materials.

Photocopy Authorization Policy:
Authorization to photocopy items for internal or personal use, or the internal or personal use of specific clients, is granted by Humana Press Inc., provided that the base fee of US $25.00 per copy is paid directly to the Copyright Clearance Center at 222 Rosewood Drive, Danvers, MA 01923. For those organizations that have been granted a photocopy license from the CCC, a separate system of payment has been arranged and is acceptable to Humana Press Inc. The fee code for users of the Transactional Reporting Service is: [0-89603-706-1/04 $25.00].

Printed in the United States of America. 10 9 8 7 6 5 4 3 2 1

E-ISBN: 1-59259-817-X

Library of Congress Cataloging-in-Publication Data

Biology and management of multiple myeloma / edited by James R. Berenson.
      p. ; cm. -- (Current clinical oncology)
   Includes bibliographical references and index.
   ISBN 0-89603-706-1 (alk. paper)
   1. Multiple myeloma.
   [DNLM: 1. Multiple Myeloma. WH 540 B6148 2004] I. Berenson, James. II. Series:
Current clinical oncology (Totowa, N.J.)
   RC280.B6B55 2004
   616.99'418--dc22

2003028089

Dedication

*I dedicated this book to my wife, Debra,
and my children, Shira and Ariana.*

*Also, a special thanks to Christine Pan James
for her assistance in the preparation and editing of this volume*

Preface

Biology and Management of Multiple Myeloma is intended to serve as an authoritative, comprehensive, and detailed interpretation of published studies related to this B cell malignancy.

The book, written by a group of international experts on this disease, should provide insights into the newest breakthroughs—from the basic pathogenesis to the clinical aspects of myeloma. The first part of the book is devoted to the biology of myeloma, where important discoveries have been made in the last few years, many of which are clinically relevant. The characteristics of the malignant cell are shown, and the important roles of oncogenic changes, chromosomal anomalies, Kaposi's sarcoma herpes virus, and cytokines are described. New epidemiological findings and prognostic factors are analyzed in subsequent chapters. The increasing importance of renal disease, anemia, and bone disease has provided a basis for the inclusion of chapters devoted to the etiology and treatment of these complications. A thorough analysis of conventional treatment regimens is provided, as well as discussion of newer experimental approaches involving immunologic targeting, inhibitors of drug resistance, and new anti-tumor agents. The role of high-dose therapy is discussed in the chapters on allogeneic and autologous transplantation.

We have tried to provide a thorough, objective overview of each area. We hope that this book provides the reader with a thorough understanding of where
myeloma research is in the clinic and research laboratory.

James R. Berenson, MD

Contents

Contributors

JUTTA ACKERMANN • *Clinical Division of Oncology, Department of Medicine I, University Hospital Vienna, Vienna, Austria*

KENNETH C. ANDERSON, MD • *Department of Adult Oncology, Dana-Farber Cancer Institute, Harvard Medical School, Boston, MA*

MICHEL ATTAL, MD • *Hematology Department, Centre Hospitalier Universitaire Purpan, Toulouse, France*

WILLIAM BENSINGER, MD • *Fred Hutchinson Cancer Research Center, Seattle, WA*

MAURIZIO BENDANDI, MD • *Department of Experimental Transplantation and Immunology, Division of Clinical Sciences, Medicine Branch, National Cancer Institute, Frederick, MD*

JAMES R. BERENSON, MD • *Institute for Myeloma & Bone Cancer Research, Los Angeles, CA*

DANIEL E. BERGSAGEL, MD • *Department of Medicine, Ontario Cancer Institute, Toronto, Ontario, Canada*

WILLIAM S. DALTON, PhD, MD • *H. Lee Moffitt Cancer Center and Research Institute, Tampa, FL*

JOHN DE VOS, MD, PhD • *INSERM U475 and Unit for Cellular Therapy, University Hospital Saint-Eloi, Montpellier, France*

MELETIOS A. DIMOPOULOS, MD • *Department of Clinical Therapeutics, University of Athens School of Medicine, Athens, Greece*

JOHANNES DRACH, MD • *Clinical Division of Oncology, Department of Medicine I, University Hospital Vienna, Vienna, Austria*

BRIAN G. M. DURIE, MD • *Division of Hematology/Oncology, Department of Medicine, Cedars-Sinai Comprehensive Cancer Center, Cedars-Sinai Medical Center, Los Angeles, CA*

GÖSTA GAHRTON, MD, PhD • *Departments of Medicine and Hematology, Huddinge University Hospital and Karolinska Institute, Stockholm, Sweden*

JEAN-LUC HAROUSSEAU, MD • *Hematology Department, CHU Hotel Dieu, Nantes, France*

GUILLERMO A. HERRERA, MD • *Departments of Pathology, Medicine, Cellular Biology, and Anatomy, Louisiana State University, Shreveport, LA*

DOUGLAS E. JOSHUA, MBBS, DPhil • *Myeloma Research Unit, Institute of Hematology, Royal Prince Alfred Hospital, Sydney, Australia*

HANNES KAUFMANN, MD • *Clinical Division of Oncology, Department of Medicine I, University Hospital Vienna, Vienna, Austria*

BERNARD KLEIN, PhD • *INSERM U475 and Unit for Cellular Therapy, University Hospital Saint-Eloi, Montpellier, France*

LARRY W. KWAK, MD, PhD • *Department of Lymphoma/Myeloma, M.D. Anderson Cancer Center, Houston, TX*

ROBERT A. KYLE, MD • *Consultant, Division of Hematology and Internal Medicine, Mayo Clinic; Professor of Medicine and of Laboratory Medicine, Mayo Clinic College of Medicine; Rochester, MN*

TERRY H. LANDOWSKI, PhD • *Department of Medicine, Arizona Cancer Center, University of Arizona, Tucson, AZ*

HEINZ LUDWIG, MD • *Departments of Medicine I and Oncology, Wilhelminenspital, Vienna, Austria*

HAKAN MELLSTEDT, MD, PhD • *Departments of Oncology and Hematology, CancerCenterKarolinska, Karolinska University Hospital, Stockholm, Sweden*

ANDERS ÖSTERBORG, MD, PhD • *Departments of Oncology and Hematology, CancerCenterKarolinska, Karolinska University Hospital, Stockholm, Sweden*

SYDNEY E. SALMON, MD • *Deceased*

GARY J. SCHILLER, MD • *Division of Hematology-Oncology, UCLA School of Medicine, Los Angeles, CA*

SONJA SEIDL, MD • *Clinical Division of Oncology, Department of Medicine I, University Hospital Vienna, Vienna, Austria*

ALAN SOLOMON, MD • *Human Immunology and Cancer Program, Department of Medicine, University of Tennessee Graduate School of Medicine, Knoxville, TN*

ROBERT A. VESCIO, MD • *Division of Hematology/Oncology, Department of Medicine, Cedars-Sinai Comprehensive Cancer Center, Cedars-Sinai Medical Center, Los Angeles, CA*

DEBORAH T. WEISS, BS • *Human Immunology and Cancer Program, Department of Medicine, University of Tennessee Graduate School of Medicine, Knoxville, TN*

NIKLAS ZOJER, MD • *Departments of Medicine I and Oncology, Wilhelminenspital, Vienna, Austria*

1 Diagnosis of Multiple Myeloma

Robert A. Kyle, MD and Daniel E. Bergsagel, MD

1. INTRODUCTION

Multiple myeloma (MM) is a neoplastic disorder characterized by the prolif-eration of a single clone of plasma cells derived from B cells in the bone marrow. Frequently, the myeloma invades adjacent bone, destroying skeletal structures and resulting in bone pain and fractures. Occasionally, plasma cells infiltrate multiple organs and produce other symptoms. The excessive production of a monoclonal (M) protein can lead to renal failure caused by Bence Jones pro-teinuria or hyperviscosity caused by excessive amounts of M protein in the blood. The diagnosis depends on the identification of abnormal monoclonal plasma cells in the bone marrow, M protein in the serum or urine, osteolytic lesions, and a clinical picture consistent with the diagnosis.

2. CLINICAL FINDINGS

2.1. Symptoms

The most important symptom of myeloma is bone pain, which is reported by approximately two-thirds of patients at the time of diagnosis (1). The pain, which is often severe and incapacitating, occurs most often in the back or ribs and less often in the extremities. Spasms of back pain, usually induced by movement, do not occur at night, except with a change of position in bed. The pain is usually

From: *Current Clinical Oncology: Biology and Management of Multiple Myeloma*
Edited by: J. R. Berenson © Humana Press Inc., Totowa, NJ

relieved by lying down. Sudden pain in the ribs followed by localized tenderness indicates a rib fracture, even when the radiograph is negative. Sudden, severe back pain caused by a compression fracture may occur after a fall or after lifting an object. The trauma responsible for the pain is often minimal. The patient's height may decrease by 4 to 6 inches during the course of the disease as a result of vertebral collapse.

The most common symptoms are weakness and fatigue caused primarily by anemia, which occurs in approximately two-thirds of patients. Fever caused by the myeloma itself occurs much less frequently than in patients with lymphoma or acute leukemia. In patients with myeloma, fever is most often caused by a bacterial or (less frequently) viral infection. The physician must search diligently for the source of fever because myeloma is responsible in only 1% of patients. Fever is not uncommon in the patient with preterminal myeloma characterized by dedifferentiation and extramedullary disease (2). Pneumococcal pneumonia or septicemia is also not uncommon. Gross bleeding, seen in fewer than 10% of patients, most often consists of epistaxis or gastrointestinal (GI) bleeding, with thrombocytopenia frequently a contributing factor. The major symptoms may result from renal insufficiency, hypercalcemia, neurologic features, and other less common symptoms that will be discussed separately.

2.2. Physical Findings

The most frequent physical finding is pallor; skeletal deformity, pathologic fractures, bone tenderness, tumors, and purpura may also be observed. The liver is palpable in 4% of patients, and the spleen in 1% (1). Lymphadenopathy is uncommon. Extramedullary plasmacytomas, which result in large subcutaneous masses with a purplish hue, are rare at diagnosis, but are common seen late in the course of the disease.

2.3. Patient Manifestations

Patients may present with features of other organ involvement, with MM identified only after further evaluation. This disorder occurs primarily in the older patient (median age: approx 65 yr); only 3% of our patients are younger than 40 yr, and 18% are younger than 50 yr (3).

2.4. Renal Involvement

Patients with MM may present with acute or, more commonly, chronic renal failure. The serum creatinine value is 2 mg/dL or more in one-fifth of patients at diagnosis. Two major causes of renal failure are "myeloma kidney" and hypercalcemia. Myeloma kidney is characterized by the presence of large, waxy, laminated casts consisting mainly of precipitated monoclonal light chains (Bence Jones protein), which are seen in the distal and collecting tubules. The extent of cast formation correlates with the amount of free urinary light chain and the severity of renal insufficiency. Hypercalcemia, present in about 25% of patients at the initial evaluation, is a major but treatable cause of renal insufficiency.

Hyperuricemia is usually associated with renal failure. Primary amyloidosis (AL), which is seen in 10% of patients, may result in the development of nephrotic syndrome, renal insufficiency, or (more commonly) both. In fact, the occurrence of heavy albuminuria in patients with MM suggests the possibility of amyloidosis.

Acute renal failure may be the initial manifestation of MM. Patients may appear to be in good health and present with acute renal failure; the diagnosis of myeloma is not considered until the recognition of Bence Jones proteinuria or other features of MM. Acute renal failure is often precipitated by dehydration or hypotension. Intravenous urography may be the precipitating factor, but the risk is low if dehydration is avoided.

Patients may present with an acquired Fanconi syndrome or light-chain deposition disease. Acquired Fanconi syndrome is characterized by proximal tubular dysfunction that results in glycosuria, phosphaturia, and aminoaciduria. Light-chain deposition disease is characterized by proteinuria, often in the nephrotic range, or renal insufficiency *(4)*.

2.5. Neurological Involvement

Radiculopathy is the most frequently observed neurological complication. It is caused by compression of the nerve by a paravertebral plasma cell tumor or occasionally by the collapsed bone itself. Pain is aggravated by movement or change of position. Spinal cord compression may result when a myeloma arising in the marrow cavity of the vertebra extends into the extradural space. This condition occurs in about 5% of patients, mainly in the thoracic cord. Paraplegia may be the presenting event. Leptomeningeal myelomatosis is uncommon but is being recognized more frequently *(5)*. Fatigue, drowsiness, headaches, reduced mentation, and associated symptoms are features of this complication. Examination of the cerebrospinal fluid reveals abnormal monoclonal plasma cells. Sensorimotor peripheral neuropathy is rare in MM; when present, it is usually a result of primary AL. Occasionally hyperviscosity is observed, manifested by blurred vision, oronasal bleeding, headache, ataxia, and drowsiness. It is found in patients with immunoglobulin (Ig)A myeloma but rarely in those with IgG.

2.6. Hypercalcemia

Hypercalcemia may be indicated by the presence of weakness, fatigue, polydipsia, polyuria, constipation, anorexia, nausea, vomiting, confusion, stupor, or coma. It is important to keep in mind that hypercalcemia will lead to dehydration, renal insufficiency, and death unless treated promptly.

2.7. Other Organs

Other organ systems, e.g., the GI tract, may become involved. Occasionally, plasma cells infiltrate the rugal folds of the stomach or a plasmacytoma develops in the stomach, with bleeding and pain as the initial symptoms. Hepatomegaly, jaundice, ascites, and plasma cell infiltration are uncommon. Rarely, the gall-bladder, bile ducts, pancreas, and large and small bowel are involved by tumor. IgA myeloma is more likely to be present when the GI tract is involved.

The ribs and sternum are frequently involved, with such involvement often characterized by localized, painless swelling associated with plasma cell tumors; in fact, this may be the first manifestation of the disease. Pain develops when a pathological fracture occurs. Asymptomatic plasmacytomas may appear as soft tissue masses on a routine chest radiograph. Occasionally, the radiograph finding is interpreted as a primary tumor of the lung, and the rib involvement is over-looked. In some cases, extramedullary involvement of the mediastinum, medi-astinal lymph nodes, or lung is the initial finding. Pleural effusion associated with plasma cell deposits in the pleura may occur later in the disease.

Occasionally, myeloma involves the pericardium and may result in pericar-dial effusion and tamponade. Plasmacytomas have been reported in the atria. Myeloma rarely involves the orbit, although extramedullary myeloma may in-volve the base of the brain and be accompanied by destruction of the clivus, thereby producing neurological symptoms from cranial nerve involvement.

2.8. Other Forms of Systemic Involvement

Patients with MM are at increased risk for infection, particularly pneumonia, septicemia, or meningitis. *Streptococcus pneumoniae* and Gram-negative organ-isms are the most frequent pathogens in these infections (6). The propensity to infection results from an impaired antibody response, a reduction in normal polyclonal immunoglobulin levels, neutropenia, and glucocorticoid therapy.

Both excessive bleeding and thrombotic events may occur. Excessive bleed-ing may result from thrombocytopenia or qualitative platelet abnormalities, pre-sumably owing to M protein activity. Inhibitors of specific coagulation factors have been recognized, and abnormal clot retraction contributes to bleeding, along with hyperviscosity, hepatic involvement, intravascular coagulation, and amy-loid. Deep vein thrombosis and pulmonary embolism have been observed in these patients; whether they are due to older age, debilitation, or myeloma is unclear.

3. LABORATORY FINDINGS

3.1. Anemia

Normocytic normochromic anemia is present during the initial examination in about 70% of cases. Although leukocyte and neutrophil counts are usually normal, thrombocytopenia is present in about 5% of patients at diagnosis. The proportion of plasma cells is low, except in patients with plasma cell leukemia. In fact, only an occasional plasma cell is found in the Wright-stained smear in

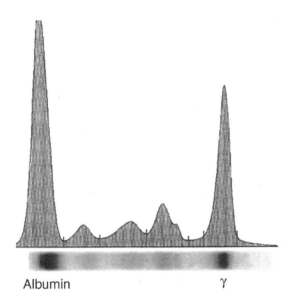

Albumin   γ

Fig. 1. *Top*, Monoclonal pattern of serum protein as traced by densitometer after electrophoresis on agarose gel: tall, narrow-based peak of γ mobility. *Bottom*, Monoclonal pattern from electrophoresis of serum on agarose gel (anode on left): dense, localized band representing monoclonal protein of γ mobility. (From ref. *6a*. By permission of Blackwell Munksgaard.)

about 15% of patients. Rouleau formation is common and found in nearly two-thirds of patients. Hypercalcemia is present in 25% of patients, and approx 20% have an increased serum creatinine value *(at least 2.0 mg/dL at diagnosis)*.

Overt hemolytic anemia is rare in patients with MM. When it does occur, it is often characterized by the presence of megaloblastoid changes associated with a folic acid or vitamin B_{12} deficiency. The erythrocyte sedimentation rate is frequently increased; however, a normal sedimentation rate does not exclude a diagnosis of myeloma. Serum alkaline phosphatase values are usually normal.

3.2. Serum and Urine M Protein

The serum protein electrophoretic pattern shows a peak or localized band in 80% of patients (Fig. 1; *6a*). Hypogammaglobulinemia is present in 10%; the rest of these patients have an equivocal abnormality or a pattern that appears normal. In our practice, IgG accounts for 52% of cases, IgA for 21%, light chain for only 16%, IgD for 2%, biclonal for 2%, and IgM for 0.5%. In 7% of cases, M protein is not detected in the serum with immunofixation; in 78%, it is detected in urine using this method *(1)*. κ Light chains are found twice as often as λ.

An M protein is found in the serum or urine at diagnosis in 97% of patients with MM. IgG and IgA myeloma have similar clinical and laboratory features at diagnosis. Patients with light-chain (Bence Jones) and IgD myeloma have a higher incidence of renal failure, lower serum M component levels, more light-chain excretion, and a higher frequency of associated AL than those with IgG and IgA myeloma.

3.3. Skeletal Findings

Conventional radiographs reveal punched-out lytic lesions, osteoporosis, and fractures in 79% of patients at diagnosis (1). The vertebrae, skull, thoracic cage, pelvis, and proximal humeri and femora are most frequently involved. Involvement of the mandible is not infrequent, and patients may suffer a pathologic fracture while eating. Osteosclerotic lesions are rare (7). Technetium (Tc) 99m bone scanning should not be used because it is inferior to conventional radiography, e.g., large lytic lesions may be overlooked because bone formation does not occur. Computed tomography (CT) is helpful in patients who have bone pain but no abnormalities on radiography (8). In one study, abnormal magnetic resonance imaging (MRI) patterns were obtained in 50 of 61 patients (82%) with MM (9). MRI in the evaluation of spinal cord compression is very useful (10).

Plasma cells usually comprise more than 10% (range: <5–100%) of all nucleated cells in bone marrow. Bone marrow involvement may be more focal than diffuse, and some patients may require repeat bone marrow examinations for diagnosis. In our experience with 1027 cases of MM in which a bone marrow aspirate and biopsy were both obtained at diagnosis, 4% had fewer than 10% plasma cells. The median plasma cell value was 50% (1).

3.4. Morphologic Appearance of Plasma Cells

Plasma cells may show striking variations on light microscopy. "Flaming" plasma cells are characterized by diffuse eosinophilic coloring of the cytoplasm resembling a sunset glow. Large flaming cells with the nucleus pushed to the side (which have been called thesaurocytes) were originally reported in patients with IgA myeloma; however, they are not specific to this type of myeloma. More often, the cytoplasm of the plasma cells is blue. It is also commonly fragmented, ragged, and extended, and may appear enormous and distended by lacunae. Some plasma cells contain Russell bodies, which are acidophilic, hyaline, crystalline, usually periodic acid-Schiff-positive structures composed of M protein that ordinarily appear as red granules within the cell, but may take the form of rods, amorphous red globs, clear crystals, or spicules resembling Auer rods. The nuclei of the plasma cells are usually eccentric and exceeded two- to threefold in volume by the cytoplasm. The chromatin pattern may be dense and either lymphoidal or reticular, with some degree of blocking or clumping. Nucleoli are common and may be large and multiple. Frequently, a relatively clear area (hof) is seen in the cytoplasm adjacent to the nucleus, representing the Golgi region.

Electron microscopy reveals a prominent, well-developed endoplasmic reticulum and a prominent, well-organized Golgi region. The endoplasmic reticulum is typically abundant and lamellar in configuration. Variations in shape and amount lead to varying degrees of endoplasmic dilation and dense body formation. Asynchrony in the nuclear and cytoplasmic maturation process in plasma cells is a prominent feature. Mature plasma cells have a relatively small, eccentrically located nucleus with a typical spoke-wheel pattern, whereas the malignant plasma cell is characterized by a large, centrally located nucleus, possibly with abundant cytoplasm and a marked perinuclear hof. The larger the nuclei and nucleoli, the greater the protein-producing capacity of the cell and the greater the likelihood of neoplasia. Cleaved, multilobulated, convoluted, or even cerebriform nuclei of variable size have been seen. The cytologic features most useful in establishing a diagnosis of myeloma are nuclear–cytoplasmic asynchrony with large nuclei and nucleoli, abnormal nuclear configuration, and variations in cell size and cytoplasmic staining.

Myeloma cells may have a very lymphoid appearance on light microscopy; this may result in myeloma being confused with lymphoma. Electron microscopy has shown a spectrum ranging from lymphocytes to plasma cells. A plasmablastic morphology is characterized by a fine reticular chromatin pattern in the nucleus, with no or minimal chromatin clumping. The nucleus must be more than 10 μm in diameter or at least one nucleolus of at least 2 μm in diameter must be seen. The cytoplasm must have little or no hof region and be less abundant in cytoplasm (<50% the volume of the nuclear area). The morphology is considered plasmablastic when plasmablasts comprise 2% or more of the plasma cells *(11)*.

The morphologic features of MM have been reviewed *(12)*. Identification of a monoclonal immunoglobulin in the cytoplasm of plasma cells using immunoperoxidase staining or immunofluorescence is helpful for recognizing polyclonal plasma cell proliferation caused by plasmacytosis owing to an autoimmune disease, metastatic carcinoma, liver disease, acquired immunodeficiency syndrome, or infection.

4. DIAGNOSIS

Suggested tests for patients in whom MM is suspected are listed in Table 1 *(13)*. The diagnosis of MM is usually not difficult, because most patients present with typical symptoms or laboratory abnormalities. Minimal criteria for the diagnosis include a substantial portion of the bone marrow composed of plasma cells (>10%) or a tissue biopsy specimen containing monoclonal plasmacytosis plus one of the following: M protein in serum (usually >3 g/dL), M protein in urine, or lytic lesions.

Table 1
Evaluation of a Patient With a Monoclonal (M) Protein

1. Obtain a complete history and perform a physical examination.
2. Measure the M protein content:
   • Serum M proteins: measure with SPEP (in g/dL)
   • Urine M proteins: measure the total protein excreted in a 24-h urine collection (g/24 h), then determine the light-chain fraction by electrophoresis of concentrated urine (UPEP) and calculate the M protein as grams per 24 h
3. Identify the light- and heavy-chain class of M protein using immunofixation.
4. Use SPEP to measure M protein levels; nephelometric immunoglobulin assays for IgG, IgA, or IgM overestimate the M protein level.
5. Measure hemoglobin, leukocyte, differential, and platelet levels.
6. Perform a bone marrow aspirate and biopsy for cytogenetic study, and plasma-cell labeling index test, if available.
7. Take needle aspirates of a solitary lytic bone lesion or extramedullary tumor(s) if the diagnosis is in doubt.
8. Evaluate renal function based on the serum creatinine value; use UPEP to distinguish proteinuria caused by glomerular lesions (urine contains an unselected mixture of all serum proteins) vs tubular lesions (urine protein consists mostly of light chains, which cannot be reabsorbed by damaged tubular cells).
9. Measure serum calcium and alkaline phosphatase levels; when indicated by clinical findings, measure serum cryoglobulin and viscosity, as well.
10. Obtain radiographs of the skull, ribs, spine, pelvis, humeri, and femora.
11. Obtain an MRI scan if a paraspinal mass is suspected or if symptoms suggest spinal cord or nerve root compression.
12. If amyloidosis is suspected, carry out needle aspiration of abdominal fat and bone marrow biopsy specimen staining for the easiest and safest ways to confirm the diagnosis.
13. Measure β_2-microglobulin, C-reactive protein, and lactate dehydrogenase levels, which are useful and independent prognostic factors.

M protein, monoclonal protein; SPEP, serum protein electrophoresis; UPEP, urine protein electrophoresis; Ig, immunoglobulin; MRI, magnetic resonance imaging.

The patient must also have the usual clinical features of MM, including end-organ damage, as defined in Table 2 (14). Connective tissue disorders, metastatic carcinoma, lymphoma, leukemia, and chronic infections must be excluded.

5. DIFFERENTIAL DIAGNOSIS

The main conditions to consider in the differential diagnosis are monoclonal gammopathy of undetermined significance (MGUS), smoldering MM (SMM), AL, and metastatic carcinoma (15). In MGUS, the M component is less than 3 g/dL, the bone marrow contains fewer than 10% plasma cells, skeletal radiography shows no osteolytic lesions or fractures, and the patient has no evidence of

Table 2
Myeloma-Related Organ or Tissue Impairment (End-Organ Damage)
Associated With the Plasma Cell Proliferative Process

Calcium levels increased: serum calcium >1.0 mg/dL above the upper limit of normal or
 > 11 mg/dL
Renal insufficiency: creatinine >2.0 mg/dL
Anemia: hemoglobin 2.0 g/dL below the lower limit of normal, or <10 g/dL
Bone lesions: lytic lesions or osteoporosis with compression fractures (use MRI or CT
 to clarify)
Other: symptomatic hyperviscosity, amyloidosis, recurrent bacterial infections (>2 episodes
 in 12 mo)

CRAB, calcium, renal insufficiency, anemia, bone lesions; MRI, magnetic resonance imaging.
(From ref. 14. By permission of Blackwell Publishing.)

anemia, hypercalcemia, renal insufficiency, or other clinical manifestations of
MM (16). Also, in asymptomatic patients, an M-protein value of more than 3 g/dL
and more than 10% of the bone marrow composed of plasma cells fulfill the
diagnostic criteria for SMM (17). Also, they have anemia, renal insufficiency,
hypercalcemia, lytic bone lesions, or other clinical manifestations related to MM.

The size of the scrum M protein, the amount of monoclonal light chain in the
urine, and the number of plasma cells in the bone marrow are helpful for distinguishing MGUS and SMM from active MM. The uninvolved (polyclonal)
immunoglobulins are usually decreased in MM, macroglobulinemia, and SMM,
but MGUS is characterized by a reduction in uninvolved immunoglobulins (as
seen in about 40% of patients with MGUS) (16,18,19). The quantitative values for
IgG and IgA obtained with nephelometry are higher than the M-protein spike and
thus overestimate the M-protein level (20). This must by taken into consideration
when following the course of MGUS. Other laboratory determinations—such as
the β_2-microglobulin level, the presence of J chains in plasma cells, increased
plasma cell acid phosphatase, reduced numbers of CD4 T lymphocytes, increased
numbers of monoclonal idiotype-bearing peripheral blood lymphocytes, and chromosome abnormalities with fluorescence in situ hybridization analysis—are
unreliable for distinguishing these conditions.

The plasma-cell labeling index may be helpful in distinguishing MGUS or
SMM from MM. The presence of a monoclonal antibody (BU-1) that is reactive
with 5-bromo-2-deoxyuridine indicates that the cell synthesizes DNA. The BU-1
antibody does not require denaturation; consequently, the presence of fluorescent
conjugated immunoglobulin antisera (κ and λ) can be used to identify monoclonal
plasma cells and plasmacytoid lymphocytes (21). The peripheral blood plasma-
cell labeling index correlates well with the bone marrow labeling index (22).

Using flow cytometric techniques, monoclonal plasma cells can be detected
in the peripheral blood of 60% of patients who have active MM and in more than

90% of those with relapsed or refractory myeloma *(23)*. Using more sensitive PCR-based methods, nearly all MM patients show the presence of malignant cells in the blood *(24,25)*. Patients with MGUS or SMM have very few or no circulating plasma cells *(23)*.

REFERENCES

1. Kyle RA, Gertz MA, Witzig TE, et al. Review of 1027 patients with newly diagnosed multiple myeloma. Mayo Clin Proc 2003; 78:21–33.
2. Suchman AL, Coleman M, Mouradian JA, Wolf DJ, Saletan S. Aggressive plasma cell myeloma: a terminal phase. Arch Intern Med 1981; 141:1315–1320.
3. Bladé J, Kyle RA. Multiple myeloma in young patients: clinical presentation and treatment approach. Leuk Lymphoma 1998; 30:493–501.
4. Heilman RL, Velosa JA, Holley KE, Offord KP, Kyle RA. Long-term follow-up and response to chemotherapy in patients with light-chain deposition disease. Am J Kidney Dis 1992; 20:34–41.
5. Leifer D, Grabowski T, Simonian N, Demirjian ZN. Leptomeningeal myelomatosis presenting with mental status changes and other neurologic findings. Cancer 1992; 70:1899–1904.
6. Savage DG, Lindenbaum J, Garrett TJ. Biphasic pattern of bacterial infection in multiple myeloma. Ann Intern Med 1982; 96:47–50.
6a. Kyle RA, Rajkumar SV. Monoclonal gammopathies of undetermined significance: a review. Immunol Rev 2003; 194:112-139.
7. Lacy MQ, Gertz MA, Hanson CA, Inwards DJ, Kyle RA. Multiple myeloma associated with diffuse osteosclerotic bone lesions: a clinical entity distinct from osteosclerotic myeloma (POEMS syndrome). Am J Hematol 1997; 56:288–293.
8. Kyle RA, Schreiman JS, McLeod RA, Beabout JW. Computed tomography in diagnosis and management of multiple myeloma and its variants. Arch Intern Med 1985; 145:1451–1452.
9. Kusumoto S, Jinnai I, Itoh K, et al. Magnetic resonance imaging patterns in patients with multiple myeloma. Br J Haematol 1997; 99:649–655.
10. Moulopoulos LA, Dimopoulos MA. Magnetic resonance imaging of the bone marrow in hematologic malignancies. Blood 1997; 90:2127–2147.
11. Greipp PR, Leong T, Bennett JM, et al. Plasmablastic morphology—an independent prognostic factor with clinical and laboratory correlates: Eastern Cooperative Oncology Group (ECOG) myeloma trial E9486 report by the ECOG Myeloma Laboratory Group. Blood 1998; 91:2501–2507.
12. Bartl R, Frisch B. Bone marrow biopsy and aspiration for diagnosis of multiple myeloma. In: Melpas JS, Bergsagel DE, Kyle RA, Anderson KC, eds. Myeloma: Biology and Management, 2nd ed. Oxford, England: Oxford University Press, 1998:89–121.
13. Kyle RA. Diagnosis of multiple myeloma. Semin Oncol 2002; 29 (suppl 17):2–4.
14. International Myeloma Working Group. Criteria for the classification of monoclonal gammopathies, multiple myeloma and related disorders: a report of the International Myeloma Working Group. Br J Haematol 2003; 121:749–757.
15. Kyle RA. Diagnosis and treatment of multiple myeloma in the elderly. Clin Geriatr 2002; 10:47–56.
16. Kyle RA, Therneau TM, Rajkumar SV, et al. A long-term study of prognosis in monoclonal gammopathy of undetermined significance. N Engl J Med 2002; 346:564–569.
17. Kyle RA, Greipp PR. Smoldering multiple myeloma. N Engl J Med 1980; 302:1347–1349.
18. Kyle RA. "Benign" monoclonal gammopathy—after 20 to 35 years of follow-up. Mayo Clin Proc 1993; 68:26–36.

19. Bladé J, Lopez-Guillermo A, Rozman C, et al. Malignant transformation and life expectancy in monoclonal gammopathy of undetermined significance. Br J Haematol 1992; 81:391–394.

20. Riches PG, Sheldon J, Smith AM, Hobbs JR. Overestimation of monoclonal immunoglobulin by immunochemical methods. Ann Clin Biochem 1991; 28:253–259.

21. Greipp PR, Witzig TE, Gonchoroff NJ, et al. Immunofluorescence labeling indices in myeloma and related monoclonal gammopathies. Mayo Clin Proc 1987; 62:969–977.

22. Witzig TE, Gonchoroff NJ, Katzmann JA, Therneau TM, Kyle RA, Greipp PR. Peripheral blood B cell labeling indices are a measure of disease activity in patients with monoclonal gammopathies. J Clin Oncol 1988; 6:1041–1046.

23. Witzig TE, Gertz MA, Lust JA, Kyle RA, O'Fallon WM, Greipp PR. Peripheral blood monoclonal plasma cells as a predictor of survival in patients with multiple myeloma. Blood 1996; 88:1780–1787.

24. Kiel K, Cremer FW, Rottenburger C, et al. Analysis of circulating tumor cells in patients with multiple myeloma during the course of high-dose therapy with peripheral blood stem cell transplantation. Bone Marrow Transplantation 1999; 23:1019–1027.

25. Rasmussen T, Jensen L, Johnsen HE. The clonal hierarchy in multiple myeloma. Acta Oncologica 2000; 39:7:765–770.

2   Epidemiology of Multiple Myeloma and Related Disease

Brian G. M. Durie, MD

1. INTRODUCTION

Plasma cell disorders include monoclonal gammopathies of undetermined significance (MGUS), smoldering/indolent myeloma, and active myeloma. Related disorders are Waldenstrom's macroglobulinemia, the heavy-chain diseases, primary systemic amyloidosis, and systemic light-chain deposition disease. The characteristic feature of these diseases is the involvement of cells that are either plasma cells or lymphocytes resembling plasma cells and typically the production of immunoglobulin (Ig) (heavy and/or light chains) in a monoclonal fashion. The most common myelomas are IgG or IgA κ or λ, and κ or λ Bence Jones-only myeloma. Waldenstrom's macroglobulinemia is IgM κ or λ in type.

There is an abundance of evidence *(1)* supporting the view that the malignant transformation in multiple myeloma (MM) occurs at a late stage of B-cell ontogeny

From: *Current Clinical Oncology: Biology and Management of Multiple Myeloma*
Edited by: J. R. Berenson © Humana Press Inc., Totowa, NJ

that precedes differentiation to the mature plasma cell, i.e., the target cell subject to malignant transformation has already been committed by antigen to the production of monoclonal IgG (κ/λ) or IgA (κ/λ), or IgM (κ/λ) in the case of Waldenstrom's macroglobulinemia. The mutation/recombination gene translation rates in antigen-driven B-cell differentiation have been variously estimated to be a million-fold higher than in somatic cells (2). Therefore, the occurrence of a transforming event that can eventuate in MM over the life span of B cells is a statistical reality. Studies of plasmacytomas in mice (3) have shown that antigenic stimulation is required for these transformation dynamics to occur. Until now, traditional epidemiology has been the major technique used to investigate the causes of this plasma cell transformation process (Fig. 1).

MM accounts for approx 1% of all cancer cases and 10 to 15% of cases of hematologic cancer specifically (4,5). Although the general incidence of MM in the United States is approx 4 to 5 per 100,000, there is broad range of incidence values for different populations, both in the United States and around the world, ranging from 1 per 100,000 or less for most Asians to 9 or more per 100,000 for populations of African origin. The basis for these racial differences is unknown. According to American Cancer Society statistics, the incidence of myeloma increased by 82% during the 1960s through the mid-1980s; the reasons for this are also unknown. The median age of patients at the time of MM diagnosis is approx 65 yr. Data from several institutions and countries around the world reflect the increasing incidence of MM during this century, as well as a decreasing median age at diagnosis (6,7). Nonetheless, myeloma remains a rare disease in individuals younger than 40 yr, with only 3 to 5% of patients falling into this age category. The extent to which a true increase in the incidence of myeloma occurs in individuals aged 40 to 65 yr remains controversial.

2. BASIC DEMOGRAPHIC PATTERNS:
INCIDENCE BY COUNTRY, AGE, GENDER, AND RACE

Tables 1 and 2 summarize incidence rates under various conditions. In Table 1, the annual age-standardized incidence rates of MM are summarized by country and by gender as high, intermediate, and low. The consistently higher incidence level in men vs women can be seen across the different groups. The much higher incidence rates for African Americans, Maoris, and Hawaiians, for example, are in sharp contrast with the very low rates for individuals from various parts of Asia, including India, Japan, the Philippines, and China. The intermediate rates are really quite consistent for the majority of the predominantly Caucasian countries, including the United States, Britain, Finland, and Germany. Similar rates apply in most other predominantly Caucasian industrialized nations, including Italy, France, Spain, and Belgium.

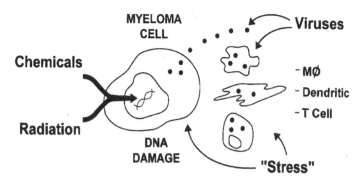

Fig. 1. The four types of causal factors for myeloma are depicted: chemicals (carcinogenic); viruses (oncogenic and/or triggering); ionizing radiation; microenvironmental stress factors (e.g., hypoxia).

Table 1
Annual Age-Standardized Incidence of Multiple Myeloma by Country

High Rates[a]	M/F	Intermediate Rates[a]	M/F	Low Rates[a]	M/F
US: African American:	10.3/7.1	US: Caucasian:	4.7/3.2	India:	1.8/1.5
New Zealand: Maori	8.4/7.8	Britain:	4.5/3.7	Japan:	2.1/1.6
Martinique:	8.3/8.0	Finland:	4.4/2.8	Philippines:	1.2/1.1
Hawaii: Hawaiian	7.4/5.6	Germany:	3.0/2.4	China:	1.1/0.5

Adapted from ref. *4*.
[a]Incidence per 100,000; listed as male/female (M/F)

Table 2
Annual Incidence of Multiple Myeloma
per 100,000 by Age, Gender, and Race

	Age Range	
Race	55–59 yr	75–79 yr
Caucasian, F/M	0.5/1.0	2.5/4.1
African American, F/M	2.0/2.0	4.5/7.9

Adapted from ref. *(8)*.

The striking effect of age is highlighted in Table 2. The very sharp increase in incidence among individuals aged 55 to 75 yr can be seen with the higher incidence for men vs women and also the substantially higher incidence for African Americans vs Caucasians. Although many explanations have been offered for the impact of age, gender, and race (discussed later in this chapter), more detailed analyses of molecular polymorphisms, human lymphocyte antigen (HLA) patterns, hormonal influences, and so on, will be required to clarify the biologic basis for these differences.

As highlighted by Schwartz *(6)* and Davis and colleagues *(7)*, analysis of multinational trends in MM can be helpful in assessing the interaction between environmental factors and the inherent predisposition of individuals of different ages, gender, and race. The broad patterns of incidence support the notion that environmental factors influenced the incidence of myeloma during the last 100 years *(8)*. Within that time frame, there has been insufficient opportunity for new generations to manifest any substantial predisposition differences.

3. RADIATION EXPOSURE AND THE RISK FOR MM AND MGUS

Evidence of an association between radiation exposure and the subsequent development of MM and MGUS is summarized in Table 3. It includes the findings of major studies that provide data from nuclear bomb survivors, nuclear facility workers, diagnostic radiation studies, as well as experimental data all indicating that ionizing irradiation can lead to the development of both MM and MGUS. Given the fact that these are relatively rare forms of cancer for which the predisposition varies by age, gender, and race, inconsistencies have been found in reported data. Because the dose and timing of radiation and additional confounding exposures are important, very detailed and careful analyses are necessary to draw any firm conclusions (*see* ref. *9*).

Nuclear bomb survivors are clearly at increased risk for MM. The association of radiation exposure to myeloma is strongly supported by a mortality study by Shimizu *(10)* and a very recent follow-up analysis by Rabitt-Roff *(11)* of UK veterans exposed to atomic radiation during nuclear tests in the Pacific Ocean. Rabitt-Roff identified 36 individuals who developed MM out of a population of approx 1500 that was exposed to the same radiation. The unique feature of the Rabitt-Roff study is the accurate ascertainment of long-term health effects among participants in nuclear weapons tests. The latency in onset of MM, especially beyond 5–10 yr, was not anticipated. Questions are raised about prior case ascertainment methods and the appropriate denominator to use for such analyses and comparisons. Additional studies are now underway (*see* NRPB web site: www.nrbp.org.uk). Of note, in this regard, follow-up data regarding US experience at Hanford, Washington and other Department of Energy (DOE) sites is available on the DOE web site *(12)*.

The data from nuclear facilities in the United States and the United Kingdom strongly support the assessment that radiation exposure can cause MM in a dose-dependent fashion. Fortunately, Gilbert *(13)* and Smith *(14)* provide information about dosing and the dramatic rise in relative risk increase with dose and duration of exposure. Likewise, Boice *(15)*, in evaluating diagnostic radiation, indicates a clear correlation between the calculated bone marrow dose and the likelihood

Table 3
Radiation Exposure and the Risk for Multiple Myeloma and MGUS

Type of Exposure	Type of Study	Relative Risk	Comments	Reference
Nuclear bomb survivors	Japan mortality	3.3	Negative incidence study unexplained	Shimuze et al., 1990 (10)
	United Kingdom incidence	36/1500 exposed[a]	Follow-up studies required	Rabbit Roff, 1998 (11)
Nuclear facility workers	US nuclear weapons plants mortality	3.3–33	Direct, increasing mortality with dose	Gilbert et al., 1989 (13)
	Sellafield, UK mortality	1.2–5.0	Increasing risk with higher exposure	Smith et al., 1986 (14)
Diagnostic radiation	Kaiser Permanente case-controlled	1.3–39	Bone marrow dose calculated and scaled	Boice et al., 1991 (15)
Thorotrast exposure	Denmark *cerebral arteriography incidence	4.6	Compared with general population	Anderson et al., 1992 (16)
MGUS Experiment in rhesus monkeys	animal	MGUS and MM seen in experimental animals	*Radiation therapy *Rescued with bone marrow transplant	Radl et al., 1991 (17)

MGUS, monoclonal gammopathy of undetermined significance; MM, multiple myeloma.
[a]This is initial report of ongoing analysis; 36 myeloma cases among 1500 exposed individuals

of the subsequent development of MM. The thorotrast exposure in Denmark is a well-established example of a special circumstance that can lead to an unexpected risk—in this case, the risk being subsequent development of MM *(16)*.

Of particular interest and relevance is the study by Radl in rhesus monkeys *(17)* in which a special technique was used that involved administering radiation to the animals then "rescuing" them by means of bone marrow transplantation. Such animal studies indicate that both MGUS and myeloma can result from high-level ionizing radiation exposure.

Overall, there is little doubt that exposure to ionizing radiation, particularly when exposure is directly to bone marrow sites, can lead to MM *(4,5)*. The risk is dose- and time-dependent. This observation, plus related observations correlating an increased likelihood of several cancers, supports the need for continued protection against potential radiation exposure. Individuals at risk must be informed and appropriate protections put in place.

4. OCCUPATIONAL EXPOSURES TO CHEMICALS AND MANUFACTURED MATERIALS AND THE RISK FOR MM

Although most now agree that radiation exposure can cause MM in particular circumstances, the risk of MM, MGUS, or both following exposure to chemicals remains controversial *(4,5)*. The challenge is to assess exposure to carcinogenic chemicals in patients developing MM and related disorders. The diversity and complexity of potential exposures *(18)* among various occupations and the subsequent correlation of such exposures with the development of a rather rare malignancy such as myeloma is a major epidemiologic challenge. It is to be expected that some results will be inconsistent. The occurrence of unintentional confounding factors and biases further complicates the situation *(9)*. Nonetheless, consistent patterns have been observed (Table 4), as well as several strong associations that provide "proof of principle" that chemical exposures can cause MM.

4.1. Pesticides

The largest number of studies of chemical exposure involves pesticides and agents used in farming occupations *(19–36)*. In 10 out of 14 studies of pesticide exposures, a substantial increase in the risk of MM was seen, with risk ratios in the range of 3.2 to 8.2 (*see* Tables 4 and 5). Of particular interest is an increased risk associated with pesticide exposure combined with exposure to other toxic chemicals, which may occur during farming. Examples of these "added risk" exposures include paints and solvents, wood treatment chemicals, and diesel engine fumes, as well as potential infections transmitted from farm animals. The risk ratio can rise from 2.1 to 7.9 with such combination exposures. This compounding of risk is a recurring theme in analyses of studies of myeloma, i.e., there is a consistent pattern or increased risk for MM with higher exposure or combined exposures.

Table 4
Occupational Exposures to Chemicals
and Manufactured Materials and Risk for Multiple Myeloma

Exposure	Risk Ratio	Comments
Pesticides	3.2–8.2	Overall: 10/14 studies positive
Pesticides alone	2.1	
Pesticides plus "farming"[a]	7.9	Other risk factors considered (e.g., paint, solvents, wood treatment chemicals, engine fumes, and infections)
Paints and solvents	1.7–5.5	Overall: 6/8 positive studies
All exposures	5.5	
"High" exposures[b]	10.0	Several studies indicate effects by dose and duration of exposure
Photographic chemicals	6.1	Single study, but supported by other data
Asbestos	1.7–61	Overall: 5/9 studies positive
"Benzene" plus petroleum refining	2.2–4.1	3/14 studies positive. Correlations complex (see text for discussion)
Weak associations:		
Hair-coloring products	1.4–4.39	• 4/7 studies positive • 4.39 risk ratio for black dyes
Miscellaneous exposures and occupations including, for example, Engine exhaust; metals (e.g., arsenic, lead); rubber and plastics industries; wood industries (esp. forestry); textile industries (incl wool spinners/weavers)	1.5–3.0	• Variable results mostly requiring further studies
Negative studies		
Alcohol		• Four negative studies
Tobacco		• Nine negative studies
		• One positive study (in Seventh Day Adventists)	Confounding factor(s) suspected (see text for discussion)

[a]"Farming" means added risks that occur while working on a farm.
[b]See ref. 38.

4.2. Paints and Solvents

The trend of increased risk with combined exposures is also noted in eight studies of myeloma risk with exposure to paints and solvents in various occupations (4,5,37–42). The risk ratio range is from 5.5 to 10 in individuals with average to high exposure to various components of paints and solvents. Six out of eight positive studies indicate the impact of both dose and duration of exposure.

Table 5
Epidemiologic Studies of Multiple Myeloma Among Farmers

Author (19–35)	Location	Relative Risk	95% CI	Comments
Boffetta	United States	3.4	(1.5–7.5)	
Cantor	Wisconsin	1.4	(1.0–1.8)	
Tollerud	North Carolina	0.06	NA	
Gallagher	Vancouver	2.2	(1.2–4.0)	
Nandakumar	Australia	1.4	(0.8–2.5)	
Steineck	Sweden	1.2	(1.1–1.3)	
Pearce	New Zealand	2.2	(1.3–3.8)	Aged 20–64 yr
		1.2	(0.8–2.0)	Aged 65+ yr
Burmeister	Iowa	1.5	NA*	
Brownson	Missouri	1.0	0.4–2.3	
Milham	Oregon/Washington	1.8	NA*	
Giles	Tasmania	0.8	NA	Men
		1.7	NA	Women
La Vecchia	Italy	2.0	(1.1–3.5)	
Fasal	California	1.0	NA	Men
		1.0	NA	Women
Flodin	Sweden	1.9	(1.1–1.9)	Men and Women
McLaughlin	Sweden	1.2	NA*	
Cuzick	England/Wales	1.6	NA	Risk calculated from % in paper

Adapted from ref. *36*.

Studies of paints and solvents highlight several other potential confounding factors, including the fact that the composition of the toxic material has changed over the decades. For example, benzene has been excluded from many products over the years. Other precautions have resulted in variations in risk, including the occasional increase in risk for MM in various occupations.

4.3. Photographic Chemicals

A study of exposure to photographic chemicals, which revealed a risk ratio of 6.1 for subsequent myeloma, raised many of the issues addressed in the studies of paint and solvent exposure *(35)*. The components of photographic chemicals have changed over the years, as have the facilities and precautions used by professional and amateur photographers. Patients presenting with myeloma during the 1980s and 1990s who had been exposed to photographic chemicals 20 or 30 yr earlier were potentially exposed to products prior to exclusion of known carcinogens. Also, the general precautions and use of ventilated dark rooms by photographers has increased substantially over the years. This highlights a problem with follow-up studies that is frequently overlooked. After an initial observation (e.g., myeloma in photographers), follow-up studies may fail to show such high levels of association, in part because the chemical composition and protective measures changed following early observations.

4.4. Asbestos

The correlations between asbestos exposure and MM are particularly interesting, (4,5) with five out of nine published studies providing evidence of a significantly increased risk. Again, much of the data suggests that co-exposures may account for variations among analyses.

4.5. Benzene and Other Petrochemicals

The correlation of benzene exposure with the incidence of myeloma in petroleum refining industries has led to particularly controversial data and conclusions (43). In several reports, investigators concluded that there is a correlation between benzene exposure and the risk for myeloma. In a recent comprehensive review, however, the authors concluded that although benzene and benzene related products can lead to leukemia, MDS, and related disorders, there is not enough evidence to establish an association with MM. A recent meta-analysis of case-controlled studies assessing the relationship between occupational chemical exposures (including benzene) and the risk for myeloma provided helpful information (44). A major source of benzene exposure in the studies analyzed was engine exhaust, and a strong correlation was found between myeloma and engine exhaust exposure, but not with benzene exposure. The authors proposed that several harmful chemicals present in engine exhausts—e.g., benzopyrene, ethylene, toluene, xylene, formaldehyde, and suspended particulate material— are potential culprits in these various studies, rather than the benzene itself. This can partly explain the conflicting study results and conclusions. More detailed molecular analyses designed to identify correlations between chemical levels in body tissues with the direct assessment of DNA damage will be helpful (9,45). Carefully studied cases of high-level benzene or petroleum product exposure in individuals who developed MM have been informative. For example, in a case involving a patient who developed a plasmacytoma in the jaw (followed by widespread myeloma), this occurred at the site of chronic exposure to a petrochemical-containing dental adhesive since childhood. Specific studies confirmed local absorption of that carcinogen through buccal mucosa.

4.6. Miscellaneous Chemical Associations

Borderline associations and negative studies should also be reviewed for less common exposure relationships (Table 4). Borderline associations can reflect the variability of exposure more than the danger of the chemicals or exposures involved. Four out of seven studies indicated a positive relationship between exposure to hair-coloring products and an increased risk for MM *(46–51)*. This is particularly true for exposure to black dyes *(46)*. Obviously, exposure to hair-coloring products includes individuals working in hairdressing and related industries, as well as product consumers. Because exposure varies among individuals, more detailed studies of individual cases at a molecular and tissue level will be required to document specific characteristics of potential exposure and the subsequent development of plasma cell disorders. Other exposures that increase the risk for MM include engine exhaust (see above) and metals (e.g., arsenic and lead), and exposures in the rubber and plastics industries, wood industry (especially in forestry workers), and various textile industries *(4,42,52,53)*.

4.7. Alcohol and Tobacco

It is unlikely that alcohol or tobacco use contributes to the development for MM. One of 10 studies indicated a positive relationship for the use of tobacco in Seventh Day Adventists. However, this finding is in such contrast to those of the other nine studies that it is felt that some other confounding factor(s) may account for it *(54,55)*.

4.8. Summary: Chemical and Industrial Exposures

Multiple studies in a wide variety of settings now support the evidence of principle that exposure to carcinogenic chemicals results in an increased likelihood of MM. Genetic susceptibility impacts the risk of specific exposures. There are enough data to recommend reduced exposures to potentially carcinogenic chemicals.

5. INFLAMMATORY AND AUTOIMMUNE DISORDERS ASSOCIATED WITH MM AND MGUS

5.1. Rheumatoid Arthritis

There is a long-standing notion that immune stimulation is an important pathogenic factor in the evolution of MM. Numerous studies have investigated the relationship of a variety of inflammatory and autoimmune diseases and the likelihood of developing MM or MGUS. It has proved very difficult to adequately assess the information generated. Studies have involved a broad range of patient and control populations. Multiple questions have been asked as part of the same study. Nonetheless, a number of comments can be made identifying several potentially important associations (Table 6). Perhaps the most striking associations have been with rheumatoid arthritis *(56–59)*. Four cohort studies have highlighted a strong relationship with MM (RR range: 3.3–9.5). These values are obviously highly relevant, but have been counterbalanced by other population- and hospital-based studies, which failed to reveal any relationship. Since there

Table 6
Inflammatory and Autoimmune Disorders
Associated With Multiple Myeloma and MGUS

Risk Ratio Observed/Expected	Condition	Study Findings
Multiple Myeloma	**High Risk**	
3.5		Rheumatoid arthritis • 4 cohort studies: • RR: 3.3, 5.0, 8.1 and 9.5 • Separate hospital- and population-based studies
2.5–<3.5		• History of allergies • Shingles • Pneumonia • BCG immunization • Eczema • RR 0.6–3.1 • RR 0.7–2.7 • RR 1.1–2.6 • RR 1.0–3.0 • Variable results
	Lower Risk Disorder	
1.5–<2.5		Multiple conditions, including: • Pernicious anemia • Hypothyroidism • Hyperthyroidism • Diabetes mellitus • Chronic disk disease • Various infections, including • chronic bronchitis • osteomyelitis • pelvic infection • urinary tract infection • ear nose and throat infections • scarlet/rheumatic fever • hepatitis • Diphtheria vaccination
MGUS		• Leishmaniasis • Cytomegalovirus infection

are important pathogenetic relationships between rheumatoid arthritis and MM, it is particularly relevant that high levels of interleukin-6 are observed in both disease. Recent studies have highlighted the possible pathogenic relationship between plasma cell disorders and the infectious process in rheumatoid arthritis, which will be discussed later in this chapter. Identifying the common predisposition, triggering factor(s), or both will be helpful in clarifying the relationships reported thus far.

5.2. Other Inflammatory Conditions

Several other relationships have been noted that pose a slightly lower level for MM (RR range: 2.5–3.5) *(4,5)*. The disease categories include a history of allergies—particularly to drugs, but also to household products—eczema, prior bacillus Calmette-Guérin immunization, and a prior history of shingles or pneumonia. Again, the results are not entirely consistent with various risk ratios reported in different types of studies and different populations. Nonetheless, there is enough of a positive correlation that a pathogenic relationship should be suspected for a subset of patients. Of note, the interest in microbial infections as the cause of many malignancies is on the rise *(60)*.

The role of infection as a trigger for MM is particularly difficult to assess, because patients with myeloma have a reduced immune response and, therefore, are susceptible to infection. Does this mean that patients with MM develop infections of different sorts because the immune system is already compromised, or, conversely, are the various infections part of the initial triggering process? As highlighted under the list of conditions associated with a lower risk (RR range: 1.5–2.5), a broad range of infections have been identified in this category. The infections involve most of the major organ systems: ear, nose, and throat, lungs, bone, urinary tract, cardiac, pelvic organs, and liver. Positive findings in such a diversity of studies strengthens the likelihood of a true pathogenic involvement. Of note, MGUS has also been associated with infections, specifically, Leishmaniasis and cytomegalovirus infection *(61)*.

5.3. Classification of Factors Involved in the Pathogenesis of MM and MGUS

The five categories of factors involved in the pathogenesis of MM are summarized in Table 7. Although familial or predisposing factors correlate with the evolution of myeloma and related disorders, remarkably little is known about them *(62)*. It is known that there are substantial racial variations in the rate of toxin metabolism and HLA differences that influence susceptibility to viruses, as well as deviations in DNA repair capability and the level of response to immune triggers (i.e., cytokines and hormones). How these factors vary among patients with myeloma is almost completely unknown *(62–67)*. Without this

Table 7
Factors Involved in the Pathogenesis of Multiple Myeloma and MGUS

Familial/predisposing factors:	Variations in toxin metabolism • P450 system polymorphisms • glutathione *S*-synthetase polymorphisms HLA differences influencing • viral susceptibility • IFN-α • IFN-γ Susceptibility to DNA injury • radiation sensitivity • DNA repair Intrinsic cytokine/hormone response patterns • cytokines: IL-6, IL-4, IL-10 • hormones: sex and pituitary
Residential/social factors	Local pesticide spraying/contamination Socioeconomic status • poor living conditions Recreational/hobby exposures • garden chemicals Personal habit risk factors • hair dyes
Occupational exposures	Variations in toxin metabolism: • P450 system polymorphisms • glutathione *S*-synthetase polymorphisms HLA differences: influence susceptibility to • viral infection • IFN-α • IFN-γ Susceptibility to DNA injury • radiation sensitivity • DNA repair mechanisms Radiation • Chemicals, metals, other
Antigenic challenges	Infections Allergies
Inflammatory disease Autoimmune disease	
Stress factors	Tissue stress/injury from implants, fractures, trauma
Psychological stress	Secondary neuroendocrine/immune effects of psychological stress

HLA, human lymphocyte antigen; IL, interleukin; IFN, interferon.

information, it will be impossible to move forward with molecular epidemiology to identify specific factors that are causally linked to myeloma. The residential, occupational, recreational, and stress factors identified also vary from patient to patient.

The potential complexity at the level of the individual patient is astounding. How can one assess an individual with a complex family and exposure history? Consider, for example, a patient who experienced all of the following prior to the onset of MM: a well-documented family history of hematologic cancer; lived in a farming community where pesticide spraying was common; regular use of black hair dye; infectious mononucleosis as child and hepatitis C as an adult; experienced a broken leg in a skiing accident that required the insertion of a pin; psychological stress when a child died tragically in an automobile accident. The existence of such a multitude of risks in a single individual creates a daunting analytical problem.

In an effort to clarify and assess such patients, this author has analyzed demographic data since 1992, both in clinical practice at the Cedars-Sinai Comprehensive Cancer Center as well as through demographic questionnaires supplied to all myeloma patients who become members of the International Myeloma Foundation (IMF). This has resulted in a database of more than 1500 personal patients and more than 50,000 patient IMF members. Controlled data analysis is clearly a challenge (Table 8). First of all, it involves a relatively rare cancer for which multiple predisposing factors exist. Multiple exposures may have occurred with varying patterns of timing, dose, and duration in different residential and occupational settings. Basic parameters may be confounded by additional cofactors as basic as socioeconomic status, alcohol intake, and tobacco use.

Some possible solutions to this dilemma are listed in Table 9 *(6,8)*. The overriding assessment to be accepted is that multiple factors can be involved in a multistep process. Ideally, a small number of patients can be studied in great detail to assess the genetic predisposition and tissue sampling, as well as to obtain a detailed exposure history and provide follow-up. With such information available as a baseline, well-defined populations can then be studied in more detail, e.g., in terms of specific places of residence, occupations, and hobbies. Larger databases (e.g., those now available to the IMF) can be used to evaluate the initial observations more critically and ask highly focused questions (e.g., to determine the impact of a family history of myeloma, cancer, or both). It is obviously important to take advantage of ethnic, gender, and age differences in all planned registry, cohort, or population studies *(69,70)*.

6. GEOGRAPHIC CLUSTERS OF MM

One method of assessing risk factors for MM is to investigate clusters of myeloma. Although epidemiologists tend to roll their eyes at the mere mention

Table 8
Difficulties in Identifying Causal Factors for Myeloma and MGUS

Relatively rare diseases	Difficult to obtain meaningful statistics
Multiple predisposing factors	Family history
	Sex
	Race
	Age
Multiple toxic/trigger exposures involved (*see* Fig. 1)	Toxin
	Antigenic trigger
	Stressor
Timing, "dosing," duration of exposures critical	Level of intrinsic susceptibility
	Level of combined cellular impact
Similar exposures achieved in many different residences, occupations, hobbies, and infections/stressor	
Multiple potential confounders/biases	

Table 9
Solutions to Causal Analysis for Multiple Myeloma and MGUS

- Use multfactorial/multistep process as model
- Study patients on case-by-case basis, especially small (e.g., family) groups. This allows:
  - Genetic analysis e.g., P450, glutathione *S*-synthetase, DNA adducts
  - Tissue sampling
  - Detailed exposure history
  - Careful follow-up
- Focus on defined populations by
  - Residence: e.g., associated with dioxins
  - Occupation: e.g., high-risk occupations such as firefighters
  - Hobbies: e.g., use of toxic chemicals
- Use large databases to confirm initial observations
- Take advantage of ethnic, gender, age differences to study mechanisms

of "clusters," clusters do occur. Thus far, eight carefully studied myeloma clusters have been published in the medical literature (Table 10). Obviously, the methodology for studying clusters is difficult. In his analysis of the published data, Schwartz used a variety of techniques to correlate the reported clusters with exposure to environmental dioxins (71–76). He noted, for example, that the reported clusters are consistently close to bodies of water or rivers. Using a unique statistical method, Schwartz was able to show that the eight clusters were more likely than not to be located adjacent to bodies of water (i.e., lakes, rivers, or seas) rather than in random geographic locations. Additionally, he was able to

Table 10
Reported Geographic Clusters of Multiple Myeloma

Location	Year	Number of patients	Comments
Thief River Falls	1970	7	Crude incidence: 10.6/100,000 No explanation
Aberdeen Scotland	1973	153	Evaluated NE Scotland 1960–1969 Crude incidence: 3.8 (vs 1.8)
Western Ireland	1985	117 MM 296 MGUS	Crude incidence: 4.5 (vs 1.1) High, but ? comparison
Petersburg Virginia	1979	21	Crude incidence: 11–12.5/100,000
Walney Island, UK	1992	7	Population: 11,000; therefore crude incidence very high
Baglan Bay, Wales	1992	42	42 myeloma deaths vs 28.3 expected
T Town, Japan	1991	7	Age-adjusted incidence: 7.3/100,000
Okechobee, Florida	1997	37	Age-adjusted incidence: 7.9/100,000

Data from ref. 72.

show that dioxin exposure was more likely to occur near water and was associated with an increased risk for MM. Examples used for this analysis included the increased incidence of myeloma in fisherman eating dioxin-contaminated fish on a regular basis in several locations around the world, including Alaska, the Baltic Sea, waters around the United Kingdom, and Lake Okeechobee, Florida. Further support comes from studies of individuals exposed to high levels of dioxins secondary to the industrial explosion in Seveso, Italy, as well as the increased incidence in myeloma in obese patients (owing to the accumulation of dioxins in fatty tissue). All of the gathered data support the hypothesis that dioxin exposure significantly increases the risk for myeloma.

These cluster analyses provide enough background information to recommend more detailed analyses in the future. New techniques for analyzing clusters have been developed which show great promise for statistical robustness in classifying and evaluating clusters (77).

7. THE INFORMATION GAP: PROBLEMS ABOUT SOURCES OF DATA ON TOXIC EXPOSURE

The preceding comments are based on data published in standard biomedical publications, including materials developed by the International Agency for Research on Cancer (IARC) of the World Health Organization (WHO), the most respected source of information on carcinogenic risk. The IARC updates data (e.g., on dioxins) regularly (78) and susceptibility (79). However, even the IARC has been subject to criticism for failing to classify known human carcinogens appropriately because of the possibility of industry backlash *(80)*. Researcher Lorenzo Tomatis was recently banned from setting foot in the IARC building in Lyon, France, because he accused the IARC of "soft-pedaling the risks of industrial chemicals." A new director was appointed in 2003.

Even more troubling is the lack of access to industrial or corporate medical data. Because toxic exposure can represent a source of potential litigation, much critical information exists in court documents and sealed corporate files. A recent book published by the The Center for Public Integrity highlights this issue and addresses the financial and geopolitical problems involved *(81)*. *Living Down Stream*, *(82)* by an ecologist, addresses the relationship between cancer and the environment, as well as public health concerns that arise because all information relevant to public safety and policy is not integrated for the common good.

Therefore, it is important to keep an open mind. Maybe "scientific" data and reviews do not always provide the full picture *(43)*. Vigilant, detailed, ongoing research is required to assess the nuances of relationships among chemicals and other toxins, the environment, and the risk for MM and other types of cancer. Does the metabolism of chemicals in the soil *(75)* pose a new unexpected risk? Are there occupations that unexpectedly confer an excessive risk for myeloma (e.g., elementary school teaching) *(83)*? Is there a possibility of myeloma clusters developing in Silicon Valley as a result of exposure to exotic chemicals in the computer industry or some other unexplained environmental hazard? *(84,85)* Are breast implants a new risk factor for myeloma and MGUS? A recent large case-control study shows that patients with MM are more likely to have breast implants *(85a)*. Why does Nogales, Arizona have 5 to 10 times the expected incidence of MM? Is it related to toxic dumping *(85)* and the water supply *(86)*? Only further studies will answer these and many more questions.

7.1. Viruses and MM and MGUS

As already discussed, many types of infection have been linked to myeloma. Viruses such as herpes zoster, bacterial infections such as pneumococcal pneumonia, plus other infections such as Leishmaniasis and syphilis have all been linked to the evolution of plasma cell disorders. Microbial infection has been linked to cancer overall *(60)*. Recently, questions were posed concerning whether infection plays a role beyond that of triggering the expansion of the abnormal clone via cytokine and other related mechanisms. Is myeloma the result of an aberrant idiotypic response to a specific infection or several types of infection? It has been demonstrated that the specificity of myeloma protein in patients with acquired immunodeficiency syndrome (AIDS) is against the gag protein region of the human immunodeficiency virus envelope *(86)*. Several reports have linked monoclonal gammopathies with hepatitis C infections *(87)*.

The increased incidence of myeloma in AIDS underscores the potential role of viruses in the pathogenesis of myeloma *(88)*. However, major reactivation of interest in this area stemmed from the observation that Kaposi's sarcoma (KS) virus HHV-8 is present in the bone marrow of patients with MM and MGUS *(89,90)*. HHV-8 does not occur in myeloma cells but rather in accessory cells, e.g., dendritic and other such cells in the bone marrow. The initial observation of the KS virus in bone marrow led to a series of attempts by groups around the world to document the frequency with which HHV-8 appears in bone marrow and other tissue samples, as well as the level of HHV-8 antibody response in serum *(90)*. Conflicting results have been obtained. Several groups confirmed the presence of HHV-8 in MM bone marrow specimens using polymerase chain reaction (PCR), whereas others failed to do so using a variety of techniques. The search for serum antibodies to HHV-8 has been largely negative results. Explanations for this have included the generally immunosuppressed state of patients with myeloma, as well as the possibility of genetic heterogeneity in the HHV-8 involved in plasma cell disorders. A recent report documenting the molecular heterogeneity of HHV-8 supports the notion that a mutation of HHV-8 that does not trigger a strong antibody response may be involved *(91)*. Further studies are necessary to clarify the role of HHV-8 in MM.

Another series of studies indicated a possible role for the simian virus 40 (SV-40) or related viruses capable of producing SV-40 T-antigen in patients with MM *(93–96)*. In a study of patients with active myeloma, RNA found in the plasma of 89% of patients experiencing a relapse was studied by PCR and found to contain RNA with SV-40 T-antigen-binding sites. This raises the possibility that the SV-40 (or Epstein-Barr virus, various adenoviruses, human papilloma virus, and other viruses containing antigens with similar binding potential) may have a role in the pathogenesis of the active disease. Additional studies have measured the amount of the RNA with SV-40 T-antigen specificity. Initial results indicate that blood obtained from patients with active myeloma contains substantial RNA levels, as well as microvesicles evident on electron microscopy and can produce an in vitro a cytopathologic effect characteristic of that of the "stealth virus" (truncated cytomegalovirus). Further investigations are necessary to clarify the implications of these observations.

In summary, recent observations of viruses point to a strong likelihood that viral triggers may in some fashion be one of the multiple factors involved in the causation of MM.

8. THE POTENTIAL FOR PREVENTION OF MM AND MGUS

The accumulated data strongly support the notion that various types of environmental exposures—including chemicals, radiation, and viruses—significantly increase the risk for MM and related plasma cell disorders. The remarkable diversity of exposures makes prevention planning a challenging prospect. It is rather easy to suggest that prevention strategies designed to reduce toxic exposures of known carcinogenic risk will help reduce the future incidence of myeloma. Many of the exposures discussed above are clearly carcinogenic. Appropriate precautions are only judicious at this point, not just for myeloma, but in general, because many individuals at risk for myeloma have already been exposed. What can be done for them? A recent report illustrating that Olestra can dramatically accentuate the excretion of dioxins highlights the possibility that high-risk individuals can be screened and receive short-term treatment to remove toxins that are present at elevated levels *(97)*. If DNA injury has already occurred, appropriate steps can be taken to reduce any potential for additional DNA injury or trigger factors such as a viral infection and local or systemic stressors. The more we learn, the better we can reduce the incidence of myeloma, which remains difficult to treat and is as yet impossible to cure.

REFERENCES

1. Warburton P, Josua DE, Gibson J, Brown RD. CD10-(Calla)-positive lymphocytes in myeloma: evidence that they are a malignant precursor population and are of germinal centre origin. Leuk Lymphoma 1989; 1:11–12.
2. Harris CC, Hollstein M. Clinical implications of the p53 tumor-suppressor gene. N Engl J Med 1992; 329:1318–1326.
3. Potter M. The developmental history of neoplastic plasma cell in mice. Sem Haematol 1973; 10:19–31.
4. Herrington LJ, Weiss NS, Olshan AD: Multiple myeloma. In: Schottenfeld D, Fraumerni JF Jr, eds. Cancer Epidemiology and Prevention. 2nd ed. New York, NY: Oxford University Press; 1996:946–970.
5. Riedel DA, Pottern LM. The epidemiology of multiple myeloma. Hematol Oncol Clin N Am 1992; 6:225–247.
6. Schwartz J. Multinational trends in multiple myeloma. Annals NY Acad Sci 1990; 63:215–244.
7. Davis DL, Hoel D, Fox J, Lopez A. International trends in cancer mortality in France, West Germany, Italy, Japan, England and Wales, and the USA. Lancet 1990; 336:474–481.
8. Miller BA, Ries LAG, Hankey BF, et al. 1993 SEER Cancer Statistics: Review. 1973–1990. National Cancer Institute; NIH Publication No. 93-2789, Washington, DC.
9. Taubes G. Epidemiology faces its limits. Science 1999; 269:164–169.
10. Shimizu Y, Kato II, Schull WJ. Studies of the mortality of A-bomb survivors: 1950–1985. Part 2. Cancer mortality based on the recently revised doses (DS86). Radiat Res 1990; 121:120–141.
11. Rabbitt-Roff S. Incidence of multiple myeloma in UK veterans exposed to atomic radiation in Pacific Nuclear tests. Occup and Environ Med 2003; 60:e18–e36.
12. US Department of Energy (DOE) Web site: http://www.hanford.go~safety/myelomaindex/htm. Posted 02/05/98.
13. Gilbert ES, Fry SA, Wigs LD, Voelz GL, Cragle DL, Petersen GR. Analyses of combined mortality data on workers at the Hanford site, Oak Ridge National Laboratory, and Rocky Flats Nuclear Weapons Plant. Radiat Res 1989; 120:19–35.
14. Smith PG, Douglas AJ. Mortality of workers at the Sellafield plant of British Nuclear Fuels. BMJ 1986; 293:845–854.
15. Boice JD, Morin MM, Glass AG, et al. Diagnostic x-ray procedures and risk of leukemia, lymphoma, and multiple myeloma. JAMA 1991; 265:1290–1294.
16. Andersson M, Sotrm HH. Cancer incidence among Danish Thorotrast-exposed patients. J Natl Cancer Inst 1992; 84:1318–1325.

17. Radl J, Liu M, Hoogeveen CM, et al. Monoclonal gammopathies in long-term surviving Rhesus monkeys after lethal irradiation and bone marrow transplantation. Clin Immunol Immunopathol 1991; 60:305–309.

18. Arcos J, Argus M, Woo Y, eds. Chemical Induction of Cancer Modulation and Combination Effects: An Inventory of the Many Factors Which Influence Carcinogenesis. Boston, Mass: Birkhauser; 1995.

19. Boffetta P, Stellman SD, Garfinkel L. A case-control study of multiple myeloma nested in the American Cancer Society prospective study. Int J Cancer 1989; 43:554–559.

20. Cantor KP, Blair A. Farming and mortality from multiple myeloma: a case-control study with the use of death certificates. J Natl Cancer Inst 1984; 72:251–255.

21. Tollerud DJ, Brinton LA, Stone BJ, Tobacman JK, Blattner WA. Mortality from multiple myeloma among North Carolina furniture workers. J Natl Cancer Inst 1985; 74:799–801.

22. Gallagher RP, Spinelli JJ, Elwood JM, Skippen DH. Allergies and agricultural exposure as risk factors for multiple myeloma. Br J Cancer 1983; 48:853–857.

23. Nandakumar A, English DR, Dougan LE, Armstrong BK. Incidence and outcome of multiple myeloma in Western Australia, 1960 to 1984. Aust N Z Med 1988; 18:774–779.

24. Steineck G, Wiklund K. Multiple myeloma in Swedish agricultural workers. Int J Epidemiol 1986; 15:321–325.

25. Pearce NE, Smith AH, Fisher DO. Malignant lymphoma and multiple myeloma linked with agricultural occupations in a New Zealand cancer registry-based study. Am J Epidemiol 1985; 121:225–237.

26. Pearce NE, Smith AH, Howard JK, Sheppard RA, Giles HJ, Teague CA. Case-control study of multiple myeloma and farming. Br J Cancer 1986; 54:493–500.

27. Burmeister LF. Cancer in Iowa farmers: recent results. Am J Ind Med 1990; 18:295–301.

28. Brownson RC, Reif JS, Chang JC, Davis JR. Cancer risks among Missouri farmers. Cancer 1989; 64:2381–2386.

29. Milham S. Leukemia and multiple myeloma in farmers. Am J Epidemiol 1971; 94:307–310.

30. Giles GG, Lickiss JN, Baikle MJ, et al. Myeloproliferative and lymphoproliferative disorders in Tasmania, 1972-1980: occupational and familial aspects. JNCI 1984; 72:1233–1240.

31. La Vecchia C, Negri E, D'Avanzo B, Franceschi S. Occupation and lymphoid neoplasms. Br J Cancer 1989; 60:385–388.

32. Fasal E, Jackson EW, Klauber MR. Leukemia and lymphoma mortality and farm residence. Am J Epidemiol 1968; 87:267–274.

33. Flodin U, Fredriksson M, Persson B. Multiple myeloma and engine exhausts, fresh wood, and creosote: a case-reference study. Am J Ind Med 1987; 12:519–529.

34. McLaughlin JK, Linet MS, Stone BJ, et al. Multiple myeloma and occupation in Sweden. Arch Environ Health 1988; 43:7–10.

35. Cuzick J, De Stavola B. Multiple myeloma: a case-control study. Br J Cancer 1988; 57:516–520.

36. Blair A, Zahm SH. Cancer among farmers. Occupational Med 1991; 3:335–354.

37. Bethwaite PB, Pearce N, Fraser J. Cancer risks in painters: study based on the New Zealand cancer registry. Br J Ind 1990; 47:742–746.

38. Lundberg L. Mortality and cancer incidence among Swedish paint industry workers with long-term exposure to organic solvents. Scand J Work Environ Health 1986; 12:108–113.

39. Demers PA, Vaughan TL, Koepsell TD, et al. A case-control study of multiple myeloma and occupation. Am J Ind Med 1992; 23:629–639.

40. Friedman GD. Multiple myeloma: relation to propoxyphene and other drugs, radiation and occupation. Int J Epidemiol 1986; 15:423–425.

41. Pottern LM, Heineman EF, Olsen JH, Raffn E, Blair A. Multiple myeloma among Danish women: employment history and workplace exposure. Cancer Causes Control 1992; 3:427–432.

42. Heineman EF, Olsen JH, Pottern LM, Gomez M, Raffn E, Blair A. Occupational risk factors for multiple myeloma among Danish men. Cancer Causes Control 1992; 3:555–568.

43. Bergsagel DE, Wong O, Bergsagel PL, et al. Benzene and multiple myeloma: appraisal of the scientific evidence. Blood 1999; 94:1174–1182.
44. Sonada T, Nagata Y, Mori M, Ishida T, Imai, K. Meta-analysis of multiple myeloma and benzene exposure. J Epidemiol 2001; 11:249–254.
45. Ambrosone CB, Kadlubar FF. Toward an integrated approach to molecular epidemiology. Am J Epidemiol 1997; 146:912–918.
46. Thun MJ, Altekruse SF, Namboodiri MM, Calle EE, Myers DG, Heath CW Jr. Hair dye use and risk of fatal cancers in US women. J Natl Cancer Inst 1994; 86:210–215.
47. Zahm SH, Weisenburger DD, Babbitt PA, Saal RC, Vaught JB, Blair A. Use of hair coloring products and the risk of lymphoma, multiple myeloma, and chronic lymphocytic leukemia. Am J Public Health 1992; 82:990–997.
48. Herrington LJ, Weiss NS, Koepseli TD, et al. Exposure to hair-coloring products in relation to the risk of multiple myeloma. Am J Public Health 1994; 84:1142–1144.
49. Brown LM, Everett GD, Burmfister LF, Blair A. Hair dye use and multiple myeloma in white men. Am J Public Health 1992; 82:1673–1674.
50. Teta JM, Walrath J, Meigs JW, Flannery JT. Cancer incidence among cosmetologists. J Natl Cancer Inst 1984; 72:1051–1057.
51. Eriksson M, Karisson M. Occupational and other environmental factors and multiple myeloma: a population-based case-control study. Br J Ind Med 1992; 49:95–103.
52. Hansen ES. A follow-up study on the mortality of truck drivers. Am J Ind Med 1993; 23:811–821.
53. Kawachi I, Pearce N, Fraser J. A New Zealand cancer registry-based study of cancer in wood workers. Cancer 1989; 64:2609–2613.
54. Linet MS, McLaughlin JK, Hsing AW, et al. Is cigarette smoking a risk factor for non-Hodgkin's lymphoma or multiple myeloma? Results from the Lutheran Brotherhood Cohort Study. Leuk Res 1992; 16:621–624.
55. Mills PK, Newell GR, Beeson WL, Fraser GE, Phillips RLP. History of cigarette smoking and risk of leukemia and mycloma: results form the Adventists Health Study. J Natl Cancer Inst 1990; 82:1832–1836.
56. Isomarki HA, Hakulinen U. Excess risk of lymphomas, leukemia and myeloma in patients with rheumatoid arthritis. J Chron Dis 1978; 31:691–696.
57. Katusic S, Beard CM, Kurland L, Weis JW, Bergstralh E. Occurrence of malignant neoplasm in the Rochester, Minnesota, rheumatoid arthritis cohort. Am J Med 1985; 78 (suppl 1A):50–55.
58. Matteson EL, Hickey AR, Maguire L, Tilson JJ. Urowitz MB. Occurrence of neoplasia in patients with rheumatoid arthritis enrolled in a DMARD registry. Rheumatoid Arthritis Azathioprine Registry Steering Committee. J Rheumatol 1991; 18:809–814.
59. Eriksson M. Rheumatoid arthritis as a risk factor for multiple myeloma: a case-control study. Eur J Cancer 1993; 29A:259–263.
60. J Parsonnet, ed. Microbes and Malignancy: Infection as a Cause of Human Cancers. New York, NY: Oxford University Press; 1999.
61. Haas H, Anders S, Bornkamm, GW, et al. Do infections induce monoclonal immunoglobulin components? Clin Exper Immunol 1990; 81:435–440.
62. Brown L, Linet M, Greenberg R, et al. Multiple myeloma and family history of cancer among blacks and whites in the US. 1999; 85:2385–2390 Cancer (Am Ca Soc).
63. Santella R. Immunological methods for detection of carcinogens: DNA damage in humans. Cancer Epidemiology, Biomarkers & Prevention 1999; 8:733–739.
64. Perera FP. Environment and cancer: who is susceptible? Science 1997; 278:1068–1073.
65. Chen S, Liu Q, Piu C, et al. Higher frequency of glutathione S-transferase deletions in black children with acute lymphoblastic leukemia. Blood 1997; 89:1701–1707.
66. Spencer D, Masten S, Lanier K, et al. Quantitative analysis of constitutive and 2,3,7,8-tetrachlorodibenzo-p-dioxin-induced cytochrome P450 1B1 expression in human lymphocytes. Cancer Epidemiology, Biomarkers & Prevention 1999; 8:139–146.

67. Roberts S, Spreadborough A, Bulman B, Barber J, Evans D, Scott D. Heritability of cellular radiosensitivity: a marker of low-penetrance predisposition genes in breast cancer? Am J Hum Genet 1999; 65:784–794.
68. I dos Santos Silva, ed. Cancer epidemiology: principles and methods. International Agency for Research on Cancer, World Health Organization; 1999; Lyon, France, Oxford University Press.
69. Miller BA, Bolonel LN, Bernstein L, et al, eds. Racial/Ethnic Patterns of Cancer in the United States: 1988-1992. Bethesda, Md: National Cancer Institute; 1996. NIH Pub. No. 96-4104.
70. Tajima K, Sonoda S, eds. Ethnoepidemiology of Cancer. Tokyo, Japan: Japan Scientific Societies Press; 1996.
71. Huff J, Lucier G, Tritscher A. Carcinogenicity of TCDD: experimental, mechanistic, and epidemiologic evidence. Ann Rev Pharmacol Toxicol 1999; 34:343–372.
72. Schwartz G. Multiple myeloma: clusters, clues, and dioxins. Cancer Epidemiology, Biomarkers & Prevention 1997; 6:49–56.
73. Bertazzi P, Pesatori A, Bernucci I, Landi M, Consonni D. Dioxin exposure and human leukemias and lymphomas: lessons from the Seveso accident and studies on industrial workers. Leukemia 1999; 13 (suppl 1):S72–S74.
74. Cranor CF, Davis D, Defur PL, et al. Brief Amici Curiae of the Lymphoma Foundation of America. The Supreme Court of the United States. No. 02-271: Dow Chemical Company, Monsanto Company, et al v Daniel Raymond Stephenson, Susan Stephenson, Daniel Anthony Stephenson, Emily Elizabeth Stephenson, Joe Isaacson, and Phyllis Lisa Isaacson. Counsel Press, 2003.
75. Lewis D, Garrison A, Wommack K, Whittemore A, Steudler P, Melillo J. Influence of environmental changes on degradation of chiral pollutants in soils. Nature 1999; 401:898–901.
76. Davis D, Magee B. Cancer and industrial chemical production. Science 1979; 206: 1356–1357.
77. Methods for investigating localized clustering of disease. In: Alexander FE, Boyle P, eds. IARC Scientific Publications No. 135. Lyon, France: Oxford University Press; 1996.
78. Polychlorinated dibenzo-para-dioxins and polychlorinated dibenzofurans. In: IARC Monographs on the Evaluation of Carcinogenic Risks to Humans. Vol 69. Lyon, France: Oxford University Press; 1997.
79. Vineis P, Malat N, Lang M, et al, eds. IARC Metabolic Polymorphisms and Susceptibility to Cancer. Lyon, France. Oxford University Press. Publication Number 148, 1999.
80. Ferber D. Carcinogens: IARC, lashed by critics, WHO's cancer agency begins a new regime. Science 2003; 301:36–37.
81. Fagin D, Lavelle M, and the Center for Public Integrity. Toxic Deception: How the Chemical Industry Manipulates Science, Bends the Law and Endangers Your Health. 2nd ed. Monroe, Me: Common Courage Press; 1999.
82. Steingraber S. Living Downstream: An Ecologist Looks at Cancer and the Environment. Reading, Mass: Addison-Wesley Publishing Company, Inc; 1997.
83. Figgs LW, Doscemeci M, Blair A. Risk of multiple myeloma by occupation and industry among men and women: a 24-state death certificate study. J Occup Med 1994; 36:1210–1221.
84. Herbert B. "Sick and suspicious." The New York Times. September 4, 2003, p. A25.
85. Herbert B. "Clouds in Silicon Valley." The New York Times. September 8th 2003, p. A24.
85a. Vescio RA, Hamilton AS, Silverman SL, Berenson JR. Breast implant exposure is more prevalent in women with multiple myeloma: a case-control study. Blood 2002; 100:11:605a.
86. Price R. Nogales: something is very wrong. USA Today. October 27, 1993.
87. Sanchez R. Water quality problems in Nogales, Sonora. Tijuana, Mexico: Department of Urban and Environmental Studies, El Colegio De La Frontera Norte; 1995, p. 2.
88. Konrad R, Kricka L, Goodman DBP, Goldman J, Silberstein L. Myeloma-associated paraprotein directed against the HIV-1 p24 antigen in an HIV-1 seropositive patient. N Eng J Med 1993; 328:1817–1820.

89. Beld M, Penning M, van Putten M, et al. Low levels of hepatitis C virus RNA in serum, plasma, and peripheral blood mononuclear cells of injecting drug users during long anti-body-undetectable periods before seroconversion. Blood 1999; 94:1183–1191.

90. Goedert J, Coete T, Virgo P, et al, for the AIDS-Cancer Match Study Group. Spectrum of AIDS-associated malignant disorders. Lancet 1998; 351:1833–1839.

91. Retting MB, Ha HJ, Vescio RA, et al. Kaposi's sarcoma-associated herpes virus infection of bone marrow dendritic cells from multiple myeloma patients. Science 1997; 276: 1851–1854.

92. Jarrett R. Prevalence of human herpesvirus 8 in multiple myeloma patients [abstract]. Multiple Myeloma Workshop; September 1999; p 83. Abstract 154.

93. Taret K, Chang Y, Klein B. KSHV is not causally associated with multiple myeloma [abstract]. Multiple Myeloma Workshop; September 1999; p 84. Abstract 155.

93a. Yi Q, Ekman M, Anton SD, et al. Blood dendritic cells from myeloma patients are not infected with Kaposi's sarcoma-associated herpesvirus (KSHV/HHV-8) [abstract]. Multiple Myeloma Workshop; September 1999; p 85. Abstract 156.

94. Wiemer E, Van Suest P, Segever CM, Sonneveld, P. Detection of Kaposis' sarcoma-associated herpesvirus in mononuclear blood cells of patients with multiple myeloma [abstract]. Multiple Myeloma Workshop; September 1999; p 86. Abstract 157.

95. Gao S, Zhang Y, Deng J, Rabkin C, Flore O, Jensen H. Molecular polymorphism of Kaposi's sarcoma-associated herpesvirus (human herpesvirus 8) latent nuclear antigen: evidence for a large repertoire of viral genotypes and dual infection with different viral genotype. J Infect Dis 1999; 180:1466–1476.

96. Durie B, Urnovitz J. Cell and molecular biology of simian virus 40: implications for human infections and disease. J Natl Cancer Inst 1999; 91:1166–1167.

97. Durie BGM, Urnovitz HB, Murphy WH. RNA in the plasma of multiple myeloma patients. Acta Oncologica 2000; 39:789–796.

98. Martin W. Melanoma growth stimulatory activity (MGSA/GRO-()) chemokine genes incorporated into an African green monkey simian cytomegalovirus-derived stealth virus. Exp Mol Pathol 1999; 66:15–18.

99. Butel J, Arrington A, Wong C, Lednick J, Finegold M. Molecular evidence of simian virus 40 infections in children. J Infect Dis 1999; 180:884–887.

100. Hahn W, Counter C, Lundberg A, Beijersbergen R, Brooks M Weinberg R. Creation of human tumor cells with defined genetic elements. Nature 1999; 400:464–472.

101. Geusau A, Tschachler E, Meixner M, et al. Olestra increases faecal excretion of 2,3,7,8-tetrachlorodibenzo-p-dioxin. Lancet 1999; 354:1266–1267.

3 Characterization of the Myeloma Clone

Robert A. Vescio, MD
and James R. Berenson, MD

CONTENTS

1. INTRODUCTION

Multiple myeloma (MM) is characterized by the accumulation of malignant plasma cells in the bone marrow compartment. These terminally differentiated B lymphocytes all produce an identical immunoglobulin known as a monoclonal protein, the laboratory hallmark of this malignancy. Because MM is typically disseminated throughout the body at diagnosis, malignant cells must also exist, even if transiently, within the circulation as well. Although plasma cells are rarely noted phenotypically within the blood of patients, flow cytometric and molecular techniques have recently been used to document their presence in substantial numbers (1–9). These circulating cells have been proposed to be responsible for the proliferative component of the malignancy, based on the observation that the identifiable myeloma cells within the bone marrow have a low proliferative rate (10). Indeed, early studies had suggested that a less mature B lymphocyte or even a primordial stem cell might be clonal (11,12). In this proposed model, these precursor cells could then sustain the plasma cell pool through differentiation in a manner akin to the process that occurs in chronic myelogenous leukemia. Recent advances in molecular biological techniques

From: *Current Clinical Oncology: Biology and Management of Multiple Myeloma*
Edited by: J. R. Berenson © Humana Press Inc., Totowa, NJ

have allowed investigators to address this question using immunoglobulin gene analysis. Immunoglobulin gene rearrangement occurs at set time points during B-cell maturation. Consequently, analysis of immunoglobulin gene sequences within malignant myeloma cells has clarified the timing of oncogenesis in myeloma. Because myeloma cell immunoglobulin gene sequences have evidence of somatic mutation and prior antigenic selection (13–15), the final oncogenic event must have occurred within a B cell that had passed through these steps during differentiation. This implies that MM oncogenesis occurs in a nearly terminally differentiated plasma cell. Whether the B-cell precursor that underwent this final event was abnormal as well remains an area of intensive research. Furthermore, the immunoglobulin gene locus appears responsible for a significant proportion of the translocations that occur within the myeloma cell. The characterization of these translocations has led to the identification of a number of potential oncogenes that may play a major role in the disease development. Thus, a clear understanding of normal immunoglobulin gene rearrangement is needed to understand myeloma pathophysiology.

2. NORMAL IMMUNOGLOBULIN GENE REARRANGEMENT

Antibodies are proteins that bind to cellular, bacterial, or viral antigens and, thus, signal their need for removal by the immune system. The normal antibody protein is a dimer composed of a set of heavy- and light-chain proteins. Given the wide range of exposures to infection, millions of unique antibodies are thus required to protect an individual from infection. However, each antibody-producing B cell produces only a single antibody protein. For this antibody diversity to occur, millions of unique B cells are produced and those that produce a useful antibody survive and eventually differentiate into a plasma cell that secretes its particular antibody protein in large quantities. These antibody genes are not directly encoded within the germline genome. The amount of DNA that would be required within every cell to produce the millions of unique antibody proteins would be prohibitive and would not permit further antibody protein development. Instead, the antibody or immunoglobulin gene loci are composed of numerous gene fragments, which are rearranged in a seemingly random fashion to generate the initial repertoire of antibody proteins (Fig. 1). As previously stated, the immunoglobulin molecule is comprised of heavy- and light-chain proteins. The heavy chain contains the most diversity and, like the light chain, is composed of two regions: the variable region, which directly binds antigen; and the constant region, which determines the class and eventual function of the antibody (e.g., C_μ for immunoglobulin M [IgM], C_γ for IgG, C_α for IgA). Early in the course of normal B-cell development, rearrangement of four separate gene segments leads to the development of the heavy-chain portion of a unique functional antibody. Three gene segments are used to encode the variable region of

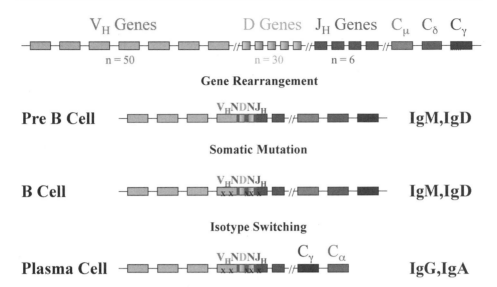

Fig. 1. Schematic diagram of the process of immunoglobulin gene rearrangement and immunoglobulin isotype switching that occurs during B-cell development. Exons are denoted by boxes and introns by thin lines. The Xs represent mutations that occur within the immunoglobulin gene sequence during the process of somatic mutation.

the heavy chain: the variable (VH), diversity (D), and joining (JH) gene segments. To generate the tremendous amount of antibody diversity that is required, these gene segments are recombined in apparent random fashion to make an initial VHDJH gene. The majority of a single functional heavy-chain variable region is encoded by one of approx 50 functional VH genes *(16)*. This gene segment gets juxtaposed with one of 30 functional D and six functional JH genes *(17)*. This joining is imprecise and thus leads to further antibody diversity by the insertion of non-templated (N) nucleotides. At the same time, a similar process occurs at the light-chain locus within the B cell. In this case, the κ (and, if unsuccessful, the γ) light chain undergoes a similar rearrangement of V, J, and C genes. As one might suspect, this rearrangement process can initially lead to the production of a substantial number of dysfunctional antibody-producing cells. A process termed *antigenic selection* thus ensues to select out the lymphocytes producing useful antibodies. The pre-B cell migrates from the bone marrow to the lymph node germinal center, where it is exposed to antigen. At this point, the immunoglobulin molecule produced by the B cell is present on its cell surface. If its surface immunoglobulin binds to an antigen presented within the lymph node germinal center, the lymphocyte receives a signal to proliferate and divide *(18,19)*. The remaining B lymphocytes undergo apoptosis. As the surviving B cells divide within the germinal center, a second and important process

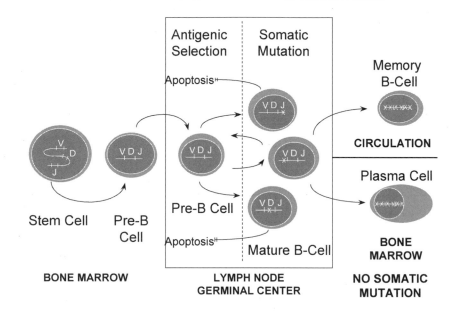

Fig. 2. Pre B cells that have undergone immunoglobulin gene rearrangement migrate to the lymph node, where they are exposed to antigens. If the B cell surface antibody binds antigen, it undergoes replication whereby mutations within the immunoglobulin gene variable region occur by chance. If the resultant antibody is dysfunctional, the B cell can no longer bind antigen and the cell undergoes apoptosis. If, however, the mutation leads to improved antibody/antigen binding, the new B cell preferentially binds to the lymph node antigens, survives, and undergoes additional cycles of replication and somatic mutation. Once a B cell has processed an antibody of high antigen affinity, the mature B cell leaves the lymph node, undergoes class switching, and differentiates into a plasma cell; at that point, no additional somatic mutation can occur.

occurs to help generate the high-affinity antibodies that are required for immunity. Somatic mutation occurs, characterized by additional mutations occurring within the immunoglobulin gene variable regions of proliferating germinal center B cells (20,21). If the resultant B cell acquires a mutation that results in antigen-binding properties superior to those of the precursor B cell, it then receives additional signals to proliferate (Fig. 2). Conversely, B cells that acquire detrimental somatic mutations undergo apoptosis because they cannot out compete with the precursor B cell for antigen binding. This stepwise process of somatic mutation and then antigenic selection occurs numerous times and is critical for the generation of high-affinity antibodies. Once an optimal antibody has been produced, the more mature B lymphocyte leaves the lymph node germinal center and migrates to the bone marrow. Along the way, most of these B cells undergo isotype switching, whereby the class of antibody produced is changed from IgM or IgD to IgG, IgA, or IgE by excision of the interceding portion of the heavy-chain gene.

Table 1
Characteristics of the VH Genes in Myeloma

• High degree of somatic mutation
• Mutations occur in antigenically driven fashion
• No clonal diversity or evolution
• Lack of VH4-21 usage

Once isotype switching occurs, no further somatic mutation occurs, presumably because no antigen is presented within the bone marrow to drive this selection process.

3. THE TIMING OF ONCOGENESIS IN MULTIPLE MYELOMA

The low proliferative rate of the phenotypically identified malignant cell and the inability of this type of cell to sustain tumor growth in vivo (as demonstrated by kinetic and other types of studies) imply that earlier precursor cells may be responsible for the proliferation of the malignant population (10). The presence of a circulating tumor component without obvious plasma cell morphology also suggests that less mature lymphocytes may be part of the clone as well, which could explain the dissemination of the disease throughout the bone marrow. Also, evidence of tumor cells at even earlier stages of hematopoietic differentiation came from studies showing the high rate of acute nonlymphoblastic leukemia in these patients and the presence of nonlymphoid surface markers on malignant plasma cells (11).

In MM, the properties of the immunoglobulin genes allow precise determination of the stage of B-cell development during which malignant transformation occurs (Table 1). Specifically, myeloma VDJ sequences have been found to contain marked somatic mutation (8–9%) (14). This degree of somatic mutation is comparable to that seen in other lymphocytes after switching class, but much higher than the 2 to 3% noted within IgM-expressing B cells. The number of replacement mutations (those leading to an amino acid change) was greater than expected by random chance in the three portions of the heavy-chain variable region that directly contributes to antigen binding, that is, the complementarity-determining regions (CDRs) (14). Because antigen binding is primarily determined by these regions, the accumulation of replacement mutations within this region implies that a process of antigenic selection occurred within the myeloma cell precursor cell. Additionally, sequence analysis has shown a relative lack of replacement mutations within the framework region of the VDJ sequence. Indeed, the ratio of replacement to silent mutations in the CDR compartment is twice that in the framework region (FR) in MM (14). This latter portion of the gene contains the codes for the overall structure of the variable region of the heavy-chain antibody. Mutations in this region often lead to marked changes in the overall structure of the antibody. The lack of mutations in the FR implies that there was a selective process prohibiting these structural mutations which, in turn, implies that a functional antibody required during the maturation of the B cell subsequently was transformed into a myeloma cell. In several additional studies, Sahota provided even stronger evidence for this antigenic selection process by analyzing both the heavy and light chains within the myeloma cells *(22)*.

Although the above findings imply that the malignant cell underwent somatic mutation and antigenic selection within the lymph node germinal center, it does not, by itself, depict the timing of the final oncogenic event in the myeloma cell. It is still possible that a malignant pre-B or B cell could go through this selection process and eventually give rise to malignant plasma cells after differentiation. Arguing against this theory is the fact that the analysis of numerous malignant clones derived from a given patient shows no diversity in the VH gene sequence *(15)*. Even sequence analysis of clones derived from different time points during the course of the disease has failed to yield evidence of VDJ sequence variation. These results differ from other B-cell tumors originating in germinal centers at earlier stages of B-cell differentiation, such as follicular non-Hodgkin's lymphoma (NHL) *(23)*. In this disease, oncogenesis occurs in a B cell that is still undergoing somatic mutation and antigenic selection. Thus, the VDJ sequence varies among the malignant clones within these patients *(24)*. These results suggest that the final oncogenic event in myeloma occurs very late in B-cell differentiation.

Although these studies imply that myelomagenesis occurs in a mature lymphocyte (e.g., a plasma cell), recent studies have found small numbers of pre-class switch monoclonal cells (C_γ-containing) in this disease *(13,25)*. Using a C_μ primer with a myeloma specific CDR2 primer, pre-class switch cells that demonstrated a CDR3 sequence identical to those seen in the myeloma clone were found in the bone marrow and blood of patients with myeloma. Similar results were obtained using a patient-specific CDR3 primer with a C_μ primer and polymerase chain reaction (PCR). From these findings, it seems likely that a pre-class switch clone persists in many patients with MM. In an attempt to quantify these cells, our group sought to find them by using colony hybridization techniques. PCR was used with a C_μ primer and a CDR1 primer matching that of patient's myeloma clone. All clones that were hybridized with an FR3 probe (to ensure that a functional VH gene was amplified) that was also hybridized to a patient-specific CDR3 probe on Southern blot were sequenced for comparison to the myeloma sequence. No matching IgM sequences were found in the five patients studied *(26)*. Because these cells were detectable by other groups only after the use of sensitive PCR techniques and in only a subset of patients, the contribution of these apparently rare cells to the malignant process remains uncertain. Multiple genetic events are probably needed before a cell becomes fully malignant, as is the case in NHL. Therefore, these rare cells may not be fully malignant in character. However, given the theory that a circulating and more proliferative component may be responsible for disease growth, there is significant interest in further analysis of these pre-class switch clonal cells.

4. USE OF SPECIFIC VH, D, AND JH GENES BY THE MALIGNANT CLONE

The approx 50 functional VH gene segments have been divided into seven families based on sequence homology ranging in size from 1 (VH6) to 22 (VH3) *(16)*. In mature B cells, use of the VH gene family is generally proportional to the number of functional genes; however, initial VDJ recombination within the heavy-chain gene does not occur in a completely random manner. Individual germ-line genes appear to be overrepresented in immature B lymphocytes owing to location and other features. Consequently, there is an overrepresentation of B lymphocytes expressing the VH4–34 gene segment in normal lymphoid tissue *(27)*. Six to eight percent of the normal B-cell repertoire contain VDJs that use this particular germ-line gene; it is also expressed at a similar rate in lymphoid malignancies arrested at early stages of B-cell ontogeny (acute lymphocytic leukemia [ALL] and chronic lymphocytic leukemia). This gene is commonly expressed in lymphocytes involved in various autoimmune phenomena (e.g., cold agglutinin disease and systemic lupus erythematosus) and appears to be a requirement for the production of anti I/i antibodies *(28,29)*. In fact, a striking 65% of diffuse large-cell lymphomas, which develop from relatively immature B cells, use the VH4 gene family, with VH4-34 being the most commonly utilized; this suggests that self-antigen recognition may stimulate oncogenesis in this neoplasm *(30)*. In contrast, circulating IgG or IgA antibodies within the serum of normal patients are rarely derived from this gene, which suggests that self-reacting pre-B cells are eventually eliminated through a process termed *clonal deletion,* or become anergic during normal B-cell development.

In myeloma, although the results of VH gene family frequency closely parallel that seen in normal B cells, VH4.21 use has almost never been observed *(31,32)*. Because this gene contains the code for antibodies that are capable of recognizing self-antigens, B cells expressing this gene prior to plasma cell development appear to be eliminated. Additionally, this may explain why auto-antibody production is less commonly found in MM than in other B-cell malignancies.

Use of specific *JH* and *D* genes in myeloma cells is quite comparable to their use in mature B lymphocytes, which further supports the late B-cell origin of myeloma (Fig. 3) *(33)*. Use of the *JH4* gene is most common, as noted in normal B cells. Use of the *DHQ52* gene was uncommon in myeloma, in contrast to findings in ALL and fetal B cells. This is the most distal *D* gene segment in the genome, which may explain its preferential rearrangement in early B-lymphocytes. In our analysis,

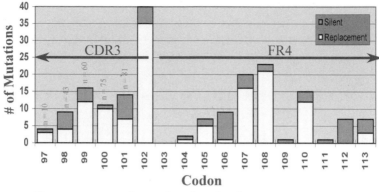

v Demonstrates prior antigenic selection

υ Replacement mutations in J_H CDR3 > expected (p <0.00001)

Fig. 3. Multiple myeloma immunoglobulin gene sequences from 83 patients were analyzed and the JH region was compared to germline JH sequences during a search for evidence of somatic mutation. Replacement mutations lead to a change in the antibody protein, whereas silent mutations do not. The framework region of JH had relatively few replacement mutations, particularly in certain key codons. In contrast, numerous replacement mutations occurred in CDR3, which encodes for the antigen-binding portions of the antibody.

CDR3 lengths in myeloma VDJ sequences were comparable to those reported in normal B cells but fusion of multiple *D* genes was much more common in myeloma. In myeloma CDR3s N-region insertion was minimal compared to that in normal B cells. Because studies of normal plasma cells have not been completed, it is unknown whether this increased frequency of *D–D* fusion and lack of N-region addition is specific to myeloma. These differences may also be explained by differing techniques of analysis, even though we used similar assignment criteria.

5. THE SURFACE PHENOTYPE OF THE MYELOMA CELL

Early studies using aneuploidy as a basis of malignant plasma cell determination suggested the existence of myeloid, megakaryocytic, and T-cell markers on the malignant clone in myeloma *(11)*. However, the use of these so-called "lineage-specific" markers was problematic because it was later learned that normal plasma cells can aberrantly express these same antigens to some degree *(34)*. Consequently, the use of flow cytometric markers to phenotype malignant cells is problematic when rare cells are being analyzed. Nevertheless, recent improvements in flow cytometric technique have been helpful for delineating the proteins expressed by the malignant clone. In addition, the coupling of flow cytometric

Table 2
Surface Phenotype of Malignant Cells

Marker	Features
CD10	Expressed by a subset (? more proliferative component)
CD19	Level of expression controversial
CD20	Expressed by a subset (? More proliferative component)
CD28 and CD86	Occurs with progressive disease
CD34	Typically not expressed by malignant clone
CD38	High expression on most but not all malignant cells
CD56 (N-CAM)	Absent in MGUS and plasma cell leukemia
CD95 (Fas antigen)	Mutations associated with lack of expression
CD13	Expressed by most myeloma cells

MGUS, monoclonal gammopathies of undetermined significance.

results with molecular studies that can be used to verify the presence of the unique myeloma cell marker (the immunoglobulin gene expressed by the malignant clone), has allowed a more precise determination of surface markers present on the malignant clone (Table 2).

5.1. Myeloma Cells and the CD34 Antigen

The CD34 antigen is expressed by the earliest hematopoietic precursor cells, including the pluripotent stem cell (35). Consequently, devices were developed that can enrich cells bearing this protein as a means of collecting populations of self-replenishing hematopoietic cells from sources contaminated with malignant cells for autologous transplantation. It has been shown that the re-infusion of hematopoietic cells selected for CD34 can support rapid and sustained engraftment following myeloablative chemotherapy (36,37). However, this process will only be of benefit if the CD34 antigen is not expressed by the malignant cell. Unfortunately, some immature B cells also express this surface marker. Because several authors previously demonstrated the presence of tumor cells in not only the bone marrow but also the blood of patients with myeloma, it became both biologically and clinically important to determine whether any malignant cells expressed this stem cell marker in these patients. To accomplish this, CD34-positive cells were purified from the bone marrow of these patients using a combination of an immunoadsorption column and flow sorting. This dual-enrichment step was important because it reduced any contamination with CD34-negative cells to a negligible level. A sensitive PCR-based assay with primers derived from the unique CDRs expressed by the patient's malignant clone was then used to search for contaminating CD34-positive myeloma cells. We found no evidence of the myeloma clone within the CD34-expressing cell population *(38)*. Several other groups have confirmed this initial report, although Pilarski and colleagues reported conflicting results *(39)*. These differences may be explained by the different antibodies and definitions used to define a CD34-positive cell. Nevertheless, from a clinical standpoint, CD34 selection of peripheral blood stem-cell products using an immunoadsorption column (Ceprate, Cellpro Inc., Bothell, WA) led to a reduction in autograft tumor burden by more than 3 logs *(37)*. This process did not significantly impede patient engraftment; thus, the use of a CD34 selection procedure to exclude malignant myeloma cells from an autograft is safe and effective *(40)*.

5.2. CD10 Expression on a Subset of Myeloma Cells

CD10, also known as the common acute lymphoblastic leukemia antigen (CALLA), was originally described as a surface antigen present on some human acute lymphoblastic leukemia cells *(41)*. Subsequently, it has been shown that CD10 is expressed on a wide variety of hematopoietic cells, including B cells, at early and late stages of differentiation *(42)*. A recent analysis using aneuploidy as a marker of malignancy found no evidence of CD10 expression in 26 patients with MM *(43)*. This is in contrast to other studies of CD10 expression in myeloma that revealed that CD10-expressing myelomatous plasma cells exist in a small percentage of patients (mean: 25%; range: 10–60%) *(44–46)*. Nevertheless, even when present, myeloma cells expressing this antigen comprised only a small fraction of the malignant population in latter studies. The distinction is important, however, because CD10-expressing cells are commonly found in patients with an aggressive disease, e.g., plasma cell leukemia *(47–49)*. Because CD10 is expressed on germinal center B cells with highly proliferative activity, this malignant subpopulation in myeloma may represent the part of the clone that leads to growth and disease progression. In support of this, some investigators have shown that the appearance of CD10-expressing tumor cells in the circulation occurs at the time of progression of myeloma *(50)*. To address this question using more sensitive molecular techniques, we searched for CD10-bearing malignant cells using patient-specific VH gene primers. Using the immunoglobulin gene as a marker for the malignancy, we found a small CD10-bearing malignant population in all cases studied *(51)*. This subpopulation of cells may play an important role in the pathogenesis of myeloma if expression of this protein correlates with the immaturity of the cell.

5.3. CD19

The CD19 molecule is expressed on the surface of B lymphocytes early during their differentiation *(52)*. It contains an immunoglobulin-like extracellular domain and can participate in B-cell proliferation by binding to surface immunoglobulin *(53)*, thereby reducing the threshold for antigen receptor stimulation of the B cell *(54)*. CD19 expression is typically diagrammed in textbooks to be lost on the more well-differentiated plasma cells. In fact, many cell lines derived from patients with myeloma do not express CD19. Nevertheless, its expression on myeloma cells remains controversial. Plasma cells derived from normal individuals were shown by Kawano and colleagues to express CD19 but not CD56 *(55)*. In contrast, myeloma cells derived from patients were uniformly CD19-negative and frequently CD56-positive. Most studies have also corroborated the lack of CD19 expression on bone marrow myeloma cells *(43,56,57)*. The presence of the protein on circulating cells remains more controversial. Pilarski and associates demonstrated the presence of CD19-expressing cells that are clonally related to their malignant bone marrow-based counterparts using immunoglobulin gene PCR *(58,59)*. They also found evidence of a substantial population of circulating B lymphocytes bearing this marker within the circulation (40–50% of all mononuclear cells) with evidence of aneuploidy *(60)*. Other investigators have found conflicting results. Using CDR3 immunoglobulin gene amplification, Chen and Epstein found only small numbers of circulating B cells in patients with multiple myeloma (median: 6%), with few of these cells related to the malignant clone *(57)*. Additionally, another study using aneuploidy as a marker for malignancy failed to detect clonal cells within the CD19 population of circulating cells *(43)*. Recent work suggests that a lack of CD19 expression by myeloma cells could improve the growth rate of these cells, because CD19 transfectants of myeloma cell lines impaired their proliferation *(61)*.

5.4. CD28 and CD28 Ligand (CD86)

Although CD28 was originally identified as an antigen present on T lymphocytes and responsible for T-cell activation, it has also been found on both malignant and nonmalignant plasma cells *(62,63)*. Its presence on the malignant plasma cells in patients with myeloma is associated with disease progression and treatment failure *(64)*. Interestingly, when CD28 is present on the malignant cells, it is accompanied by the presence of its ligand, CD86 *(63)*. By contrast, there is an inverse correlation between CD28 and the expression of the neural cell adhesion molecule marker CD56 (N-CAM CD56) *(65)*.

5.5. CD38

Previous studies have demonstrated the high expression of CD38 on normal and malignant plasma cells *(45,55,66)*. Although this antigen is not expressed on the pluripotent stem cell *(67)*, it is expressed weakly on early lineage-committed cells. If CD38 where to be expressed on all malignant cells, it could be possible to select for CD38-negative cells in autografts and render these products tumor-free. In addition, humanized anti-CD38 antibodies have been developed for potential therapeutic benefit *(68)*. However, most studies of CD38 expression in myeloma have relied on insensitive immunohistochemical techniques, which cannot be used to identify an infrequent CD38 negative tumor population in patients with myeloma. Using flow sorting with anti-CD38 antibodies on peripheral blood mononuclear cells from these patients, we identified a CD38-negative tumor cell population with aPCR-based assay in all myeloma patients (69). However, the frequency of these circulating CD38 cells was markedly less than for the CD38-expressing tumor cells in all cases. Thus, although tumor cells lacking CD38 exist in myeloma, they represent a relatively minor component of the malignant population. Because CD38 is not expressed on B cells prior to the plasma cell stage, these malignant cells may be less mature and have a more proliferative capability.

5.6. N-CAM CD56

The neural cell adhesion molecule (N-CAM) CD56 is a member of the immunoglobulin superfamily and, as the name implies, was originally detected on a wide variety of neural cells (70). It has also been recently identified on hematopoietic cells, especially natural killer cells and, more recently, on malignant plasma cells in the majority of myeloma patients and to a lesser extent on the monoclonal plasma cells from patients with monoclonal gammopathies of undetermined significance (MGUS) (55,71,72). The antigen is lacking on plasma cells derived from normal individuals and on the circulating clonal cells within patients with plasma cell leukemia. Because most myeloma lines are derived from these latter patients, many also lack CD56 expression. These cell lines were found to lack CD56 expression due to decreased DNA transcription (73). These studies suggest that this adhesion molecule helps keep the plasma cell within the bone marrow microenvironment. Alternatively, with autonomous growth (i.e., plasma cell leukemia development), its presence is no longer required and cells can traverse to the bloodstream. The lack of CD56 expression by the myeloma clone has been found to correlate with current and future development of plasma cell leukemia (65). In this study, 40% of patients with CD56-negative or weak expression of this antigen by malignant cells developed a leukemic phase compared with only a 15% incidence in patients in whom myeloma cells express this antigen. More recent studies suggest that serum levels of NCAM can be used to predict the outcome in these patients, with higher levels associated with a poor clinical outcome (74). Moreover, it has been shown that low levels (>20 U/mL) can be used to distinguish patients with MGUS from those patients with myeloma.

5.7. CD138

Syndecan-1 (CD138) is a transmembrane heparin sulfate proteoglycan that is expressed primarily on pre-B cells and immunoglobulin-producing plasma cells (75,76). The majority of myeloma cells within patients bears this surface antigen. Monoclonal antibodies against this protein are being developed for therapeutic use (77). Functional studies of myeloma reveal that syndecan-1 can mediate cell–

cell adhesion and bind these cells to type I collagen *(78)*. In vitro studies have demonstrated that circulating syndecan-1 can inhibit myeloma cell growth and induce apoptosis *(79)*. Paradoxically, patients with elevated levels of circulating syndecan-1 were found to have shortened survival times (20 mo) compared with the remaining patients (median survival: 44 mo; $p < 0.0001$) *(80)*.

6. CONCLUSIONS

Recent advances in molecular biology have clarified that the final malignant event in MM must occur in a terminally differentiated B cell or plasma cell. Nevertheless, a circulating component of clonal cells is detectable in the majority of patients with this disease. These cells have been differentially described as either less-differentiated B lymphocytes with more aggressive features of proliferation or as merely the circulatory plasma cell component of this bone marrow-based disease. This distinction is important, because these circulatory cells could represent the proliferative reservoir of the malignancy. Further studies aimed at analyzing the features of the proliferative compartment of malignant cells in MM will certainly aid investigators in their search for more effective therapeutic options.

REFERENCES

1. Berenson J, Wong R, Kim K, Brown N, Lichtenstein A. Evidence for peripheral blood B lymphocyte but not T lymphocyte involvement in multiple myeloma. Blood 1987; 70: 1550–1553.
2. Corradini P, Voena C, Omede P, et al. Detection of circulating tumor cells in multiple myeloma by a PCR-based method. Leukemia 1993; 7:1879–1882.
3. Jensen GS, Mant MJ, Belch AJ, Berenson JR, Ruether BA, Pilarski LM. Selective expression of CD45 isoforms defines CALLA+ monoclonal B lineage cells in peripheral blood from myeloma patients as late stage B cells. Blood 1991; 78:711–719.
4. Kiel K, Cremer FW, Rottenburger C, et al. Analysis of circulating tumor cells in patients with multiple myeloma during the course of high-dose therapy with peripheral blood stem cell transplantation. Bone Marrow Transplant 1999; 23:1019–1027.
5. Rawstron AC, Owen RG, Davies FE, et al. Circulating plasma cells in multiple myeloma: characterization and correlation with disease stage. Br J Haematol 1997; 97:46–55.
6. Rottenburger C, Kiel K, Bosing T, et al. Clonotypic CD20+ and CD19+ B cells in peripheral blood of patients with multiple myeloma post high-dose therapy and peripheral blood stem cell transplantation. Br J Haematol 1999; 106:545–552.
7. Szczepek AJ, Seeberger K, Wizniak J, Mant MJ, Belch AR, Pilarski LM. A high frequency of circulating B cells share clonotypic immunoglobulin heavy-chain VDJ rearrangements with autologous bone marrow plasma cells in multiple myeloma, as measured by single-cell and in situ reverse transcriptase-polymerase chain reaction. Blood 1998; 92:2844–2855.
8. Van Riet I, Heirman C, Lacor P, De Waele M, Thielemans K, Van Camp B. Detection of monoclonal B lymphocytes in bone marrow and peripheral blood of multiple myeloma patients by immunoglobulin gene rearrangement studies. Br J Haematol 1989; 73:289–295.
9. Vescio RA, Han EJ, Schiller GJ, et al. Quantitative comparison of multiple myeloma tumor contamination in bone marrow harvest and leukoapheresis autografts. Bone Marrow Transplant 1996; 18:103–110.

10. Grogan TM, Durie BG, Lomen C, et al. Delineation of a novel pre-B cell component in plasma cell myeloma: immunochemical, immunophenotypic, genotypic, cytologic, cell culture, and kinetic features. Blood 1987; 70:932–942.

11. Epstein J, Xiao HQ, He XY. Markers of multiple hematopoietic-cell lineages in multiple myeloma [see comments]. N Engl J Med 1990; 322:664–668.

12. Kubagawa H, Vogler LB, Capra JD, Conrad ME, Lawton AR, Cooper MD. Studies on the clonal origin of multiple myeloma. Use of individually specific (idiotype) antibodies to trace the oncogenic event to its earliest point of expression in B-cell differentiation. J Exp Med 1979; 150:792–807.

13. Bakkus MH, Van Riet I, Van Camp B, Thielemans K. Evidence that the clonogenic cell in multiple myeloma originates from a pre-switched but somatically mutated B cell. Br J Haematol 1994; 87:68–74.

14. Vescio RA, Cao J, Hong CH, et al. Myeloma immunoglobulin heavy chain V region sequences reveal prior antigenic selection and marked somatic mutation but no intraclonal diversity. J Immunol 1995; 155:2487–2497.

15. Ralph QM, Brisco MJ, Joshua DE, Brown R, Gibson J, Morley AA. Advancement of multiple myeloma from diagnosis through plateau phase to progression does not involve a new B-cell clone: evidence from the immunoglobulin heavy chain gene. Blood 1993; 82:202–206.

16. Cook GP, Tomlinson IM, Walter G, et al. A map of the human immunoglobulin VH locus completed by analysis of the telomeric region of chromosome 14q. Nat Genet 1994; 7:162–168.

17. Sanz I. Multiple mechanisms participate in the generation of diversity of human H chain CDR3 regions. J Immunol 1991; 147:1720–1729.

18. Arpin C, Dechanet J, Van Kooten C, et al. Generation of memory B cells and plasma cells in vitro. Science 1995; 268:720–722.

19. Choe J, Kim HS, Zhang X, Armitage RJ, Choi YS. Cellular and molecular factors that regulate the differentiation and apoptosis of germinal center B cells: anti-Ig down-regulates Fas expression of CD40 ligand-stimulated germinal center B cells and inhibits Fas-mediated apoptosis. J Immunol 1996; 157:1006–1016.

20. Berek C, Berger A, Apel M. Maturation of the immune response in germinal centers. Cell 1991; 67:1121–1129.

21. Jacob J, Kelsoe G, Rajewsky K, Weiss U. Intraclonal generation of antibody mutants in germinal centres. Nature 1991; 354:389–392.

22. Sahota SS, Leo R, Hamblin TJ, Stevenson FK. Myeloma VL and VH gene sequences reveal a complementary imprint of antigen selection in tumor cells. Blood 1997; 89:219–226.

23. Zelenetz AD, Chen TT, Levy R. Clonal expansion in follicular lymphoma occurs subsequent to antigenic selection. J Exp Med 1992; 176:1137–1148.

24. Ottensmeier CH, Thompsett AR, Zhu D, Wilkins BS, Sweetenham JW, Stevenson FK. Analysis of VH genes in follicular and diffuse lymphoma shows ongoing somatic mutation and multiple isotype transcripts in early disease with changes during disease progression. Blood 1998; 91:4292–4299.

25. Corradini P, Boccadoro M, Voena C, Pileri A. Evidence for a bone marrow B cell transcribing malignant plasma cell VDJ joined to C mu sequence in immunoglobulin (IgG)- and IgA-secreting multiple myelomas. J Exp Med 1993; 178:1091–1096.

26. Berenson JR, Vescio RA, Hong CH, et al. Multiple myeloma clones are derived from a cell late in B lymphoid development. Curr Top Microbiol Immunol 1995; 194:25–33.

27. Kraj P, Friedman DF, Stevenson F, Silberstein LE. Evidence for the overexpression of the VH4-34 (VH4.21) immunoglobulin gene segment in the normal adult human peripheral blood B cell repertoire. J Immunol 1995; 154:6406–6420.

28. Miller JJ 3rd, Bieber MM, Levinson JE, Zhu S, Tsou E, Teng NN. VH4-34 (VH4.21) gene expression in the chronic arthritides of childhood: studies of associations with anti-lipid A antibodies, HLA antigens, and clinical features. J Rheumatol 1996; 23:2132–2139.

29. van Vollenhoven RF, Bieber MM, Powell MJ, et al. VH4-34 encoded antibodies in systemic lupus erythematosus: a specific diagnostic marker that correlates with clinical disease characteristics. J Rheumatol 1999; 26:1727–1733.

30. Hsu FJ, Levy R. Preferential use of the VH4 immunoglobulin gene family by diffuse large-cell lymphoma. Blood 1995; 86:3072–3082.

31. Rettig MB, Vescio RA, Cao J, et al. VH gene usage is multiple myeloma: complete absence of the VH4.21 (VH4- 34) gene. Blood 1996; 87:2846–2852.

32. Kiyoi H, Naito K, Ohno R, Naoe T. Comparable gene structure of the immunoglobulin heavy chain variable region between multiple myeloma and normal bone marrow lymphocytes. Leukemia 1996; 10:1804–1812.

33. Kunkel LA, Vescio R, Cao J, et al. Analysis of multiple myeloma third complementarity-determining regions reveals characteristics of prenatal B cells. Ann N Y Acad Sci 1995; 764:519–522.

34. Terstappen LW, Johnsen S, Segers-Nolten IM, Loken MR. Identification and characterization of plasma cells in normal human bone marrow by high-resolution flow cytometry. Blood 1990; 76:1739–1777.

35. Berenson RJ, Andrews RG, Bensinger WI, et al. Antigen CD34+ marrow cells engraft lethally irradiated baboons. J Clin Invest 1988; 81:951–955.

36. Shpall EJ, Jones RB, Bearman SI, et al. Transplantation of enriched CD34-positive autologous marrow into breast cancer patients following high-dose chemotherapy: influence of CD34-positive peripheral blood progenitors and growth factors on engraftment. J Clin Oncol 1994; 12:28–36.

37. Schiller G, Vescio R, Freytes C, et al. Transplantation of CD34+ peripheral blood progenitor cells after high- dose chemotherapy for patients with advanced multiple myeloma. Blood 1995; 86:390–397.

38. Vescio RA, Hong CH, Cao J, et al. The hematopoietic stem cell antigen, CD34, is not expressed on the malignant cells in multiple myeloma. Blood 1994; 84:3283–3290.

39. Szczepek AJ, Bergsagel PL, Axelsson L, Brown CB, Belch AR, Pilarski LM. CD34+ cells in the blood of patients with multiple myeloma express CD19 and IgH mRNA and have patient-specific IgH VDJ gene rearrangements. Blood 1997; 89:1824–1833.

40. Vescio R, Schiller G, Stewart AK, et al. Multicenter phase III trial to evaluate CD34(+) selected versus unselected autologous peripheral blood progenitor cell transplantation in multiple myeloma. Blood 1999; 93:1858–1868.

41. Brown G, Hogg N, Greaves M. Candidate leukaemia-specific antigen in man. Nature 1975; 258:454–456.

42. Greaves MF, Hariri G, Newman RA, Sutherland DR, Ritter MA, Ritz J. Selective expression of the common acute lymphoblastic leukemia (gp 100) antigen on immature lymphoid cells and their malignant counterparts. Blood 1983; 61:628–639.

43. McSweeney PA, Wells DA, Shults KE, et al. Tumor-specific aneuploidy not detected in CD19+ B-lymphoid cells from myeloma patients in a multidimensional flow cytometric analysis. Blood 1996; 88:622–632.

44. Hamilton MS, Ball J, Bromidge E, Franklin IM. Surface antigen expression of human neoplastic plasma cells includes molecules associated with lymphocyte recirculation and adhesion. Br J Haematol 1991; 78:60–65.

45. Leo R, Boeker M, Peest D, et al. Multiparameter analyses of normal and malignant human plasma cells: CD38+, CD56+, CD54+, cIg+ is the common phenotype of myeloma cells. Ann Hematol 1992; 64:132–139.

46. Ruiz-Arguelles GJ, San Miguel JF. Cell surface markers in multiple myeloma. Mayo Clin Proc 1994; 69:684–690.

47. Wearne AJ, Joshua DE, Brown RD, Kronenberg H. Multiple myeloma: the relationship between CALLA (CD10) positive lymphocytes in the peripheral blood and light chain isotype suppression. Br J Haematol 1987; 67:39–44.

48. Sakalova A, Holomanova D, Mikulecky M, Mistrik M, Lipsic T, Steruska M. Prognostic value of plasma-cell immunophenotype in patients with multiple myeloma. Neoplasma 1993; 40:351–354.

49. Caligaris-Cappio F, Bergui L, Tesio L, et al. Identification of malignant plasma cell precursors in the bone marrow of multiple myeloma. J Clin Invest 1985; 76:1243–1251.

50. Durie BG, Grogan TM. CALLA-positive myeloma: an aggressive subtype with poor survival. Blood 1985; 66:229–232.

51. Cao J, Vescio RA, Rettig MB, et al. A CD10-positive subset of malignant cells is identified in multiple myeloma using PCR with patient-specific immunoglobulin gene primers. Leukemia 1995; 9:1948–1953.

52. Nadler LM, Anderson KC, Marti G, et al. B4, a human B lymphocyte-associated antigen expressed on normal, mitogen-activated, and malignant B lymphocytes. J Immunol 1983; 131:244–250.

53. Stamenkovic I, Seed B. CD19, the earliest differentiation antigen of the B cell lineage, bears three extracellular immunoglobulin-like domains and an Epstein-Barr virus-related cytoplasmic tail. J Exp Med 1988; 168:1205–1210.

54. Carter RH, Fearon DT. CD19: lowering the threshold for antigen receptor stimulation of B lymphocytes. Science 1992; 256:105–107.

55. Harada H, Kawano MM, Huang N, et al. Phenotypic difference of normal plasma cells from mature myeloma cells. Blood 1993; 81:2658–2663.

56. Zandecki M, Facon T, Bernardi F, et al. CD19 and immunophenotype of bone marrow plasma cells in monoclonal gammopathy of undetermined significance. J Clin Pathol 1995; 48:548–552.

57. Chen BJ, Epstein J. Circulating clonal lymphocytes in myeloma constitute a minor subpopulation of B cells [see comments]. Blood 1996; 87:1972–1976.

58. Billadeau D, Quam L, Thomas W, et al. Detection and quantitation of malignant cells in the peripheral blood of multiple myeloma patients. Blood 1992; 80:1818–1824.

59. Bergsagel PL, Smith AM, Szczepek A, Mant MJ, Belch AR, Pilarski LM. In multiple myeloma, clonotypic B lymphocytes are detectable among CD19+ peripheral blood cells expressing CD38, CD56, and monotypic Ig light chain. Blood 1995; 85:436–447.

60. Pilarski LM, Belch AR. Circulating monoclonal B cells expressing P glycoprotein may be a reservoir of multidrug-resistant disease in multiple myeloma. Blood 1994; 83:724–736.

61. Mahmoud MS, Fujii R, Ishikawa H, Kawano MM. Enforced CD19 expression leads to growth inhibition and reduced tumorigenicity. Blood 1999; 94:3551–3558.

62. Zhang XG, Olive D, Devos J, et al. Malignant plasma cell lines express a functional CD28 molecule. Leukemia 1998; 12:610–618.

63. Robillard N, Jego G, Pellat-Deceunynck C, et al. CD28, a marker associated with tumoral expansion in multiple myeloma. Clin Cancer Res 1998; 4:1521–1526.

64. Pellat-Deceunynck C, Bataille R, Robillard N, et al. Expression of CD28 and CD40 in human myeloma cells: a comparative study with normal plasma cells. Blood 1994; 84:2597–2603.

65. Pellat-Deceunynck C, Barille S, Jego G, et al. The absence of CD56 (NCAM) on malignant plasma cells is a hallmark of plasma cell leukemia and of a special subset of multiple myeloma. Leukemia 1998; 12:1977–1982.

66. Hata H, Matsuzaki H, Matsuno F, et al. Establishment of a monoclonal antibody to plasma cells: a comparison with CD38 and PCA-1. Clin Exp Immunol 1994; 96:370–375.

67. Kinniburgh D, Russell NH. Comparative study of CD34-positive cells and subpopulations in human umbilical cord blood and bone marrow. Bone Marrow Transplant 1993; 12:489–494.

68. Ellis JH, Barber KA, Tutt A, et al. Engineered anti-CD38 monoclonal antibodies for immunotherapy of multiple myeloma. J Immunol 1995; 155:925–937.

69. Rettig M, Hong C, Vescio R, et al. Reduction of tumor cells in multiple myeloma (MM) peripheral blood using a CD38 immunoadsorption column. Proc Am Soc Clin Onc 1995; 14:1351.

70. Walsh FS, Doherty P. Neural cell adhesion molecules of the immunoglobulin superfamily: role in axon growth and guidance. Ann Rev Cell Dev Biol 1997; 13:425–456.
71. Kaiser U, Auerbach B, Oldenburg M. The neural cell adhesion molecule NCAM in multiple myeloma. Leuk Lymphoma 1996; 20:389–395.
72. Sonneveld P, Durie BG, Lokhorst HM, Frutiger Y, Schoester M, Vela EE. Analysis of multidrug-resistance (MDR-1) glycoprotein and CD56 expression to separate monoclonal gammopathy from multiple myeloma. Br J Haematol 1993; 83:63–67.
73. Remels L, Bakkus M, Van Riet I, Van Camp B, Thielemanns K. Molecular characterization of N-CAM (CD56, Leu-19) expression in multiple myeloma. In: Radl J, van Camp B, eds. Monoclonal Gammopathies III: Clinical Significance and Basic Mechanisms. Eurage, Leiden, The Netherlands, 1991:67–71.
74. Ong F, Kaiser U, Seelen PJ, et al. Serum neural cell adhesion molecule differentiates multiple myeloma from paraproteinemias due to other causes. Blood 1996; 87:712–716.
75. Ridley RC, Xiao H, Hata H, Woodliff J, Epstein J, Sanderson RD. Expression of syndecan regulates human myeloma plasma cell adhesion to type I collagen. Blood 1993; 81:767–774.
76. Chilosi M, Adami F, Lestani M, et al. CD138/syndecan-1: a useful immunohistochemical marker of normal and neoplastic plasma cells on routine trephine bone marrow biopsies. Mod Pathol 1999; 12:1101–1106.
77. Post J, Vooijs WC, Bast BJ, De Gast GC. Efficacy of an anti-CD138 immunotoxin and doxorubicin on drug-resistant and drug-sensitive myeloma cells. Int J Cancer 1999; 83:571–576.
78. Dhodapkar MV, Sanderson RD. Syndecan-1 (CD 138) in myeloma and lymphoid malignancies: a multifunctional regulator of cell behavior within the tumor microenvironment. Leuk Lymphoma 1999; 34:35–43.
79. Dhodapkar MV, Abe E, Theus A, et al. Syndecan-1 is a multifunctional regulator of myeloma pathobiology: control of tumor cell survival, growth, and bone cell differentiation. Blood 1998; 91:2679–2688.
80. Seidel C, Sundan A, Hjorth M, et al. Serum syndecan-1: a new independent prognostic marker in multiple myeloma. Blood 2000; 95:388–392.

4 Oncogenesis of Multiple Myeloma

Johannes Drach, MD, Sonja Seidl, MD, Jutta Ackermann, and Hannes Kaufmann, MD

CONTENTS

1. INTRODUCTION

Multiple myeloma (MM) represents a malignancy of differentiated B lymphocytes, which accumulate as clonal plasma cells in the bone marrow. Novel insights into the biology and molecular pathology of the disease have suggested that MM originates from a somatically mutated and isotype-switched follicle-center B cell that has retained its ability to differentiate into a plasma cell homing to the bone marrow. Initiation and progression of the disease is associated with multiple genetic and molecular aberrations, which are summarized in this chapter.

From: *Current Clinical Oncology: Biology and Management of Multiple Myeloma*
Edited by: J. R. Berenson © Humana Press Inc., Totowa, NJ

2. MULTIPLE MYELOMA CONSISTS
OF TWO MAJOR CYTOGENETIC CATEGORIES

Cytogenetic and molecular genetic investigations of MM cells have provided evidence that virtually all cases of MM are characterized by chromosomal abnormalities *(1)*. Karyotypes from MM cells are usually very complex, but careful analyses of large series have demonstrated that MM can be subdivided into two cytogenetic categories *(2,3)*: hyperdiploid nonhyperdiploid (consisting of hypodiploid, pseudodiploid, and near-tetraploid karyotypes). The hyperdiploid subtype is defined by the presence of multiple trisomic chromosomes (most commonly chromosomes 3, 5, 7, 9, 11, 15, and 19) that are associated with a gain of DNA and indicated by evidence of DNA-aneuploidy using flow cytometry. The number of structural abnormalities per cell was lower in the hyperdiploid group (mean: 5.1) compared with the hypodiploid group (mean: 9.1), and the types of abnormalities were similar in both groups *(3)*. Furthermore, interphase fluorescent *in situ* hybridization (FISH) analyses have shown that translocations of 14q32 are relatively infrequent in hyperdiploid MM cells (>40%), but occur in more than 80% of nonhyperdiploid MM cells *(4)*. The association between 14q32 translocations and nonhyperdiploid MM was seen predominantly in patients with recurrent chromosome partners to the 14q32 chromosomal region (11q13, 4p16, and 16q23). Likewise, chromosome 13 monosomy is more common in patients with nonhyperdiploid karyotypes *(2–4)*

Recognition of hypodiploid MM is also of clinical significance, because patients with this type of MM have a particularly unfavorable prognosis *(2,3)*. This may at least in part be explained by the observation that some of the prognostically adverse chromosomal aberrations [translocations t(4;14) and t(14;16), deletion of 13q; see below] are overrepresented in patients with hypodiploid MM.

3. IMMUNOGLOBULIN HEAVY-CHAIN TRANSLOCATIONS
IN MM AND THEIR MOLECULAR CONSEQUENCES

One of the structural abnormalities most frequently observed in MM karyotypes involves the immunoglobulin (Ig) heavy-chain (*IgH*) gene locus on 14q32, which is usually part of a translocation. Already under physiological conditions, the *IgH* gene locus is a genetically unstable region, because it undergoes active hypermutation and so-called switch recombination when an antigen-stimulated B lymphocyte passes through the follicular center of lymph nodes. These events result in the selection of a particular B-cell clone exposing a high-affinity immunoglobulin and in a switch from the production of mostly IgM to mostly IgG and IgA. Unlike the physiological process whereby Ig gene sequences are brought together during switch recombination, 14q32 translocations in MM are charac-

Table 1
14q32 Translocations in Multiple Myeloma: Partner Chromosomes

	Chromosome	Gene	Incidence, % (approx)
Primary translocations			
	11q13	cyclin-d1	15–20
	4p16.3	fgfr3/mmset	12
	16q23	c-maf	5–7
	6p21	cyclin-d3	5
Secondary translocations			
	8q24	c-myc	>10
	6p25	mum/irf4	>5
	20q11	mafB	>5
	1q21	irta 1/irta 2	Rare

terized by the juxtaposition of *IgH* gene sequences with non-immunoglobulin DNA sequences (so-called illegitimate switch rearrangements) *(5)*. These translocations are an almost universal event in MM cell lines *(6)*. Based on interphase FISH analyses, investigators have reported that *IgH* translocations are present in approx 50% of patients with monoclonal gammopathies of undetermined significance (MGUS), in 50 to 60% of patients with MM, and in more than 80% of patients with plasma cell leukemia *(7–10)*. Heterogeneous translocation partners have been described (Table 1), with 11q13, 4p16.3, 16q23, and 6p21 being recurrent in 14q32 translocations in primary MM tumor specimens. These four types of *IgH* translocations, which are mutually exclusive, comprise approx 60% of all *IgH* translocations and are mediated primarily by errors occurring during *IgH* switch recombination. These reciprocal translocations result in the activation of oncogenes, because they fall under the influence of the following enhancer regions at the *IgH* gene locus:

11q13. A t(11;14)(q13;q32) can be found in approx 15% of patients with MM and may lead to overexpression of *cyclin D1*. In contrast to mantle cell lymphoma, breakpoints on 11q13 in MM are not clustered in the major translocation cluster, but are scattered over a relatively large genomic region *(11)*. Probably as a result of this heterogeneity, a t(11;14) may also result in dysregulation of a second gene (myeloma overexpressed gene, *myeov*), which is located centromeric to *cyclin D1 (12)*. Because of yet unknown reasons, a t(11;14) is particularly common in IgM, IgE, and nonsecretory MM cells (but not in IgD MM cells), with a fivefold increase in incidence compared with IgG and IgA MM cells *(13)*

4p16.3. A t(4;14)(p16;q32), which can only be detected by molecular cytogenetics—owing to the telomeric breakpoint on chromosome 4—is present in approx

15% of MM cases *(14)*. This translocation results in dysregulated expression of two genes, fibroblast growth factor receptor 3 (*fgfr3*) on the derivative chromosome 14 and the multiple myeloma SET (*mmset*) domain on the derivative chromosome 4 *(14)* fgfr3, which is not expressed by normal plasma cells, is overexpressed as a consequence of the translocation, and in some cases, activating mutations have also been found on the translocated allele. Observations that expression of *fgfr3* promotes myeloma cell proliferation and prevents apoptosis, and that activation of *fgfr3* is a transforming event in hematopoietic cells further substantiate an oncogenic role for *fgfr3* in MM *(15,16)*. Thus, the FGFR3 protein could represent a specific therapeutic target in MM cases carrying a t(4;14). In addition, the presence of a t(4;14) could influence the choice of cytotoxic agent, because in the murine myeloma cell line B9, cells overexpressing *fgfr3* were resistant to treatment with dexamethasone but not to exposure with anthracyclines or alkylating agents *(17)*. As with *fgfr3, mmset* overexpression only occurs in the presence of a t(4;14). Recent data suggest that presence of a *mmset/IgH* fusion transcript and expression of MMSET protein and lack of *fgfr3* expression may occur in up to one-third of MM cases with a t(4;14) *(18)*. These cases may be characterized by the loss of one copy of *fgfr3* In another study, expression of *fgfr3* transcripts was observed in only 23 of 31 MM cases (74%) carrying the t(4;14) *(19)*. Collectively, these data suggest that activation of *mmset* may be the critical transforming event in at least part of the development of MM cells with a t(4;14), although the role of the mmset protein for MM pathogenesis awaits further characterization.

16q23. The t(14;16)(q32;q23), which is present in approx 5% of patients with MM, results in the expression of *c-maf* in MM cells at a high level *(20)*. *c-maf* has been identified as a transcription factor in lymphoid cells involved in regulation of the expression of interleukin (IL)-4, but its role in the molecular pathology of MM still needs to be determined.

6p21. A rare recurrent translocation is the t(6;14)(p21;q32), which has been observed in 1 of 30 MM cell lines examined and in approx 4% of primary MM specimens *(21)*. The t(6;14) results in overexpression of *cyclin D3*.

3.1. IgH Translocations With Unknown Partner Chromosomes

In the remaining 40% of MM tumors with evidence of a 14q32 translocation, the translocation partner has remained unidentified. Several translocations have been described in cell lines [e.g., t(6;14)(p25;q32)], but there is lack of evidence that these abnormalities are recurrent translocations in primary MM specimens. Most likely, they represent secondary translocations that occur during the progression of the disease.

3.2. Prognostic Implications of IgH Translocations

The analysis of recurrent IgH translocations in the context of clinical data strongly suggests that distinct subgroups of MM patients can be defined according to their genomic alterations: Presence of a t(4;14) and t(14;16) is indicative for a poor prognosis *(10,22)*, whereas a t(11;14) is associated with a rather favorable outcome *(10,23)*. Patients with an IgH translocation with an unknown translocation partner represent an intermediate prognostic group, which can be further subdivided according to the status of chromosome 13q (favorable outcome with normal chromosome 13; poor prognosis with deletion of 13q) *(10)*

Primary IgH translocations are not only present in MM cells, but may also be found in MGUS plasma cells (discussed later in this chapter). It has been hypothesized that such IgH translocations represent an immortalizing event in plasma cells and are thus considered early events in myelomagenesis. However, because IgH translocations specific for other B-cell malignancies, for example, the t(14;18)(q32;q21) and t(8;14)(q24;q32) translocations, have also been described at low levels in healthy individuals, additional genetic events may be required to transform a B lymphocyte into a cell with full malignant potential *(24)*

4. DELETION OF CHROMOSOME 13Q

Partial or complete loss of chromosome 13q has been observed as the chromosomal region that is most frequently recurrently deleted in MM karyotypes. Using metaphase cytogenetics, investigators have determined that a chromosome 13q abnormality can be found in approx 15% of patients with MM at the time of diagnosis, *(1,3,17,25)*, whereas interphase FISH studies have shown a higher frequency of 13q deletions in MM cells, occurring in 39 to 54% of newly diagnosed cases *(8,26–28)*.

This abnormality has gained considerable interest since several studies reported a strong association of a deletion 13q with an unfavorable prognosis for patients with MM *(25–30)*. However, the negative effect on prognosis may not only be limited to loss of chromosome 13, because it has also been found with the loss of other chromosomes, as reflected by a hypodiploid karyotype: in the report by Fassas and colleagues, both deletion 13 and the presence of a hypodiploid karyotype were independent predictors of a poor outcome *(32)*. In contrast, investigators in two other cytogenetic studies concluded that a chromosome 13 deletion does not add independent prognostic significance to that provided by karyotypic hypodiploidy *(2,3)*.

Information regarding candidate genes, which are lost as a consequence of the deletion, is still limited. In the majority of cases involving a 13q deletion, a large proportion of the 13q arm is deleted, indicating a loss of the entire chromosome arm or even monosomy 13 *(28)*. However, interstitial deletions mainly involving band 13q14—as well as dual loss at 13q14 and 13q34, with an intact intervening region *(33)*—have also been observed recurrently. In a recent study, it has been suggested that a commonly deleted region that includes the *D13S319* locus is located at 13q14 between the *RB-1* and *D13S25* gene loci *(33)*. This genomic region encompasses an area rich in expressed sequence-tagged sites and contains *DLEU1*, *DLEU2*, and *RFP2* genes. Direct sequencing of the *RFP2* gene did not reveal any mutations in six patients and four cell lines exhibiting a 13q14 deletion. It has not yet been determined whether *RFP2* may be involved in the pathogenesis of MM by means of other mechanisms of inactivation (e.g. haploinsufficiency).

A chromosome 13 abnormality may be associated with specific 14q translocations: *(10)* Data obtained thus far indicate that there are significant associations between t(4;14) and the presence of a deletion 13q (>80%), as well as t(14;16) and deletion 13q (100% in the few reported cases). In contrast, patients lacking any 14q translocation displayed significantly less frequent abnormalities of chromosome 13q (approx 25% of cases). No correlations were found between t(11;14) and deletion 13q; likewise, there is no apparent association between a 14q32 translocation with an unknown partner chromosome and deletion 13q.

5. CHROMOSOMAL ABERRATIONS IN MGUS PLASMA CELLS

Because of the low number of clonal bone marrow plasma cells and their low proliferative rate, virtually no informative karyotypes are available from individuals with MGUS. FISH studies, however, have demonstrated that chromosomal aneuploidy is a common finding that is already present at the level of MGUS: Plasma cells from individuals with MGUS may exhibit not only numerical changes (trisomies of chromosomes 3, 7, 9, and 11)*(34)*, but also structural aberrations, e.g., 14q translocations and deletions of 13q *(8,9,35)*.

Translocations involving the *IgH* locus have been reported to occur in 46% of patients with MGUS, as determined by interphase FISH analysis (36 of 79 patients in the study by Avet-Loiseau and colleagues; *(8)* 27 of 59 patients in the study by Fonseca and colleagues) *(9)*. A t(11;14)(q13;q32) was found to be the most common translocation in MGUS. The t(4;14) can also be detected in MGUS (as determined by FISH or by a reverse transcriptase PCR for the *IgH-MMSET* transcript), but was reported to occur in fewer than 10% of cases *(8,9,36)*. As in MM, the presence of a t(4;14) can result in the expression of the FGFR3 protein. Thus, all 14q translocations observed in MM also appear to be present in MGUS, including the t(14;16) *(9)*. So far, no association of a specific translocation with progression of MGUS to MM has been reported.

Several studies also show the presence of a chromosome 13q deletion in the clonal plasma cells of patients with MGUS, with a prevalence ranging between 15 and 50% *(8,9,35,37)*. With respect to 14q translocations, approx 50% of patients with a t(11;14) had a concomitant deletion of 13q, whereas there was a strong association between t(4;14) and deletion 13q (similar to observations in

MM) *(8,9)*. It is at present unknown whether an IgH translocation or a deletion 13q may occur earlier during the development or existence of MGUS. There is some evidence that a chromosome 13 abnormality may be important for the progression of MGUS to MM, *(37,38)* but this issue needs to be addressed in larger cohorts of patients.

6. ONCOGENIC EVENTS ASSOCIATED WITH DISEASE PROGRESSION

6.1. Translocations Involving c-myc

Chromosomal aberrations of 8q24 (*c-myc* gene locus) have only rarely been reported by classical karyotypic analyses of MM. Similarly, a t(8;14)(q24;q32) determined by interphase FISH was present in only 3 of 140 primary MM tumors *(8)*. However, multicolor FISH studies of metaphase chromosomes obtained from 38 patients with advanced MM indicated that complex translocations involving *c-myc* occur in approx 40% of these cases *(39)*. In contrast to Burkitt's lymphoma, where *c-myc* is rearranged with *Ig* gene loci as a primary molecular event, translocations with *c-myc* in MM mostly involve non-Ig gene sequences with complex aberrations often affecting more than two chromosomes. A *c-myc* aberration represents a late event in the pathogenesis of MM and one that is unlikely to have a significant prognostic impact.

6.2. Mutations of N- and K-ras

Whereas activating point mutations of N-*ras* and K-*ras* (codons 12, 13, and 61) are rare events in MGUS, solitary plasmacytoma, and indolent MM, they have been reported to occur in 10 to 40% of patients with MM at diagnosis and with even greater frequency in patients in an advanced and terminal stage of MM *(40)*

However, earlier studies have underestimated the frequency of *ras*-mutation positive cases, because a recent study employing a sensitive PCR restriction fragment length polymorphism strategy on enriched plasma cell populations has reported N-*ras* codon 61 mutation in all of 34 MM cases at presentation *(41)*. Of note, *ras* mutation-positive cells comprised only a subpopulation of the total plasma cell population. Similarly, Bezieau and colleagues, using a sensitive allele-specific amplification method, detected N-*ras* and/or K-*ras* mutations in 55% of MM cases at diagnosis (and in 81% of cases at relapse) *(42)*. Overall, these recent findings suggest that *ras* mutations play a major role in the oncogenesis of MM and are mainly associated with disease progression, because as mutations they appear to be rare in MGUS.

6.3. Abnormalities of p53

p53 Mutations are rare in patients with MM at diagnosis, but may be found with increasing frequency in patients with relapse or plasma cell leukemia *(43)*.

Deletions of 17p13, including the *p53* gene, may also be present in MM at diagnosis; however, because these abnormalities often involve small interstitial deletions, molecular cytogenetic techniques are required for their detection *(44)*. The presence of a 17p13 deletion has been associated with shortened survival *(22,44)*. Deletions of 17p13 have not been observed in MGUS plasma cells.

7. EPIGENETIC ABNORMALITIES OF CELL CYCLE REGULATORS AND TUMOR SUPPRESSOR GENES

Epigenetics is the study of modifications in gene expression that do not involve changes in DNA nucleotide sequences. Modifications in gene expression through the methylation of DNA and remodelling of chromatin via histone proteins are believed to be the most important epigenetic changes. Current interest in the role of methylation has focused on the potential of aberrant methylation in silencing tumor suppressor genes.

In MM, hypermethylation of genes such as *death-associated protein (DAP)-kinase, SOCS-1,* and the cell cycle regulators *p15* and *p16* has been associated with gene inactivation. The p15 and p16 proteins are cell-cycle regulator proteins involved in the inhibition of G_1 phase progression. They compete with cyclin D1 for binding to CDK4/CDK6 and, therefore, inhibit CDK4/6 complex kinase activity, resulting in dephosphorylation of pRb and related G_1 arrest. Frequencies of *p16* or *p15* gene methylation of up to 75% have been reported in MM and in myeloma-derived cell lines *(45)*, and *p16* methylation was associated with an increased proliferation rate for plasma cells and a poor prognosis *(46)*. Methylation of *p16* and *p15* was also detected in MGUS, which suggests that methylation of these genes is an early event and not associated with the transition from MGUS to MM *(47)*

Loss of *DAP-kinase* expression has been associated with promoter hyper-methylation in 67% of MM cases. *DAP-kinase* is a gene that regulates apoptosis induced by interferon-α. Preliminary findings suggest prognostic implications for *DAP kinase* in MM *(45)*. The SOCS-1 protein has been shown to be involved into the Jak/STAT pathway. It suppresses signalling by a wide variety of cytokines, including IL-6, IL-4, leukemia inhibitory factor, oncostatin M, and interferons. It has been shown that regulation of cytokine signaling by SOCS-1 is important in normal lymphocyte development and differentiation. *SOCS-1* was inactivated by hypermethylation in almost 63% of MM patient samples *(48)*.

The frequent demonstration of aberrant gene-promotor methylation in MM and MGUS provides not only new insights into the biology of MM, but also suggests that this pathway may be a potential target for novel therapeutic interventions. Hypermethylation-associated gene silencing is a potentially reversible phenom-enon, and demethylating agents such as 5-aza-2' deoxycytidine have been shown to exert clinical activity in patients with myelodysplastic syndromes *(49)*

8. GENETIC EVENTS DEFINED BY GLOBAL
GENE EXPRESSION PROFILING OF MM

Global gene expression profiling utilizes arrays that contain thousands of oligonucleotide probes packed at extremely high density. By exploiting the complementary base pairing of nucleic acids, a large number of genes can be monitored in a single experiment. The initial results obtained with this new technique indicated that MM plasma cells can be differentiated from normal plasma cells by using approximately 120 genes, whereas MGUS plasma cells and MM cells are currently indistinguishable using this approach *(50)*. Among MM plasma cells, genes associated with B-cell differentiation may be highly variable, and based upon the pattern of expression of early and late differentiation antigens, four MM subgroups could be identified *(50)*. The MM_1 subgroup contained samples resembling normal plasma cells and MGUS plasma cells, whereas the MM_4 subgroup contained samples resembling MM cell lines. The most significant gene expression patterns differentiating MM_1 and MM_4 were cell-cycle control and DNA metabolism genes. Furthermore, the MM_4 subgroup was more likely to have abnormal cytogenetics, elevated serum β_2 microglobulin, elevated creatinine, and deletions of chromosome 13, which suggests that the MM_4 subgroup may represent a high-risk clinical entity. This system represents the framework for a new MM molecular classification system and identifies the genetic differences associated with these distinct subgroups. Thus, knowledge of the molecular genetics of this particular subgroup should provide insight into its biology and possibly provide a rationale for appropriate subtype-specific therapeutic interventions.

In another approach, cDNA arrays were used to identify genes that are overexpressed in MM cells compared with autologous B-lymphoblastoid cell lines. The overexpressed genes included an oncogenic tyrosine kinase receptor (*Tyro3*), an autocrine growth factor (heparin-binding epidermal growth factor-like growth factor), a cell invasion protease (thrombin receptor), chemokine receptors (CCR1 and CCR2), and the Notch receptor ligand Jagged2 *(51)*. Thus, several pathways that have not yet been linked with MM biology could play a role in the pathogenesis of MM.

9. MM PATHOGENESIS AS A MULTISTEP PROCESS

From cytogenetic and molecular studies in MM and MGUS, one can conclude that critical chromosomal abnormalities leading to karyotypic instability already occur in MGUS plasma cells and that additional genetic events take place during the evolution of MM and progression to advanced stages of the disease. A model has been proposed that implicates multiple genetic events in the pathogenesis of monoclonal gammopathies (Fig. 1) *(52)*. One of the earliest chromosomal events may be the occurrence of a 14q32 translocation with

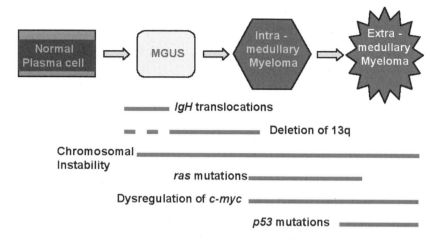

Fig. 1. Multistep molecular pathogenesis of monoclonal gammopathies (modified from ref. *52*). The approximate timing of some specific oncogeneic events is indicated by horizontal lines.

consecutive activation of an oncogene at one of the various translocation partner regions, which results in immortalization of the plasma cell clone. Karyotypic instability becomes apparent in MGUS plasma cells and may be even more pronounced as soon as the disease begins to progress. Acquisition of additional chromosomal changes (including deletion 13q), as well as activation of oncogenes, may then lead to transformation and the development of MM. Factors produced by MM cells generate a milieu in bone marrow that supports proliferation of the malignant clone. During this phase of the disease, MM cells remain growth factor-dependent and thus are localized to bone marrow. Late-occurring genetic and molecular events (e.g., secondary translocations, dysregulation of additional oncogenes) characterize MM cell growth that becomes more and more independent of the supportive role of bone marrow stroma cells. This phase is clinically characterized by an aggressive course, with frequent extramedullary manifestations.

10. FUTURE DIRECTIONS

From a clinical perspective, it has long been recognized that MM is characterized by a heterogeneous group of entities with distinct biological behavior. We are now at the beginning of the development of a molecular classification of MM. At present, it can be concluded that distinct MM entities can be defined by specific chromosomal abnormalities. In the context of 14q32 translocations, it will be important to resolve the question of yet unknown translocation partners and their contribution to biology and clinical behavior. Likewise, it will be relevant to study molecular events in the group of MM patients who do not exhibit a 14q32 translocation. Also, genes that are dysregulated by a 13q deletion and other chromosomal losses need to be defined. Finally, molecular events leading to the transition from MGUS to MM are still poorly characterized.

It is anticipated that systematic use of novel molecular techniques, in particular global gene expression profiling *(50,53)*, may lead to new insights into molecular changes in MM. It can also be envisioned that the elucidation of fundamental genetic events in monoclonal gammopathies may lead to the definition of specific targets for more effective therapeutic interventions in the future, in particular for MM patients with unfavorable cytogenetic features.

REFERENCES

1. Zandecki M, Lai JL, Facon T. Multiple myeloma: almost all patients are cytogenetically abnormal. Br J Haematol 1996; 94:217-227.
2. Debes-Marun CS, Dewald GW, Bryant S, et al. Chromosome abnormalities clustering and its implications for pathogenesis and prognosis in myeloma. Leukemia 2003; 17:427–436.
3. Smadja NV, Bastard C, Brigaudeau C, Leroux D, Fruchart C. Hypodiploidy is a major prognostic factor in multiple myeloma. Blood 2001; 98:2229–2238.
4. Fonseca R, Debes-Marun CS, Picken EB, et al. The recurrent IgH translocations are highly associated with non-hyperdiploid variant multiple myeloma. Blood 2003; 102:2562–2567.
5. Willis TG, Dyer MJ. The role of immunoglobulin translocations in the pathogenesis of B-cell malignancies. Blood 2000; 96:808–822.
6. Bergsagel PL, Chesi M, Nardini E, Brents LA, Kirby SL, Kuehl WM. Promiscuous translocations into immunoglobulin heavy chain switch regions in multiple myeloma. Proc Natl Acad Sci U S A 1996; 93:13931–13936.
7. Avet-Loiseau H, Daviet A, Brigaudeau C, et al. Cytogenetic, interphase, and multicolor fluorescence in situ hybridization analyses in primary plasma cell leukemia: a study of 40 patients at diagnosis, on behalf of the Intergroupe Francophone du Myelome and the Groupe Francais de Cytogenetique Hematologique. Blood 2001; 97:822–825.
8. Avet-Loiseau H, Facon T, Daviet A, et al. 14q32 translocations and monosomy 13 observed in monoclonal gammopathy of undetermined significance delineate a multistep process for the oncogenesis of multiple myeloma. Intergroupe Francophone du Myelome. Cancer Res 1999; 59:4546–4550.
9. Fonseca R, Bailey RJ, Ahmann GJ, et al. Genomic abnormalities in monoclonal gammopathy of undetermined significance. Blood 2002; 100:1417–1424.
10. Moreau P, Facon T, Leleu X, et al. Recurrent 14q32 translocations determine the prognosis of multiple myeloma, especially in patients receiving intensive chemotherapy. Blood 2002; 100:1579–1583.
11. Ronchetti D, Finelli P, Richelda R, et al. Molecular analysis of 11q13 breakpoints in multiple myeloma. Blood 1999; 93:1330–1337.
12. Janssen JW, Vaandrager JW, Heuser T, et al. Concurrent activation of a novel putative transforming gene, myeov, and cyclin D1 in a subset of multiple myeloma cell lines with t(11;14)(q13;q32). Blood 2000; 95:2691–2698.
13. Avet-Loiseau H, Garand R, Lode L, Harousseau JL, Bataille R. Translocation t(11;14)(q13;q32) is the hallmark of IgM, IgE, and nonsecretory multiple myeloma variants. Blood 2003; 101:1570–1571.

14. Chesi M, Nardini E, Brents LA, et al. Frequent translocation t(4;14)(p16.3;q32.3) in multiple myeloma is associated with increased expression and activating mutations of fibroblast growth factor receptor 3. Nat Genet 1997; 16:260–264.
15. Plowright EE, Li Z, Bergsagel PL, et al. Ectopic expression of fibroblast growth factor receptor 3 promotes myeloma cell proliferation and prevents apoptosis. Blood 2000; 95:992–998.
16. Chesi M, Brents LA, Ely SA, et al. Activated fibroblast growth factor receptor 3 is an oncogene that contributes to tumor progression in multiple myeloma. Blood 2001; 97:729–736.
17. Pollett JB, Trudel S, Stern D, Li ZH, Stewart AK. Overexpression of the myeloma-associated oncogene fibroblast growth factor receptor 3 confers dexamethasone resistance. Blood 2002; 100:3819–3821.
18. Santra M, Zhan F, Tian E, Barlogie B, Shaughnessy J. A subset of multiple myeloma harboring the t(4;14)(p16;q32) translocation lack FGFR3 expression but maintain an IGH/MMSET fusion transcript. Blood 2002; 14:14.
19. Keats JJ, Reiman T, Maxwell CA, et al. In multiple myeloma, t(4;14)(p16;q32) is an adverse prognostic factor irrespective of FGFR3 expression. Blood 2003; 101:1520–1529.
20. Chesi M, Bergsagel PL, Shonukan OO, et al. Frequent dysregulation of the c-maf proto-oncogene at 16q23 by translocation to an Ig locus in multiple myeloma. Blood 1998; 91:4457–4463.
21. Shaughnessy J Jr, Gabrea A, Qi Y, et al. Cyclin D3 at 6p21 is dysregulated by recurrent chromosomal translocations to immunoglobulin loci in multiple myeloma. Blood 2001; 98:217–223.
22. Fonseca R, Blood E, Rue M, et al. Clinical and biologic implications of recurrent genomic aberrations in myeloma. Blood 2003; 101:4569–4575.
23. Soverini S, Cavo M, Cellini C, et al. Cyclin D1 overexpression is a favorable prognostic variable for newly diagnosed multiple myeloma patients treated with high-dose chemotherapy and single or double autologous transplantation. Blood 2003; 102:1588–1593.
24. Janz S, Potter M, Rabkin CS. Lymphoma- and leukemia-associated chromosomal translocations in healthy individuals. Genes Chromosomes Cancer 2003; 36:211–223.
25. Tricot G, Barlogie B, Jagannath S, et al. Poor prognosis in multiple myeloma is associated only with partial or complete deletions of chromosome 13 or abnormalities involving 11q and not with other karyotype abnormalities. Blood 1995; 86:4250–4256.
26. Perez-Simon JA, Garcia-Sanz R, Tabernero MD, et al. Prognostic value of numerical chromosome aberrations in multiple myeloma: a FISH analysis of 15 different chromosomes. Blood 1998; 91:3366–3371.
27. Zojer N, Konigsberg R, Ackermann J, et al. Deletion of 13q14 remains an independent adverse prognostic variable in multiple myeloma despite its frequent detection by interphase fluorescence in situ hybridization. Blood 2000; 95:1925–1930.
28. Fonseca R, Oken MM, Harrington D, et al. Deletions of chromosome 13 in multiple myeloma identified by interphase FISH usually denote large deletions of the q arm or monosomy. Leukemia 2001; 15:981–986.
29. Desikan R, Barlogie B, Sawyer J, et al. Results of high-dose therapy for 1000 patients with multiple myeloma: durable complete remissions and superior survival in the absence of chromosome 13 abnormalities. Blood 2000; 95:4008–4010.
30. Fonseca R, Harrington D, Oken MM, et al. Biological and prognostic significance of interphase fluorescence in situ hybridization detection of chromosome 13 abnormalities (delta13) in multiple myeloma: an eastern cooperative oncology group study. Cancer Res 2002; 62:715–720.
31. Facon T, Avet-Loiseau H, Guillerm G, et al. Chromosome 13 abnormalities identified by FISH analysis and serum beta 2-microglobulin produce a powerful myeloma staging system for patients receiving high-dose therapy. Blood 2001; 97:1566–1571.
32. Fassas AB, Spencer T, Sawyer J, et al. Both hypodiploidy and deletion of chromosome 13 independently confer poor prognosis in multiple myeloma. Br J Haematol 2002; 118:1041–1047.

33. Elnenaei MO, Hamoudi RA, Swansbury J, et al. Delineation of the minimal region of loss at 13q14 in multiple myeloma. Genes Chromosomes Cancer 2003; 36:99–106.
34. Drach J, Angerler J, Schuster J, et al. Interphase fluorescence in situ hybridization identifies chromosomal abnormalities in plasma cells from patients with monoclonal gammopathy of undetermined significance. Blood 1995; 86:3915–3921.
35. Konigsberg R, Ackermann J, Kaufmann H, et al. Deletions of chromosome 13q in monoclonal gammopathy of undetermined significance. Leukemia 2000; 14:1975–1979.
36. Sibley K, Fenton JA, Dring AM, Ashcroft AJ, Rawstron AC, Morgan GJ. A molecular study of the t(4;14) in multiple myeloma. Br J Haematol 2002; 118:514–520.
37. Avet-Loiseau H, Li JY, Morineau N, et al. Monosomy 13 is associated with the transition of monoclonal gammopathy of undetermined significance to multiple myeloma. Intergroupe Francophone du Myeloma. Blood 1999; 94:2583–2589.
38. Kaufmann H, Ackermann J, Nösslinger T, et al. Deletion of chromosome 13q is a frequent abnormality in multiple myeloma evolving from a preexisting monoclonal gammopathy of undetermined significance. Blood 2002; 100:103a.
39. Shou Y, Martelli ML, Gabrea A, et al. Diverse karyotypic abnormalities of the c-myc locus associated with c-myc dysregulation and tumor progression in multiple myeloma. Proc Natl Acad Sci U S A 2000; 97:228–233.
40. Liu P, Leong T, Quam L, et al. Activating mutations of N- and K-ras in multiple myeloma show different clinical associations: analysis of the Eastern Cooperative Oncology Group Phase III Trial. Blood 1996; 88:2699–2706.
41. Kalakonda N, Rothwell DG, Scarffe JH, Norton JD. Detection of N-Ras codon 61 mutations in subpopulations of tumor cells in multiple myeloma at presentation. Blood 2001; 98:1555–1560.
42. Bezieau S, Devilder MC, Avet-Loiseau H, et al. High incidence of N and K-Ras activating mutations in multiple myeloma and primary plasma cell leukemia at diagnosis. Hum Mutat 2001; 18:212–224.
43. Neri A, Baldini L, Trecca D, Cro L, Polli E, Maiolo AT. p53 gene mutations in multiple myeloma are associated with advanced forms of malignancy. Blood 1993; 81:128–135.
44. Drach J, Ackermann J, Fritz E, et al. Presence of a p53 gene deletion in patients with multiple myeloma predicts for short survival after conventional-dose chemotherapy. Blood 1998; 92:802–809.
45. Ng MH, To KW, Lo KW, et al. Frequent death-associated protein kinase promoter hypermethylation in multiple myeloma. Clin Cancer Res 2001; 7:1724–1729.
46. Mateos MV, Garcia-Sanz R, Lopez-Perez R, et al. Methylation is an inactivating mechanism of the p16 gene in multiple myeloma associated with high plasma cell proliferation and short survival. Br J Haematol 2002; 118:1034–1040.
47. Guillerm G, Gyan E, Wolowiec D, et al. p16(INK4a) and p15(INK4b) gene methylations in plasma cells from monoclonal gammopathy of undetermined significance. Blood 2001; 98:244–246.
48. Galm O, Yoshikawa H, Esteller M, Osieka R, Herman JG. SOCS-1, a negative regulator of cytokine signaling, is frequently silenced by methylation in multiple myeloma. Blood 2002; 27:27.
49. Wijermans P, Lubbert M, Verhoef G, et al. Low-dose 5-aza-2'-deoxycytidine, a DNA hypomethylating agent, for the treatment of high-risk myelodysplastic syndrome: a multicenter phase II study in elderly patients. J Clin Oncol 2000; 18:956–962.
50. Zhan F, Hardin J, Kordsmeier B, et al. Global gene expression profiling of multiple myeloma, monoclonal gammopathy of undetermined significance, and normal bone marrow plasma cells. Blood 2002; 99:1745–1757.
51. De Vos J, Couderc G, Tarte K, et al. Identifying intercellular signaling genes expressed in malignant plasma cells by using complementary DNA arrays. Blood 2001; 98:771–780.
52. Hallek M, Bergsagel PL, Anderson KC. Multiple myeloma: increasing evidence for a multi-step transformation process. Blood 1998; 91:3–21.
53. Claudio JO, Masih-Khan E, Tang H, et al. A molecular compendium of genes expressed in multiple myeloma. Blood 2002; 100:2175–2186.

5 Cytokines in Multiple Myeloma

John De Vos, MD, PhD and Bernard Klein, PhD

CONTENTS

INTRODUCTION
MECHANISMS CONTROLLING NORMAL PLASMA CELL GENERATION
SURVIVAL AND GROWTH FACTORS IN MM
CONCLUSION
REFERENCES

1. INTRODUCTION

Multiple myeloma (MM) is a neoplasm characterized by the clonal accumulation of malignant plasma cells. Myeloma cells localize in the bone marrow, where their survival is strongly dependent on the normal stromal cells that secrete cytokines and interact with the malignant cells through adhesion molecules. This chapter briefly summarizes the main features of normal plasma cell development. It will then consider recent information on the cytokines that control myeloma cell growth and survival and discuss the pathobiological relevance of these data.

2. MECHANISMS CONTROLLING NORMAL PLASMA CELL GENERATION

Virgin B cells that are activated in a T-cell-independent or primary T-cell-dependent response may differentiate into immunoglobulin (Ig) M-secreting plasma cells in peripheral lymphoid organs. These plasma cells are short-lived and are not somatically hypermutated. By contrast, a secondary T-cell-dependent immune response leads to the production of either memory B cells or plasmablastic cells that differentiate further into long-lived IgG- or IgA-secreting plasma cells. Antigen-activated B cells undergo rapid and intense proliferation in the germinal center (GC) of peripheral lymphoid organs in association

From: *Current Clinical Oncology: Biology and Management of Multiple Myeloma*
Edited by: J. R. Berenson © Humana Press Inc., Totowa, NJ

with somatic mutations of the antigen receptor. GC B cells die by apoptosis unless they receive survival signals. Two essential survival signals have to be delivered to GC cells: high-affinity interaction of B-cell membrane immunoglobulin with the antigen found on follicular dendritic cells, and activation of B cell CD40 ligand molecules expressed on antigen-activated GC CD4 T cells (reviewed in ref. *1*). In addition, two cytokines—interleukin (IL)-2 and IL-4—play an important role in the proliferation of GC B cells *(2)*. CD40 stimulation leads to antibody class switching and differentiation into memory B cells. Conversely, the generation of plasmablastic cells requires interruption of CD40 signaling and the presence of IL-10, the most potent B-cell differentiation factor at this stage *(3–5)*. Recent data suggest that CD27—another member of the tumor necrosis factor (TNF) receptor family—could play a role opposite to that of CD40 by inducing plasma cell differentiation *(6)*.

Little is known about the terminal maturation of low-rate secreting plasmablastic cells into high-rate immunoglobulin-secreting plasma cells owing to the low frequency of these cells in vivo. However, the concept of proliferating early plasmablastic cells has been clearly demonstrated in in vitro B-cell differentiation systems (Pokeweed mitogen or T-cell activation) *(7,8)* in patients with reactive plasmacytosis *(9,10)* and in the polyclonal plasmablastic cell (PPC) model we recently developed *(11)*. In some patients with acute inflammation, plasmablasts undergo a brief but considerable in vivo expansion that leads to reactive plasmacytosis. These plasmablastic cells—which consist of immature CD138/syndecan-1⁻ plasmablastic cells and more mature CD138⁺ plasmablastic cells *(10)*—are highly proliferative and short-lived. IL-6 is likely to be a main factor controlling the proliferation, survival, or both of these normal plasmablastic cells, because an anti-IL-6 antibody can block the proliferation and differentiation of these cells in samples from patients with reactive polyclonal plasmacytosis or cardiac myxomas *(10,12)*. IL-6, however, is not sufficient for plasmablast survival. Indeed, we recently developed an in vitro model of the generation of PPCs, starting with peripheral blood B cells obtained from healthy donors or patients with MM. In this model, memory B cells are cultured with a CD40 ligand transfectant, IL-4, IL-2, IL-10, and IL-12 for 4 d. Plasma cell differentiation is induced by removing CD40 stimulation and changing the cytokine combination, i.e., removing IL-4 and adding IL-6 *(11)*. These plasmablastic cells are highly proliferating but inevitably undergo apoptosis at days 7 through 8 in culture, despite the addition of IL-6. This model is therefore well suited for use in determining the mechanisms that control the survival of plasmablastic cells, in addition to IL-6 signaling.

Bone marrow is the main location of immunoglobulin production in humans *(13,14)*. Among the mononucleated cells in bone marrow, plasma cells comprise 0.2 to 0.4%. Most of these plasma cells are long-lived, which suggests that they have found microenvironmental niches that sustain their survival. Their survival is antigen-independent and could be mediated in part by cytokines *(15)*. Additional lines of evidence point to an important role of IL-6 in the survival and proliferation of normal plasma cells. Massive polyclonal plasmacytosis develops in mice bearing an IL-6 transgene driven by the Eμ promoter, and they die within 7 wk *(16)*. IL-6 is also a major plasma-cell differentiation factor controlling immunoglobulin production. Antibodies against IL-6 inhibit the generation of cells producing immunoglobulin at high rates in vitro *(17–19)*. In addition, cell–cell contact and interactions with the extracellular matrix are considered essential for the survival and further differentiation of plasmablasts *(15,20,21)*; the interaction of fibronectin with the receptor VLA-4 on plasma cells has been shown to be essential for this process. Neither IL-6 nor fibronectin alone exerted any effect, but the combination of both factors induced optimal in vitro immunoglobulin secretion by plasma cells *(22)*. More recently, Cassese and colleagues demonstrated that IL-5, IL-6, TNF-α, stromal cell-derived factor-1α and signaling via CD44 support the survival of isolated bone-marrow plasma cells, whereas the early B-cell development, cytokine IL-7 and stem cell factor did not support plasma cell survival *(23)*.

The fully differentiated plasma cell is a nondividing cell that has lost most of its B-cell markers, including major histocompatibility class II and surface immunoglobulin. This cell expresses high levels of *CD38* and *syndecan-1* and secretes large amounts of specific antibody (hourly rate: up to 10^8 molecules/cell) *(14)*. An important emerging feature of normal plasma cells recently demonstrated in mice models is a marked, long-term survival and a half-life exceeding 90 d in mouse and resulting in the secretion of antibodies for extended periods of time (>1 y) in the absence of detectable memory B cells *(24–26)*. It is noteworthy that a very low proliferation rate and marked in vivo survival resemble characteristics of the pathobiology of the malignant counterpart of plasma cells, i.e., myeloma cells.

3. SURVIVAL AND GROWTH FACTORS IN MM

Myeloma cells and normal plasma cells share common survival and growth factors. Particularly, IL-6 plays a major role in MM. Interactions with bone marrow cells seem equally essential, although details on these interactions are still poorly understood.

3.1. IL-6 Cytokines

3.1.1. IL-6

IL-6 is a cytokine with pleiotropic effects on hematopoietic and nonhematopoietic cells *(27)*. This cytokine binds with the membrane receptor IL-6R, forming an IL-6/IL-6R complex that binds with and induces the dimerization of a membrane transducer chain termed gp130. Interestingly, cells may produce a soluble IL-6R agonist—sIL-6R—that activates membrane gp130 when it binds with IL-6. As described above, IL-6 is the only proliferation factor and the main differentiation factor identified for normal plasmablastic cells. It is also the major growth factor in the malignant counterparts of these cells in mice, i.e., mouse plasmacytomas, B-cell hybridomas, and MM. Several lines of evidence suggest a central role for IL-6 in MM pathobiology.

IL-6 is the major cytokine promoting the proliferation of primary human myeloma cells (28,29). This proliferation is weak, resulting in a small percentage of malignant cells in the cell cycle, and transient, lasting 1 to 2 wk in vitro. For patients with fulminant disease and extramedullary proliferation, IL-6-dependent myeloma cell lines have been obtained (30). When IL-6 is removed, these cell lines stop proliferating and progressively die by apoptosis. Accordingly, myeloma cells spontaneously express IL-6R. Antibodies against IL-6R or gp130 block the proliferation of either primary plasma cell or MM IL-6-dependent cell lines (29,31). In contrast, agonist antibodies against anti-gp130 agonists that induce gp130 dimerization can replace IL-6 and support the survival and growth of these cell lines (32).

The role of IL-6 in multiple myeloma disease is also supported by in vivo data. High plasma levels of this cytokine have been found in MM patients and are associated with a poor prognosis (33,34). It has also been shown that levels of plasma C-reactive protein, an acute-phase reactant produced by the liver under the control of IL-6 (35), are often increased in patients with multiple myeloma. Serum C reactive protein correlates with IL-6 levels and is a powerful prognostic factor (36). In most studies, investigators have shown that IL-6 is produced in vivo by nonmalignant bone marrow cells and not by myeloma cells (reviewed in ref. 37). IL-6 synthesis is triggered both by adhesion of myeloma cells to bone marrow stromal cells (38,39) and by IL-1 (40). The central role of IL-1 will be described in detail later in this chapter. Finally, the contention that IL-6 plays a pivotal role in MM in vivo is also demonstrated by clinical improvement in patients treated with anti-IL-6 monoclonial antibody (MAb) (35). This type of therapy can inhibit myeloma cell proliferation, induce a decrease in tumor cell mass, and reduce tumor-associated toxicity (fever, bone pain, and cachexia). These effects have been observed only in patients in whom the overall IL-6 production in vivo is low enough to be neutralized by anti-IL-6 MAb activity (41–43). Only in the low IL-6 producers can IL-6 be neutralized by the antagonist antibodies.

A major role for IL-6 in malignant plasma cell development has also been demonstrated in murine models. The BALB/c mouse strain has a genetic susceptibility to the development of plasmacytomas. Intraperitoneal injection of pristane (or silicone gels) induces plasma cell tumor formation in 40 to 60% of the mice. It has been demonstrated that these tumors develop exclusively from cells in oil-induced granulomatous tissue, which have been found to produce elevated concentrations of plasmacytoma growth factor(s) (44). The mouse plasmacytoma growth factor was purified, and cloning of its cDNA showed that it is the murine homologue of human IL-6 (45). Indeed, when BALB/c mice are backcrossed with animal knockouts for the IL-6 gene (IL-6 –/–), they fail to develop plasmacytomas after pristane injections *(46)*. On the contrary, introduction of BALB/c genetic background into Eμ/IL-6 transgenic mice resulted in the spontaneous occurrence of plasmacytomas *(47)*. Another murine model uses a retrovirus bearing the *raf* and *myc* oncogenes that induce plasmacytoma and myeloid neoplasm formation in mice homozygous (+/+) or heterozygous (+/–) for the wild-type *IL-6* allele. Mice homozygous for the *IL-6-null* allele (–/–) are completely resistant to plasma cell tumor development, although they still present myeloid tumors with the expected incidence *(48)*.

3.1.2. OTHER IL-6-TYPE CYTOKINES

IL-6 is part of a family of broadly acting cytokines whose receptors share the common signal-transducing component, gp130 *(27)*. This family consists of IL-11, leukemia inhibitory factor (LIF), oncostatin M (OSM), ciliary neurotrophic factor (CNTF), and cardiotrophin-1. The various gp130 cytokines share some biological functions and accordingly they can stimulate some MM cell lines that depend on the expression of the specific chain of the cytokine receptor *(30)*. LIF-, OSM-, IL-11-, or CNTF-dependent myeloma cell lines have been obtained *(49)*. Unlike cell lines that are sensitive to IL-6 only, these cell lines produce autocrine IL-10, which, by up-regulating the LIF receptor (LIFR) expression, confers sensitivity on cytokines that require this second receptor chain *(50)*. However, the relative importance of these gp130 cytokines in the control of the proliferation of myeloma cells in vivo has not yet been clarified. In fact, we have found that these IL-6-type cytokines are poorly produced by malignant samples in vitro and are barely detected in the plasma in MM patients compared with IL-6 (unpublished data). Thus, IL-6 is likely to be the major gp130-activating cytokine involved in MM biology.

3.1.3. VIRAL IL-6

It has been suggested that the herpes virus KSHV could play an essential role in MM pathophysiology by infecting dendritic cells in the medullary microenvironment *(51)*. The infected dendritic cell would synthesize viral IL-6 (vIL-6), thereby promoting and sustaining MM growth. It has been shown that vIL-6 is able to activate gp130 and, thus, is able to sustain the survival and proliferation of an IL-6-dependent MM cell line *(52)*. However, some studies have shown a lack of KSHV infection in patients with MM as initially stated by our group *(52a)* in agreement with data on KSHV serology and epidemiology in MM *(53)*.

3.2. Other Growth Factors

3.2.1. IL-10

As discussed previously, normal plasma cell differentiation is controlled mainly by two cytokines: IL-6 and IL-10. In MM, IL-6 has lost its differentiation properties, yet retains its survival and proliferation potential. Likewise, IL-10 is a proliferation factor but not a differentiation factor for human MM cells, i.e., IL-10 does not induce cytologic differentiation or increase immunoglobulin synthesis in IL-6-dependent MM cell lines *(54)*. It can stimulate the proliferation of two out of four IL-6-dependent MM cell lines in the absence of IL-6, however; this is not affected by anti-IL-6 or anti-IL-6R antibodies. IL-10-dependent MM cell lines have been obtained. Moreover, IL-10 can stimulate the proliferation of freshly explanted myeloma cells in IL-6-deprived cultures of tumor cells obtained from patients with active MM. However, the myeloma cell growth factor activity if IL-10 is abrogated by an antibody to the gp130 IL-6 transducer, indicating that IL-10 effects are mediated through an IL-6 family cytokine, yet are different from IL-6 *(50)*. This IL-10 growth activity is explained by an autocrine production of OSM by the myeloma cells. In the absence of IL-10, OSM is inactive as a result of the lack of the coreceptor to OSM, which is necessary to activate the gp130 transducer. IL-10, by inducing LIFR or possibly the other OSM receptor, induces a functional autocrine OSM loop *(50)*. IL-10 also induces IL-11R expression and autocrine IL-10 production; this explains the IL-11 responsiveness of some MM cell lines (Table 1) *(55)*. IL-10 is found in low concentrations in the supernatant of cultures of malignant cells obtained from patients with active disease. Accordingly, IL-10 is infrequently detected in the plasma of patients with MM, except for patients with plasma cell leukemia *(54)*.

3.2.2. IL-1

The proinflammatory cytokine IL-1 is a potent inducer of IL-6 production in monocytes, fibroblasts, and endothelial cells *(56,57)*. Human bone marrow myeloma cells spontaneously produce IL-1—mainly IL-1β—and this cytokine has been shown to contribute to the high levels of IL-6 production in the MM-malignant environment *(58)*. The IL-1 producer cell in MM has been a controversial subject because several groups have shown that myeloma cells are the major producers of IL-1 *(59,60)*, whereas others have reported that purified myeloma cells fail to express the IL-1 gene *(61)*. We recently reinvestigated this issue by means of in situ hybridization and immunocytochemistry *(40)*. Both techniques showed that bone marrow myeloid and megakaryocytic cells expressed high levels of the IL-1β gene and produced IL-1β. Myeloma cells also expressed IL-1β, although to a lesser extent. For two patients with plasma cell leukaemia, *IL-1β* gene expression was detected in bone marrow myeloma cells, unlike circulating myeloma cells, suggesting that IL-1β expression in myeloma cells is not constitutive but, rather, induced by the bone marrow environment. Furthermore, 9 myeloma cell lines failed to express the IL-1β gene. Many IL-1-induced effects are mediated by prostaglandins *(57)*, and prostaglandin E_2 (PGE2) plays a major role in the production of IL-6 in the malignant environment in the BALB/C mouse model *(62)*. We demonstrated that IL-1-induced IL-6 produc-

Table 1
Cytokine Production and Cytokine Receptor Expression in Myeloma Cell Lines

Multiple cyeloma cell line	XG-1	XG-2	XG-4	XG-6	XG-7
Cell growth dependent	Yes	Yes	Yes	Yes	No
Cytokines produced					
IL-6	−	−	−	−	+
IL-10	−	−	+	+	+
OSM	+	+	−	−	+
IL-11	−	−	−	−	−
LIF	−	−	−	−	−
Receptors expressed					
gp130	+	+	+	+	+
IL-6R	+	+	+	+	+
LIFR	− (IL-10 → +)	− (IL-10 → +)	+	+	+
IL-11R	− (IL-10 → +)	− (IL-10 → +)	+	+	ND
Growth response to exogenous cytokines					
IL-6	+	+	+	+	+
IL-10	+	+	−	−	ND
OSM	− (IL-10 → +)	− (IL-10 → +)	+	+	+
IL-11	− (IL-10 → +)	− (IL-10 → +)	+	+	+
LIF	− (IL-10 → +)	− (IL-10 → +)	+	+	+

Note. XG-1 and XG-2 cell lines respons to IL-10 by inducing LIF receptor (LIFR) expression and conferring on them sensitivity to OSM. An autocrine OSM loop is not observed in XG-4 and XG-6 owing to the lack of OSM production. XG-7 is an autonomously growing MM cell line that produces IL-6 and OSM.

tion in MM malignant samples through a PGE2 loop. Both the IL-1 receptor antagonist IL-1RA and the cyclooxygenase inhibitor indomethacin that blocks PGE2 synthesis were able to inhibit IL-6 production by 80%. Taken together, these data suggest a central role for IL-1 in MM pathobiology. In addition, it should be noted that IL-1β is a major osteoclast-activating factor (OAF) and is thereby believed to contribute to the lytic bone lesions observed in mycloma (63,64).

3.2.3. IL-15

IL-15 is a proliferation and a survival factor for human T and B lymphocytes, natural killer cells, and neutrophils. A receptor for IL-15 was reported to be expressed by myeloma cell lines and on primary myeloma cells (65). Recombinant IL-15 promoted proliferation and survival of myeloma cells; these effects were not mediated by the gp130 receptor chain, because IL-15-induced proliferation is not blocked by anti-gp130 neutralizing antibodies (65,66). Blocking autocrine IL-15 in myeloma cell lines increased the rate of spontaneous apoptosis.

IL-15 transcripts and the IL-15 protein were detected in some myeloma cell samples, suggesting that IL-15 could stimulate myeloma cells either in an autocrine or paracrine fashion *(65,66)*.

3.2.4. GRANULOCYTE-MACROPHAGE COLONY-STIMULATING FACTOR

Normal plasma cells, as well as myeloma cells, express the granulocyte-macrophage colony-stimulating factor (GM-CSF) receptor *(67, 68)*, which is functional in MM cell lines, as indicated by its ability to activate the mitogen-activated protein kinase (MAPK) cascade. We and other researchers have shown that GM-CSF induces primary myeloma cells and MM cell line proliferation *(68,69)*. This stimulation is abrogated by anti-IL-6R antibodies, however, which suggests that GM-CSF has no direct growth factor activity in human myeloma cells, but increases the IL-6 responsiveness of myeloma cells *(69)*. GM-CSF is produced in short-term cultures of unfractionated bone marrow mononucleated cells obtained from patients with MM, but not in highly purified MM cells nor in MM cell lines. Accordingly, the GM-CSF gene is not expressed in tumor samples, and its serum levels are low or undetectable in MM patients *(69–71)*.

This cytokine has been used mainly to mobilize and collect hematopoietic stem cells in MM patients. No major deleterious in vivo stimulation of the malignant growth by this cytokine has yet been reported.

3.2.5. INTERFERON-α

The usefulness of interferon (IFN)-α in myeloma therapy is still a much debated subject *(72)*. The controversy is based on in vitro studies showing that the effects of IFN-α on primary myeloma cells might be inhibitory or stimulatory, depending on patient sample *(73,74)*. The stimulatory effect is mostly seen at low doses and the inhibitory effect at high doses *(73)*. Myeloma cell line growth can also be either inhibited or stimulated by IFN-α *(75,76)*. Two opposite features of the IFN-α effect on myeloma cells can be used to explain these discrepancies. Although IFN-α alone can induce IL-6-dependent MM cell line proliferation in the absence of IL-6—in part through an autocrine IL-6 loop *(76)* and a gp130 transactivation mediated by the JAK1 and Tyk2 kinases *(77)*—IFN-α partially inhibits IL-6-induced proliferation of myeloma cell lines (unpublished results). The mechanism involved could be a partial blockage of IL-6-induced gp130-linked SHP-2 phosphorylation and MAPkinase activation, which has been demonstrated in the U266 cell line *(78)*. Another nonexclusive molecular basis for the inhibitory effect of IFN-α on the proliferation of some MM cell lines has recently been reported by Arora and associates *(79)*, who showed that the heterogeneity in IFN-α-mediated growth effects in two autonomously growing MM cell lines correlated with the differential induction of *cyclin D2* and *p19^{INK4d}* expression. Thus, because many autonomously growing MM cell lines may function through an autocrine IL-6 loop, the gross effect of IFN-α on some cell lines may be growth inhibition. On the other hand, we and other researchers demonstrated that IFN-α is a potent survival factor for MM cell lines, in that it inhibits apoptosis induced by IL-6 deprivation or dexamethasone treatment *(31,80)*. Similarly, it has been reported that IFN-α could block Fas-induced apoptosis in lymphoblastoid cell lines and MM cell lines *(81)*. These data were challenged by Spets and colleagues, who demonstrated that IFN-α could increase or trigger Fas-induced apoptosis in myeloma cell lines *(82)*. Therefore, depending on experimental conditions or tumor samples, IFN-α can have opposing effects. These in vitro findings, as well as the pleiotropic effects of IFN-α in vivo *(83)*, might explain both the anti-malignant response in some patients and the development of plasma cell leukemia during IFN-α therapy, as reported for two patients *(84,85)*.

Another cautionary note on the clinical use of IFN-α is its inhibitory effects on immunoglobulin secretion *(74,86)*. The M protein is one of the usual malignant mass parameters taken into account when assessing treatment response. By hindering monoclonal protein synthesis, IFN-α might inaccurately suggest a treatment response without necessarily having an anti-malignant effect.

3.2.6. INTERFERON-γ

Several reports have shown that IFN-γ is a potent inhibitor of myeloma cell proliferation. This effect has been documented in freshly explanted myeloma cells as well as in IL-6-dependent myeloma cell lines *(74,87)*. This inhibition is associated with the down-regulation of the IL-6R, both at the RNA and the protein level *(87)*. Additionally, studies in other tumor models suggest that IFN-γ could directly interfere with apoptosis regulation (i.e., the induction of several caspases) and the pro-apoptotic protein Bak *(88)*.

3.2.7. TNF-α

TNF-α is a cytokine that may serve as either an apoptotic or a survival signal, depending on the cell type and the state of activation of the cell. These two opposite outcomes arise from the selective activation of different signal transduction pathways, one that activates the caspase cascade and leads to apoptosis, the other activating the NF-κB family of transcription factors and the c-jun N-terminal protein kinase (JNK) to elicit a survival signal *(89–91)*. In MM, TNF-α promotes the proliferation of myeloma cell lines and partially protects myeloma cells from IL-6 deprivation-induced apoptosis *(60,92,93)*. This activity is independent of IL-6-type cytokines, because it is not blocked by a MAb to IL-6 or gp130 *(93)*. In one IL-6-dependent MM cell line, TNF-α was able to sustain long-term growth in the absence of IL-6 *(93)*. TNF-α also up-regulates several adhesion molecules on MM 1S MM cells and enhances malignant cell-specific binding to bone marrow stromal cells *(94)*. It has been reported that TNF-α is produced by malignant cells obtained from patients with MM and could contribute to the endogenous IL-6 production in the malignant environment *(60,95)*. Indeed, TNF-α is elevated in serum from patients with MGUS and MM compared with normal controls and is a factor of poor prognosis in patients with MGUS; thus, it is associated with a higher risk of evolution to MM *(96,97)*.

3.2.8. INSULIN-LIKE GROWTH FACTORS

The importance of insulin-like growth factors (IGF-I and IGF-II) has emerged in MM. IGFs are key mitogens in many types of malignancies *(98)*, and IGF-II is an essential signal in some murine models of cancer *(99)*. Large concentrations of IGFs are found in plasma (>600 ng/mL) *(100)* bound to IGF-binding proteins (IGF-BP), mainly IGF-BP3. Of special interest in MM—a disease in which malignant cells survive and proliferate close to the bone matrix—IGFs are produced by bone cells and trapped in the bone matrix. Using autonomously growing cell lines, several groups have documented that myeloma cells express the IGF receptor and proliferate in response to IGF-I or IGF-II *(101,102)*. Using IL-6-responsive MM cell lines and bovine serum albumin-supplemented (instead of fetal calf serum-supplemented) culture media, Jelinek and colleagues demonstrated that IGFs can induce a potent proliferative response in MM cells in the absence of IL-6 *(103)*. Using myeloma cell lines whose survival and proliferation is strictly dependent on the addition of exogenous cytokines, we found that IGF-I is both a proliferation and a survival factor as potent as IL-6 for myeloma cells *(104)*. We also found that the effect of IGFs was independent of IL-6 or other gp130-activating cytokines, and vice versa. Moreover, IGF failed to activate the JAK/STAT pathway, but did induce phosphorylation of IRS-1 and activation of the PI-3 kinase/AKT pathway, unlike IL-6 *(104,105)*. In a murine model, Li and associates demonstrated that the expression of a dominant-negative mutant of IGF-IR in plasma cell lines strongly suppressed tumorigenesis in vivo *(106)*. All these data strongly suggest that IGFs are potent survival and proliferation factors for myeloma cells independent of IL-6.

IGFs could play a major role in vivo in myeloma physiopathology. It has recently been demonstrated that proteoglycan heparan sulfates can cause the dissociation of the IGF–IGF-BP complexes *(107)* that circulate abundantly in individuals with MM. Myeloma cells specifically express high levels of syndecan-1, a proteoglycan with heparan sulfate chains (discussed later in this chapter). Dissociation of the IGF–IGF-BP complexes may result in the mobilization of IGF to the myeloma cell IGF receptor.

3.2.9. FIBROBLAST GROWTH FACTORS AND SOLUBLE SYNDECAN-1

Two observations point to the role of fibroblast growth factors (FGFs) in MM pathophysiology. First, t(4;14) translocations involving *FGFR3* and immunoglobulin genes are found in 15% of patients with myeloma *(108,109)*; moreover, mutations leading to the constitutive activation of this receptor are found in some myeloma samples *(108,110)*. Second, heparan sulfate proteo-glycans are obligatory for FGF molecules to bind with FGFRs *(111)*. Syndecan-1—a heparan sulfate proteoglycan and adhesion molecule for collagen type I and fibronectin that is involved in MM cell adhesion *(112)*—is strongly expressed on myeloma cells *(113,114)*. Syndecan-1 binds with several heparin-binding growth factors, including FGF, hepatocyte growth factor (HGF), vascular endothelial growth factor (VEGF), heparin-binding (HB) EGF-like growth factor (HB-EGF), and IGF-BP; thus, it could play an important role in myeloma pathobiology.

Membrane syndecan-1 expression on IL-6-dependent myeloma cells rapidly disappears on apoptotic cells upon removal of IL-6 *(113)*. IL-6 or IFN-α can prevent the loss of syndecan-1. It is well known that syndecans can become soluble molecules by shedding their extracellular domains (ectodomains) and that this shedding is tightly regulated *(115)*. Soluble syndecan-1 is produced by myeloma cells *(116)*. Using the enzyme-linked immunosorbent assay method, we detected increased levels of soluble syndecan-1 in plasma samples obtained from patients with myeloma compared with those of age-related healthy subjects. The median value was 165 ng/mL in patients with myeloma compared with 15 ng/mL in healthy subjects. We found that soluble syndecan-1 is a powerful prognostic factor in patients with newly diagnosed myeloma *(117)*. The mean survival was 24 mo in patients with plasma syndecan-1 below 165 ng/mL compared with 48 mo for patients with plasma syndecan-1 levels below 165 ng/mL. In a mouse model, it was shown that soluble syndecan-1 promoted myeloma growth and dissemination *(118)*. Recent findings indicate that the soluble ectodomain of syndecan-1 may be a potent activator or inhibitor of FGF activity, depending on the level of poorly sulfated domains in heparan sulfate chains, which indicates that the function of circulating syndecan-1 in patients with MM requires further study *(119)*.

Basic fibroblast growth factor (bFGF) is an angiogenic growth factor that triggers neovascularization in solid tumors and some lymphohematopoietic malignancies. In MM, both myeloma cell lines and myeloma cells isolated from the marrow of patients with MM were shown to express and secrete bFGF *(120,121)*. Bone marrow stromal cells (BMSCs) obtained from patients with MM and control subjects expressed high-affinity FGF receptors R1 through R4, and stimulation of BMSCs with bFGF induced an increase in IL-6 secretion. Conversely, stimulation with IL-6 enhanced bFGF expression and secretion by myeloma cells, suggesting paracrine interactions between myeloma and marrow stromal cells involving bFGF and IL-6.

3.2.10. HGF

HGF/scatter factor is a heparin-binding growth factor known to promote cell proliferation, invasion, and motility and to cause blood vessel formation; thus, it could be involved in the growth of cancer cells and in metastasis *(122)*. HGF and its receptor, the proto-oncogene *c-met*, are expressed in both myeloma cell lines and primary MM tumor cells *(123)*. HGF is a growth factor for myeloma cell lines; its activity is blocked by the removal of heparan sulfate chains in syndecan-1 by heparitinase. These observations indicate that syndecan-1 is critical to capture heparin-binding HGF and to present it to its receptor, c-met. HGF is detected in the supernatant of primary cultures of myeloma cells. A report on 398 myeloma patients showed that serum HGF is elevated at diagnosis in 43% of myeloma patients compared with healthy controls *(124)*. The serum level of HGF is correlated with that of IL-6 in MM and was a prognostic factor in a subgroup of patients with high serum β_2 microglobulin levels. In serial analysis, it was shown that serum HGF levels are higher at diagnosis and relapse than at response. However, the precise biological significance of this finding in MM remains to be established.

HGF may also be involved in myeloma-associated osteolytic bone disease, based on the finding that it directly induces the proliferation and the activation of osteoclasts *(125)* and induces the secretion of another OAF from osteoblasts: IL-11 *(126)*.

3.2.11. HB-EGF

Using Atlas macroarrays, we found that myeloma cell lines overexpressed the HB-EGF gene compared with EBV-transformed B-cell lines or normal plasmablastic cells and that inhibitors of HB-EGF can block IL-6-dependent survival of these myeloma cell lines *(127)*. HB-EGF cooperates with IL-6 to trigger the optimal survival of myeloma cells, likely through an interaction between the transducer chains, gp130, and EGF receptors *(128)*. HB-EGF can activate two of the four members of the EGF receptor family (ErbB1 and ErbB4) that are variably expressed by myeloma cells. HB-EGF triggers the PI-3K/AKT pathway in myeloma cells but not STAT3 phosphorylation (unpublished data). Several coreceptors can enhance the binding of HB-EGF and increase its biological activity: syndecan-1, the tetraspanin CD9, and integrin $\alpha3\beta1$ *(129)*. Using Affymetrix microarrays and FACS analysis, we found that these coreceptors are overexpressed in myeloma cells compared with B cells or plasmablastic cells *(11)*. In addition, because 11 members of the EGF family are able to activate the ErbB receptors, other EGF members may be involved in myeloma cell biology. Several inhibitors of EGF activity (humanized MAbs, inhibitors of ErbB kinase activity) are investigated clinically in patients with epithelial cancers. Our recent data indicate that ErbB inhibitors can potentiate dexamethasone-induced apoptosis of myeloma cell lines and primary myeloma cells in most patients and suggest that they might improve treatment of patients with MM.

3.2.12. VEGF

MM is characterized by a significant increase in bone marrow neovascularization. There is a correlation between the extent of bone marrow angiogenesis, determined by microvessel area, and activity of the disease *(121,130)*. VEGF stimulates angiogenesis, including tumor neovascularization. Myeloma cell lines and myeloma cells isolated from the marrow of patients with MM were shown to secrete VEGF *(131)*. Myeloma cells did not express or only weakly expressed the VEGF receptors FLT-1 and FLK-1/KDR, whereas FLK-1/KDR was abundantly expressed by BMSCs *(131,132)*. Interestingly, stimulation of BMSCs with VEGF induced an increase in IL-6 secretion, and, conversely, stimulation with IL-6 enhanced VEGF secretion by myeloma cells. This mutual stimulation suggests a paracrine interaction between myeloma and marrow stromal cells that is triggered by VEGF and IL-6 and results in mutual stimulation of neoangiogenesis and tumor growth. The fact that the progression of MM is associated with an increase in angiogenesis fostered the development of clinical trials using antiangiogenic therapy and resulted in the discovery of the efficacy of thalidomide in the treatment of MM *(133)*.

3.3. Osteoclastogenic Factors

MM is characterized by bone lesions caused by the proliferation and activation of osteoclasts. This major cause of morbidity may play a central role in disease progression by increasing the amount of room required for the expansion of the malignant cells. Myeloma stimulates osteoclastogenesis by triggering a coordinated increase in the TNF-related activation-induced cytokine (TRANCE/OPGL/RANKL/TNFSF11) and a decrease in its decoy receptor, osteoprotegerin (OPG) *(134,135)*. In murine models of human myeloma, administration of a recombinant TRANCE antagonist such as RANK-Fc or OPG both prevents myeloma-induced bone destruction and interferes with myeloma progression *(134,136)*. Other osteoclastogenic factors include HGF, IL-11, macrophage inflammatory protein (MIP)-1α, and MIP-1β. Indeed, MIP-1α and MIP-1β are two C-C chemokines that are produced and secreted by a majority of MM cell lines and primary MM cells samples *(137)*. Secretion of MIP-1α and MIP-1β is correlated with the ability of myeloma cells to enhance osteoclastic bone resorption.

3.3.1. BAFF FAMILY

BAFF and APRIL belong to the TNF family and activate at least three receptors in the TNF receptor family: BAFF-R, BCMA, and TACI. BAFF proteins are critical for the survival of B cells and may be involved in systemic lupus erythematosus *(138)*. Activation of BAFF receptor family results in activation of the NF-κ B pathway and probably other unidentified pathways. Using DNA microarray, we and other investigators found an overexpression of two BAFF receptors, BCMA and TACI *(11,139)*. Looking for a role for the BAFF family in the survival and proliferation of myeloma cells, we found that BAFF or APRIL are potent survival and proliferation factors of myeloma cells, depending on the cell's expression of BAFF-R or TACI *(140)*. BAFF can also protect myeloma cells from dexamethasone-induced apoptosis. These data suggest that a BAFF inhibitor could be useful in the treatment of patients with MM in association with dexamethasone.

3.3.2. Transforming Growth Factor-β

Transforming growth factor (TGF)-β is a potent inhibitor of both human and murine hematopoiesis *(141,142)*. In B-cell development, TGF-β is a suppressor of B-cell proliferation and subsequent differentiation, as indicated by immunoglobulin secretion *(143)*. At the nonproliferation stage in plasma cells, TGF-β does not inhibit immunoglobulin production but nevertheless sensitizes the plasma cells to apoptosis *(143, 144)*. TGF-β secretion increases during the B-cell differentiation process and remains detectable in immunoglobulin-secreting cells; this suggests an autocrine-negative feedback loop for B-cell proliferation. Myeloma tumor cells and derived cell lines express TGF-β mRNA *(70)*, and elevated serum-levels have been observed in murine plasmacytoma *(145)*. Urashima and colleagues reported that both MM and MM-BMSCs secrete a greater amount of TGF-β than normal controls *(146)*. Moreover, plasma cells can directly induce TGF-β secretion by BMSCs and thus induce pre-B-cell apoptosis *(147)*. Malignant MM cells are refractory to the inhibitory effects of TGF-β *(146)*. These results should be linked with those of a recent study that showed that the TGF-β receptor expressed by murine plasmacytomas is not functional, owing to a lack of TGF-β crosslinking. Plasmacytoma cell lines are refractory to TGF-β–mediated growth inhibition and apoptosis, whereas nontransformed plasma cells that accumulate in IL-6-transgenic mice undergo accelerated apoptosis during treatment with TGF-β *(144)*. Thus, TGF-β could contribute to the impairment of humoral immunity (a characteristic of MM) without inhibiting malignant growth. In particular, the serum levels of TGF-β are elevated in patients with MM who display below-normal serum polyclonal immunoglobulin levels *(148)*.

3.4. Other Cytokines

Some cytokines have occasionally been reported to induce proliferation in myeloma tumor samples or myeloma cell lines. In one report, stem cell factor (SCF) increased proliferation in five fresh myeloma samples and in two out of three cell lines tested; it has also enhanced the proliferation of myeloma cells that are responsive to IL-6 *(149)*. A partial autocrine loop involving SCF was observed in the MT3 MM cell line. IL-3 and IL-5 have also been reported to promote myeloma cell proliferation *(150–152)*.

4. CONCLUSION

It has been proposed that myeloma pathogenesis evolves as a three-step process: (1) MGUS, (2) intramedullary myeloma, (3) extramedullary myeloma

(153). In patients with chronic disease and medullary involvement, the slight proliferation observed in short-term cultures is controlled by IL-6. However, IL-6 alone is not sufficient to trigger the survival of primary myeloma cells obtained from patients with chronic disease. Indeed, when these primary myeloma cells were highly purified, 60 to 80% died by apoptosis within 2 d in culture *(117)*. IL-6 could reduce apoptosis, but did not support a long-term survival. Other myeloma cell survival factors (e.g., IFN-α, TNF-α IGFs, and HB-EGF) independent of IL-6, also reduced apoptosis, but did not support long-term survival. Thus, BMSCs provide critical signals that support the survival of primary myeloma cells, together with IL-6. Myeloma cell lines have been obtained that require both IL-6 and the presence of a stromal cell layer. The signal delivered by the stromal cells has not yet been identified and its solubility is still a debated subject *(154,155)*. One mechanism whereby stromal cells might promote the survival of myeloma cells is the induction of a functional IL-6 receptor on tumor cells *(39)*. In patients with extramedullary proliferation, additional mutations must have occurred in malignant cells, allowing survival and proliferation of myeloma cells with IL-6 alone.

Overall, a vast amount of information has been accumulated on MM proliferation and survival factors. However, the respective role of each of the above-mentioned growth factors is not yet known. Cooperation between the signaling cascades may be a critical point, as suggested by recent findings showing a cross-talk between the gp130 IL-6 transducer IFN receptor and the IGR receptor *(77)*. Furthermore, gp130 and IGF-1R are both colocalized in caveolin-associated membrane caveolae in human myeloma cells, together with PI-3 kinase and src kinase, and abrogation of caveolae by cholesterol inhibitors blocks IL-6 or IGF-1 induced transduction, in particular the PI-3K/AKT pathway *(156)*. Of major interest, the *caveolin 1* gene is overexpressed on malignant plasma cells compared with normal B cells or plasma cells. Taken together, these data suggest that gp130 IL-6 transducers, IGF-1 receptors, and EGF receptors and eventually coreceptors (e.g., syndecan-1 and CD9) are colocalized within caveolin-associated caveolae.

The dissection of the signals controlling myeloma cell expansion will be of invaluable interest for the design of new and targeted treatments for MM.

REFERENCES

1. Liu YJ, de Bouteiller O, Fugier-Vivier I. Mechanisms of selection and differentiation in germinal centers. Curr Opin Immunol 1997; 9:256-262.
2. Choe J, Kim HS, Armitage RJ, Choi YS. The functional role of B cell antigen receptor stimulation and IL-4 in the generation of human memory B cells from germinal center B cells. J Immunol 1997; 159:3757-3766.
3. Randall TD, Heath AW, Santos-Argumedo L, Howard MC, Weissman IL, Lund FE. Arrest of B lymphocyte terminal differentiation by CD40 signaling: mechanism for lack of antibody-secreting cells in germinal centers. Immunity 1998; 8:733-742.

4. Arpin C, Dechanet J, Van Kooten C, et al. Generation of memory B cells and plasma cells in vitro. Science 1995; 268:720-722.

5. Choe J, Choi YS. IL-10 interrupts memory B cell expansion in the germinal center by inducing differentiation into plasma cells. Eur J Immunol 1998; 28:508-515.

6. Jacquot S, Kobata T, Iwata S, Morimoto C, Schlossman SF. CD154/CD40 and CD70/CD27 interactions have different and sequential functions in T cell-dependent B cell responses: enhancement of plasma cell differentiation by CD27 signaling. J Immunol 1997; 159: 2652-2657.

7. Jelinek DF, Lipsky PE. The role of B cell proliferation in the generation of immunoglobulin-secreting cells in man. J Immunol 1983; 130:2597-2604.

8. Vernino L, McAnally LM, Ramberg J, Lipsky PE. Generation of nondividing high rate Ig-secreting plasma cells in cultures of human B cells stimulated with anti-CD3-activated T cells. J Immunol 1992; 148:404-410.

9. Gavarotti P, Boccadoro M, Redoglia V, Golzio F, Pileri A. Reactive plasmacytosis: case report and review of the literature. Acta Haematol 1985; 73:108-110.

10. Jego G, Robillard N, Puthier D, et al. Reactive plasmacytoses are expansions of plasmablasts retaining the capacity to differentiate into plasma cells. Blood 1999; 94:701-712.

11. Tarte K, De Vos J, Thykjaer T, et al. Generation of polyclonal plasmablasts from peripheral blood B cells: a normal counterpart of malignant plasmablasts. Blood 2002; 100:1113-1122.

12. Jourdan M, Bataille R, Seguin J, Zhang XG, Chaptal PA, Klein B. Constitutive production of interleukin-6 and immunologic features in cardiac myxomas. Arthritis Rheum 1990; 33:398-402.

13. MacMillan R, Longmire RL, Yelenosky R, Lang JE, Heath V, Craddock CG. Immunoglobulin synthesis by human lymphoid tissues : normal bone marrow as a major site of IgG production. J Immunol 1972; 109:1386-1390.

14. Hibi T, Dosch HM. Limiting dilution analysis of the B cell compartment in human bone marrow. Eur J Immunol 1986; 16:139-145.

15. Manz RA, Radbruch A. Plasma cells for a lifetime? Eur J Immunol 2002; 32:923-927.

16. Suematsu S, Matsuda T, Aozasa K, et al. IgG1 plasmacytosis in interleukin 6 transgenic mice. Proceedings of the National Academy of Sciences of the United States of America 1989; 86:7547-7551.

17. Muraguchi A, Hirano T, Tang B, et al. The essential role of B cell stimulatory factor 2 (BSF-2/IL-6) for the terminal differentiation of B cells. J Exp Med 1988; 167:332-340.

18. Roldan E, Brieva JA. Terminal differentiation of human bone marrow cells capable of spontaneous and high-rate immunoglobulin secretion: role of bone marrow stromal cells and interleukin 6. Eur J Immunol 1991; 21:2671-1677.

19. Kawano MM, Mihara K, Huang N, Tsujimoto T, Kuramoto A. Differentiation of early plasma cells on bone marrow stromal cells requires interleukin-6 for escaping from apoptosis. Blood 1995; 85:487-494.

20. Brieva JA, Roldan E, Rodriguez C, Navas G. Human tonsil, blood and bone marrow in vivo-induced B cells capable of spontaneous and high-rate immunoglobulin secretion in vitro: differences in the requirements for factors and for adherent and bone marrow stromal cells, as well as distinctive adhesion molecule expression. Eur J Immunol 1994; 24:362-366.

21. Merville P, Dechanet J, Desmouliere A, et al. Bcl-2+ tonsillar plasma cells are rescued from apoptosis by bone marrow fibroblasts. J Exp Med 1996; 183:227-236.

22. Roldan E, Garcia-Pardo A, Brieva JA. VLA-4-fibronectin interaction is required for the terminal differentiation of human bone marrow cells capable of spontaneous and high rate immunoglobulin secretion. J Exp Med 1992; 175:1739-1747.

23. Cassese G, Arce S, Hauser AE, et al. Plasma cell survival is mediated by synergistic effects of cytokines and adhesion-dependent signals. J Immunol 2003; 171:1684-1690.

24. Manz RA, Thiel A, Radbruch A. Lifetime of plasma cells in the bone marrow. Nature 1997; 388:133-134.

25. Slifka MK, Antia R, Whitmire JK, Ahmed R. Humoral immunity due to long-lived plasma cells. Immunity 1998; 8:363-372.
26. Slifka MK, Ahmed R. Long-lived plasma cells: a mechanism for maintaining persistent antibody production. Curr Opin Immunol 1998; 10:252-258.
27. Heinrich PC, Behrmann I, Muller-Newen G, Schaper F, Graeve L. Interleukin-6-type cytokine signalling through the gp130/Jak/STAT pathway. Biochem J 1998; 334:297-314.
28. Kawano M, Hirano T, Matsuda T, et al. Autocrine generation and essential requirement of BSF-2/IL-6 for human multiple myeloma. Nature 1988; 332:83-85.
29. Klein B, Zhang XG, Jourdan M, et al. Paracrine rather than autocrine regulation of myeloma-cell growth and differentiation by interleukin-6. Blood 1989; 73:517-526.
30. Zhang XG, Gaillard JP, Robillard N, et al. Reproducible obtaining of human myeloma cell lines as a model for tumor stem cell study in human multiple myeloma. Blood 1994; 83:3654-3663.
31. Ferlin-Bezombes M, Jourdan M, Liautard J, Brochier J, Rossi JF, Klein B. IFN-alpha is a survival factor for human myeloma cells and reduces dexamethasone-induced apoptosis. J Immunol 1998; 161:2692-2699.
32. Gu ZJ, De Vos J, Rebouissou C, et al. Agonist anti-gp130 transducer monoclonal antibodies are human myeloma cell survival and growth factors. Leukemia 2000; 14:188-197.
33. Bataille R, Jourdan M, Zhang XG, Klein B. Serum levels of interleukin 6, a potent myeloma cell growth factor, as a reflect of disease severity in plasma cell dyscrasias. J Clin Invest 1989; 84:2008-2011.
34. Ludwig H, Nachbaur DM, Fritz E, Krainer M, Huber H. Interleukin-6 is a prognostic factor in multiple myeloma. Blood 1991; 77:2794-2795.
35. Klein B, Wijdenes J, Zhang XG, et al. Murine anti-interleukin-6 monoclonal antibody therapy for a patient with plasma cell leukemia. Blood 1991; 78:1198-1204.
36. Bataille R, Boccadoro M, Klein B, Durie B, Pileri A. C-reactive protein and beta-2 microglobulin produce a simple and powerful myeloma staging system. Blood 1992; 80:733-737.
37. Klein B, Zhang XG, Lu ZY, Bataille R. Interleukin-6 in human multiple myeloma. Blood 1995; 85:863-872.
38. Uchiyama H, Barut BA, Mohrbacher AF, Chauhan D, Anderson KC. Adhesion of human myeloma-derived cell lines to bone marrow stromal cells stimulates interleukin-6 secretion. Blood 1993; 82:3712-3720.
39. Bloem AC, Lamme T, de Smet M, et al. Long-term bone marrow cultured stromal cells regulate myeloma tumour growth in vitro: studies with primary tumour cells and LTBMC-dependent cell lines. Br J Haematology 1998; 100:166-175.
40. Costes V, Portier M, Lu ZY, Rossi JF, Bataille R, Klein B. Interleukin-1 in multiple myeloma: producer cells and their role in the control of IL-6 production. Br J Haematol 1998; 103:1152-1160.
41. Bataille R, Barlogie B, Lu ZY, et al. Biologic effects of anti-interleukin-6 murine monoclonal antibody in advanced multiple myeloma. Blood 1995; 86:685-691.
42. Lu ZY, Brailly H, Wijdenes J, Bataille R, Rossi JF, Klein B. Measurement of whole body interleukin-6 (IL-6) production: prediction of the efficacy of anti-IL-6 treatments. Blood 1995; 86:3123-3131.
43. Klein B, Brailly H. Cytokine-binding proteins: stimulating antagonists. Immunol Today 1995; 16:216-220.
44. Nordan RP, Potter M. A macrophage-derived factor required by plasmacytomas for survival and proliferation in vitro. Science 1986; 233:566-569.
45. Simpson RJ, Moritz RL, Rubira MR, Van Snick J. Murine hybridoma/plasmacytoma growth factor: complete amino-acid sequence and relation to human interleukin-6. Eur J Biochem 1988; 176:187-197.
46. Lattanzio G, Libert C, Aquilina M, et al. Defective development of pristane-oil-induced plasmacytomas in interleukin-6-deficient BALB/c mice. Am J Pathol 1997; 151:689-696.

47. Suematsu S, Matsusaka T, Matsuda T, et al. Generation of plasmacytomas with the chromosomal translocation t(12;15) in interleukin 6 transgenic mice. Proceedings of the National Academy of Sciences of the United States of America 1992; 89:232-235.

48. Hilbert DM, Kopf M, Mock BA, Kohler G, Rudikoff S. Interleukin 6 is essential for in vivo development of B lineage neoplasms. J Exp Med 1995; 182:243-248.

49. Gu ZJ, Zhang XG, Hallet MM, et al. A ciliary neurotrophic factor-sensitive human myeloma cell line. Exp Hematol 1996; 24:1195-1200.

50. Gu ZJ, Costes V, Lu ZY, et al. Interleukin-10 is a growth factor for human myeloma cells by induction of an oncostatin M autocrine loop. Blood 1996; 88:3972-3986.

51. Rettig MB, Ma HJ, Vescio RA, et al. Kaposi's sarcoma-associated herpesvirus infection of bone marrow dendritic cells from multiple myeloma patients. Science 1997; 276:1851-1854.

52. Burger R, Neipel F, Fleckenstein B, et al. Human herpesvirus type 8 interleukin-6 homologue is functionally active on human myeloma cells. Blood 1998; 91:1858-1863.

52a. Tarte K, Olsen SJ, Lu ZY, et al. Clinical-grade functional dendritic cells from patients with multiple myeloma are not infected with Kaposi's sarcoma-associated herpesvirus. Blood 1998; 91:1852–1857.

53. Tarte K, Chang Y, Klein B. Kaposi's sarcoma-associated herpesvirus and multiple myeloma: lack of criteria for causality. Blood 1999; 93:3159–3163.

54. Lu ZY, Zhang XG, Rodriguez C, et al. Interleukin-10 is a proliferation factor but not a differentiation factor for human myeloma cells. Blood 1995; 85:2521-2527.

55. Lu ZY, Gu ZJ, Zhang XG, et al. Interleukin-10 induces interleukin-11 responsiveness in human myeloma cell lines. FEBS Lett 1995; 377:515-518.

56. Tosato G, Jones KD. Interleukin-1 induces interleukin-6 production in peripheral blood monocytes. Blood 1990; 75:1305-1310.

57. Dinarello CA. Biologic basis for interleukin-1 in disease. Blood 1996; 87:2095-2147.

58. Kawano M, Tanaka H, Ishikawa H, et al. Interleukin-1 accelerates autocrine growth of myeloma cells through interleukin-6 in human myeloma. Blood 1989; 73:2145-2148.

59. Cozzolino F, Torcia M, Aldinucci D, et al. Production of interleukin-1 by bone marrow myeloma cells. Blood 1989; 74:380-387.

60. Carter A, Merchav S, Silvian-Draxler I, Tatarsky I. The role of interleukin-1 and tumour necrosis factor-alpha in human multiple myeloma. Br J Haematol 1990; 74:424-431.

61. Borset M, Helseth E, Naume B, Waage A. Lack of IL-1 secretion from human myeloma cells highly purified by immunomagnetic separation. Br. J Haematol 1993; 85:446-451.

62. Hinson RM, Williams JA, Shacter E. Elevated interleukin 6 is induced by prostaglandin E2 in a murine model of inflammation: possible role of cyclooxygenase-2. Proc Natl Acad Sci U S A 1996; 93:4885-4890.

63. Kawano M, Yamamoto I, Iwato K, et al. Interleukin-1 beta rather than lymphotoxin as the major bone resorbing activity in human multiple myeloma. Blood 1989; 73:1646-1649.

64. Torcia M, Lucibello M, Vannier E, et al. Modulation of osteoclast-activating factor activity of multiple myeloma bone marrow cells by different interleukin-1 inhibitors. Exp Hematol 1996; 24:868-874.

65. Tinhofer I, Marschitz I, Henn T, Egle A, Greil R. Expression of functional interleukin-15 receptor and autocrine production of interleukin-15 as mechanisms of tumor propagation in multiple myeloma. Blood 2000; 95:610-618.

66. Hjorth-Hansen H, Waage A, Borset M. Interleukin-15 blocks apoptosis and induces proliferation of the human myeloma cell line OH-2 and freshly isolated myeloma cells. Br J Haematol 1999; 106:28-34.

67. Till KJ, Burthem J, Lopez A, Cawley JC. Granulocyte-macrophage colony-stimulating factor receptor: stage-specific expression and function on late B cells. Blood 1996; 88:479-486.

68. Villunger A, Egle A, Kos M, et al. Functional granulocyte/macrophage colony stimulating factor receptor is constitutively expressed on neoplastic plasma cells and mediates tumour cell longevity. Br J Haematol 1998; 102:1069-1080.

69. Zhang XG, Bataille R, Jourdan M, et al. Granulocyte-macrophage colony-stimulating factor synergizes with interleukin-6 in supporting the proliferation of human myeloma cells. Blood 1990; 76:2599-2605.
70. Portier M, Zhang XG, Ursule E, et al. Cytokine gene expression in human multiple myeloma. Br J Haematol 1993; 85:514-520.
71. Nachbaur D, Herold M, Huber H. Endogenous circulating granulocyte-macrophage colony-stimulating factor in multiple myeloma. Blood 1991; 78:539-540.
72. Peest D, Blade J, Harousseau JL, Klein B, Osterborg A, San Miguel JF. Cytokine therapy in multiple myeloma. Br. J Haematol 1996; 94:425-432.
73. Brenning G. The in vitro effect of leucocyte alpha-interferon on human myeloma cells in a semisolid agar culture system. Scand J Haematol 1985; 35:178-185.
74. Palumbo A, Battaglio S, Napoli P, et al. Recombinant interferon-gamma inhibits the in vitro proliferation of human myeloma cells. Br J Haematol 1994; 86:726-732.
75. Jelinek DF, Aagaard-Tillery KM, Arendt BK, Arora T, Tschumper RC, Westendorf JJ. Differential human multiple myeloma cell line responsiveness to interferon-alpha: analysis of transcription factor activation and interleukin 6 receptor expression. J Clin Invest 1997; 99:447-456.
76. Jourdan M, Zhang XG, Portier M, Boiron JM, Bataille R, Klein B. IFN-alpha induces autocrine production of IL-6 in myeloma cell lines. J Immunol 1991; 147:4402-4407.
77. French JD, Walters DK, Jelinek DF. Transactivation of gp130 in myeloma cells. J Immunol 2003; 170:3717-3723.
78. Berger LC, Hawley RG. Interferon-beta interrupts interleukin-6-dependent signaling events in myeloma cells. Blood 1997; 89:261-271.
79. Arora T, Jelinek DF. Differential myeloma cell responsiveness to interferon-alpha correlates with differential induction of p19(INK4d) and cyclin D2 expression. J Biol Chem 1998; 273:11799-11805.
80. Liu P, Oken M, Van Ness B. Interferon-alpha protects myeloma cell lines from dexamethasone-induced apoptosis. Leukemia 1999; 13:473-480.
81. Egle A, Villunger A, Kos M, et al. Modulation of Apo-1/Fas (CD95)-induced programmed cell death in myeloma cells by interferon-alpha 2. Eur J Immunol 1996; 26:3119-3126.
82. Spets H, Georgii-Hemming P, Siljason J, Nilsson K, Jernberg-Wiklund H. Fas/APO-1 (CD95)-mediated apoptosis is activated by interferon-gamma and interferon- in interleukin-6 (IL-6)-dependent and IL-6-independent multiple myeloma cell lines. Blood 1998; 92:2914-2923.
83. Gutterman JU. Cytokine therapeutics: lessons from interferon alpha. Proc Natl Acad Sci U S A 1994; 91:1198-1205.
84. Blade J, Lopez-Guillermo A, Tassies D, Montserrat E, Rozman C. Development of aggressive plasma cell leukaemia under interferon-alpha therapy. Br J Haematol 1991; 79:523-525.
85. Sawamura M, Murayama K, Ui G, et al. Plasma cell leukaemia with alpha-interferon therapy in myeloma. Br J Haematol 1992; 82:631.
86. Tanaka H, Tanabe O, Iwato K, et al. Sensitive inhibitory effect of interferon-alpha on M-protein secretion of human myeloma cells. Blood 1989; 74:1718-1722.
87. Portier M, Zhang XG, Caron E, Lu ZY, Bataille R, Klein B. gamma-Interferon in multiple myeloma: inhibition of interleukin-6 (IL-6)-dependent myeloma cell growth and down-regulation of IL-6-receptor expression in vitro. Blood 1993; 81:3076-3082.
88. Ossina NK, Cannas A, Powers VC, et al. Interferon-gamma modulates a p53-independent apoptotic pathway and apoptosis-related gene expression. J Biol Chem 1997; 272:16351-16357.
89. Ashkenazi A, Dixit VM. Death receptors: signaling and modulation. Science 1998; 281:1305-1308.
90. Van Antwerp DJ, Martin SJ, Kafri T, Green DR, Verma IM. Suppression of TNF-alpha-induced apoptosis by NF-kappaB. Science 1996; 274:787-789.

91. Lee SY, Reichlin A, Santana A, Sokol KA, Nussenzweig MC, Choi Y. TRAF2 is essential for JNK but not NF-kappaB activation and regulates lymphocyte proliferation and survival. Immunity 1997; 7:703-713.

92. Borset M, Waage A, Brekke OL, Helseth E. TNF and IL-6 are potent growth factors for OH-2, a novel human myeloma cell line. Eur J Haematol 1994; 53:31-37.

93. Jourdan M, Tarte K, Legouffe E, Brochier J, Rossi JF, Klein B. Tumor necrosis factor is a survival and proliferation factor for human myeloma cells. Eur Cytokine Netw 1999; 10:65-70.

94. Hideshima T, Chauhan D, Schlossman R, Richardson P, Anderson KC. The role of tumor necrosis factor alpha in the pathophysiology of human multiple myeloma: therapeutic applications. Oncogene 2001; 20:4519-4527.

95. Lichtenstein A, Berenson J, Norman D, Chang MP, Carlile A. Production of cytokines by bone marrow cells obtained from patients with multiple myeloma. Blood 1989; 74:1266-1273.

96. Filella X, Blade J, Guillermo AL, Molina R, Rozman C, Ballesta AM. Cytokines (IL-6, TNF-alpha, IL-1alpha) and soluble interleukin-2 receptor as serum tumor markers in multiple myeloma. Cancer Detect Prev 1996; 20:52-56.

97. Blade J, Filella X, Montoto S, et al. Clinical relevance of interleukin 6 and tumor necrosis factor alpha serum levels in monoclonal gammopathy of undetermined significance [abstract]. Blood 1997; 90:351a.

98. Baserga R. The insulin-like growth factor I receptor: a key to tumor growth? Cancer Res 1995; 55:249-252.

99. Christofori G, Naik P, Hanahan D. A second signal supplied by insulin-like growth factor II in oncogene-induced tumorigenesis. Nature 1994; 369:414-418.

100. Chan JM, Stampfer MJ, Giovannucci E, et al. Plasma insulin-like growth factor-I and prostate cancer risk: a prospective study. Science 1998; 279:563-566.

101. Georgii-Hemming P, Wiklund HJ, Ljunggren O, Nilsson K. Insulin-like growth factor I is a growth and survival factor in human multiple myeloma cell lines. Blood 1996; 88:2250-2258.

102. Nishiura T, Karasuno T, Yoshida H, et al. Functional role of cation-independent mannose 6-phosphate/insulin-like growth factor II receptor in cell adhesion and proliferation of a human myeloma cell line OPM-2. Blood 1996; 88:3546-3554.

103. Jelinek DF, Witzig TE, Arendt BK. A role for insulin-like growth factor in the regulation of IL-6-responsive human myeloma cell line growth. J Immunol 1997; 159:487-496.

104. Ferlin M, Noraz N, Hertogh C, Brochier J, Taylor N, Klein B. Insulin-like growth factor induces the survival and proliferation of myeloma cells through an IL-6-independent transduction pathway. Br J Haematol 2000; 111:626-634.

105. Ge NL, Rudikoff S. Insulin-like growth factor I is a dual effector of multiple myeloma cell growth. Blood 2000; 96:2856-2861.

106. Li W, Hyun T, Heller M, et al. Activation of insulin-like growth factor I receptor signaling pathway is critical for mouse plasma cell tumor growth. Cancer Res 2000; 60:3909-3915.

107. Arai T, Parker A, Busby W, Jr., Clemmons DR. Heparin, heparan sulfate, and dermatan sulfate regulate formation of the insulin-like growth factor-I and insulin-like growth factor-binding protein complexes. J Biol Chem 1994; 269:20388-20393.

108. Chesi M, Nardini E, Brents LA, et al. Frequent translocation t(4;14)(p16.3;q32.3) in multiple myeloma is associated with increased expression and activating mutations of fibroblast growth factor receptor 3. Nature Genetics 1997; 16:260-264.

109. Onwuazor ON, Wen XY, Wang DY, et al. Mutation, SNP, and isoform analysis of fibroblast growth factor receptor 3 (FGFR3) in 150 newly diagnosed multiple myeloma patients. Blood 2003; 102:772-773.

110. Fracchiolla NS, Luminari S, Baldini L, Lombardi L, Maiolo AT, Neri A. FGFR3 gene mutations associated with human skeletal disorders occur rarely in multiple myeloma. Blood 1998; 92:2987-2989.

111. Kan M, Wang F, Xu J, Crabb JW, Hou J, McKeehan WL. An essential heparin-binding domain in the fibroblast growth factor receptor kinase. Science 1993; 259:1918-1921.
112. Ridley RC, Xiao H, Hata H, Woodliff J, Epstein J, Sanderson RD. Expression of syndecan regulates human myeloma plasma cell adhesion to type I collagen. 1993; 81:767-774.
113. Jourdan M, Ferlin M, Legouffe E, et al. The myeloma cell antigen syndecan-1 is lost by apoptotic myeloma cells. Br J Haematol 1998; 100:637-646.
114. Witzig TE, Kimlinger T, Stenson M, Therneau T. Syndecan-1 expression on malignant cells from the blood and marrow of patients with plasma cell proliferative disorders and B-cell chronic lymphocytic leukemia. Leuk Lymphoma 1998; 31:167-175.
115. Subramanian SV, Fitzgerald ML, Bernfield M. Regulated shedding of syndecan-1 and -4 ectodomains by thrombin and growth factor receptor activation. J Biol Chem 1997; 272:14713-14720.
116. Dhodapkar MV, Kelly T, Theus A, Athota AB, Barlogie B, Sanderson RD. Elevated levels of shed syndecan-1 correlate with tumour mass and decreased matrix metalloproteinase-9 activity in the serum of patients with multiple myeloma [published erratum appears in Br J Haematol 1998 May;101(2):398]. Br J Haematol 1997; 99:368-371.
117. Klein B, Li XY, Lu ZY, et al. Activation molecules on human myeloma cells. Curr Topics Microbiol Immunol 1999. In press.
118. Yang Y, Yaccoby S, Liu W, et al. Soluble syndecan-1 promotes growth of myeloma tumors in vivo. Blood 2002; 100:610-617.
119. Kato M, Wang H, Kainulainen V, et al. Physiological degradation converts the soluble syndecan-1 ectodomain from an inhibitor to a potent activator of FGF-2. Nat Med 1998; 4:691-697.
120. Bisping G, Leo R, Wenning D, et al. Paracrine interactions of basic fibroblast growth factor and interleukin-6 in multiple myeloma. Blood 2003; 101:2775-2783.
121. Vacca A, Ribatti D, Presta M, et al. Bone marrow neovascularization, plasma cell angiogenic potential, and matrix metalloproteinase-2 secretion parallel progression of human multiple myeloma. Blood 1999; 93:3064-3073.
122. Zarnegar R, Michalopoulos GK. The many faces of hepatocyte growth factor: from hepatopoiesis to hematopoiesis. J Cell Biol 1995; 129:1177-1180.
123. Borset M, Hjorth-Hansen H, Seidel C, Sundan A, Waage A. Hepatocyte growth factor and its receptor c-met in multiple myeloma. Blood 1996; 88:3998-4004.
124. Seidel C, Borset M, Turesson I, Abildgaard N, Sundan A, Waage A. Elevated serum concentrations of hepatocyte growth factor in patients with multiple myeloma. The Nordic Myeloma Study Group. Blood 1998; 91:806-812.
125. Grano M, Galimi F, Zambonin G, et al. Hepatocyte growth factor is a coupling factor for osteoclasts and osteoblasts in vitro. Proc Natl Acad Sci U S A 1996; 93:7644-7648.
126. Hjertner O, Torgersen ML, Seidel C, et al. Hepatocyte growth factor (HGF) induces interleukin-11 secretion from osteoblasts: a possible role for HGF in myeloma-associated osteolytic bone disease. Blood 1999; 94:3883-3888.
127. De Vos J, Couderc G, Tarte K, et al. Identifying intercellular signaling genes expressed in malignant plasma cells by using complementary DNA arrays. Blood 2001; 98:771-780.
128. Wang YD, De Vos J, Jourdan M, et al. Cooperation between heparin-binding EGF-like growth factor and interleukin-6 in promoting the growth of human myeloma cells. Oncogene 2002; 21:2584-2592.
129. Davis-Fleischer KM, Besner GE. Structure and function of heparin-binding EGF-like growth factor (HB-EGF). Frontiers in Bioscience 1998; 3:d288-d299.
130. Vacca A, Ribatti D, Roncali L, et al. Bone marrow angiogenesis and progression in multiple myeloma. Br. J Haematol 1994; 87:503-508.
131. Dankbar B, Padro T, Leo R, et al. Vascular endothelial growth factor and interleukin-6 in paracrine tumor-stromal cell interactions in multiple myeloma. Blood 2000; 95:2630-2636.

132. Bellamy WT, Richter L, Frutiger Y, Grogan TM. Expression of vascular endothelial growth factor and its receptors in hematopoietic malignancies. Cancer Res 1999; 59:728-733.

133. Singhal S, Mehta J, Desikan R, et al. Antitumor activity of thalidomide in refractory multiple myeloma. N Engl J Med 1999; 341:1565-1571.

134. Pearse RN, Sordillo EM, Yaccoby S, et al. Multiple myeloma disrupts the TRANCE/osteoprotegerin cytokine axis to trigger bone destruction and promote tumor progression. Proc Natl Acad Sci U S A 2001; 98:11581-11586.

135. Giuliani N, Bataille R, Mancini C, Lazzaretti M, Barille S. Myeloma cells induce imbalance in the osteoprotegerin/osteoprotegerin ligand system in the human bone marrow environment. Blood 2001; 98:3527-3533.

136. Croucher PI, Shipman CM, Lippitt J, et al. Osteoprotegerin inhibits the development of osteolytic bone disease in multiple myeloma. Blood 2001; 98:3534-3540.

137. Abe M, Hiura K, Wilde J, et al. Role for macrophage inflammatory protein (MIP)-1alpha and MIP-1beta in the development of osteolytic lesions in multiple myeloma. Blood 2002; 100:2195-2202.

138. Mackay F, Kalled SL. TNF ligands and receptors in autoimmunity: an update. Curr Opin Immunol 2002; 14:783-790.

139. Claudio JO, Masih-Khan E, Tang H, et al. A molecular compendium of genes expressed in multiple myeloma. Blood 2002; 100:2175-2186.

140. Tarte K, Moreaux J, Legouffe E, Rossi JF, Klein B. BAFF Is a survival factor for multiple myeloma cells [abstract]. Blood 2002; Abstract #3203.

141. Sitnicka E, Ruscetti FW, Priestley GV, Wolf NS, Bartelmez SH. Transforming growth factor beta 1 directly and reversibly inhibits the initial cell divisions of long-term repopulating hematopoietic stem cells. Blood 1996; 88:82-88.

142. Jansen R, Damia G, Usui N, et al. Effects of recombinant transforming growth factor-beta 1 on hematologic recovery after treatment of mice with 5-fluorouracil. J Immunol 1991; 147:3342-3347.

143. Matthes T, Werner-Favre C, Zubler RH. Cytokine expression and regulation of human plasma cells: disappearance of interleukin-10 and persistence of transforming growth factor-beta 1. Eur J Immunol 1995; 25:508-512.

144. Amoroso SR, Huang N, Roberts AB, Potter M, Letterio JJ. Consistent loss of functional transforming growth factor beta receptor expression in murine plasmacytomas. Proc Natl Acad Sci U S A 1998; 95:189-194.

145. Berg DJ, Lynch RG. Immune dysfunction in mice with plasmacytomas. I. Evidence that transforming growth factor-beta contributes to the altered expression of activation receptors on host B lymphocytes. J Immunol 1991; 146:2865-2872.

146. Urashima M, Ogata A, Chauhan D, et al. Transforming growth factor-beta1: differential effects on multiple myeloma versus normal B cells. Blood 1996; 87:1928-1938.

147. Tsujimoto T, Lisukov IA, Huang N, Mahmoud MS, Kawano MM. Plasma cells induce apoptosis of pre-B cells by interacting with bone marrow stromal cells. Blood 1996; 87: 3375-3383.

148. Kyrtsonis MC, Repa C, Dedoussis GV, et al. Serum transforming growth factor-beta 1 is related to the degree of immunoparesis in patients with multiple myeloma. Med Oncol 1998; 15:124-128.

149. Lemoli RM, Fortuna A, Grande A, et al. Expression and functional role of c-kit ligand (SCF) in human multiple myeloma cells. 1994; 88:760-769.

150. Bergui L, Schena M, Gaidano G, Riva M, Caligaris C. Interleukin 3 and interleukin 6 synergistically promote the proliferation and differentiation of malignant plasma cell precursors in multiple myeloma. 1989; 170:613-618.

151. Okuno Y, Takahashi T, Suzuki A, et al. Establishment and characterization of four myeloma cell lines which are responsive to interleukin-6 for their growth. Leukemia 1991; 5:585-591.

152. Anderson KC, Jones RM, Morimoto C, Leavitt P, Barut BA. Response patterns of purified myeloma cells to hematopoietic growth factors. Blood 1989; 73:1915-1924.

153. Hallek M, Leif BP, Anderson KC. Multiple myeloma: increasing evidence for a multistep transformation process. Blood 1998; 91:3-21.

154. Van Riet I, De Greef C, Aharchi F, et al. Establishment and characterization of a human stroma-dependent myeloma cell line (MM5.1) and its stroma-independent variant (MM5.2). Leukemia 1997; 11:284-293.

155. Degrassi A, Hibert DM, Rudikoff S, Anderson AO, Potter M, Coon HG. In vitro culture of primary plasmacytomas requires stromal cell feeder layers. Proc Nat Acad Sci U S A 1993; 90:2060-2064.

156. Podar K, Tai YT, Cole CE, et al. Essential role of caveolae in interleukin-6- and insulin-like growth factor I-triggered Akt-1-mediated survival of multiple myeloma cells. J Biol Chem 2003; 278:5794-5801.

6 Monoclonal Gammopathy of Undetermined Significance

Robert A. Kyle, MD

CONTENTS

1. INTRODUCTION

Monoclonal gammopathy is characterized by the proliferation of a single clone of plasma cells that produces a homogeneous monoclonal protein (M protein). Each M protein consists of two heavy polypeptide chains of the same class and subclass and two light polypeptide chains of the same type. The heavy polypeptide chains are γ in immunoglobulin (Ig) G, α in IgA, μ in IgM, δ in IgD, and ε in IgE. The light-chain types are κ and λ.

From: *Current Clinical Oncology: Biology and Management of Multiple Myeloma*
Edited by: J. R. Berenson © Humana Press Inc., Totowa, NJ

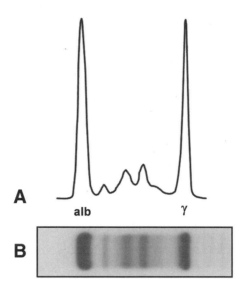

Fig. 1. (**A**) Monoclonal pattern of serum protein as traced by densitometer after electrophoresis on agarose gel: tall, narrow-based peak of γ mobility. (**B**) Monoclonal pattern from electrophoresis of serum on agarose gel (anode on left): dense, localized band representing monoclonal protein of γ mobility. (From ref. *4*. By permission of the American Society for Microbiology.)

2. DETECTION OF M PROTEINS

Agarose gel electrophoresis is the best method for detecting an M protein. After the recognition of a localized band or spike in the electrophoretogram, immunofixation should be performed to confirm the presence and determine the type of M protein that is present.

An M protein is usually visible as a discrete band on the agarose gel electrophoretic strip or as a tall, narrow spike or peak in the γ or β regions or, rarely, in the α_2 area of the densitometer tracing (Fig. 1). Two M proteins (biclonal gammopathy) are seen in 3 to 4% of sera samples containing an M protein *(1)* and, rarely, 3 M proteins are found (triclonal gammopathy) *(2)*. A small monoclonal gammopathy may be present even when the total protein; α, β, and γ components; and quantitative immunoglobulins are all within normal limits. The type of M protein is best determined by immunofixation. This should be performed whenever a sharp spike or band is found in the agarose gel. It is critical to exclude a polyclonal increase in immunoglobulins (Fig. 2). Immunofixation is particularly helpful for the recognition of biclonal and triclonal gammopathies. Some laboratories use immunoelectrophoresis to detect an M protein, but this method is not as sensitive as immunofixation. Another useful approach is capillary zone electrophoresis, which measures protein by absorption. In this method, protein stains

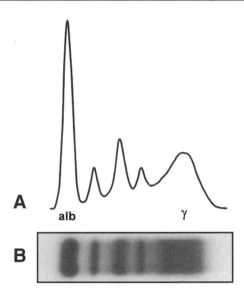

Fig. 2. (**A**) Polyclonal pattern from densitometer tracing of agarose gel: broad-based peak of γ mobility. (**B**) Polyclonal pattern from electrophoresis of agarose gel (anode on left). The band at the right is broad and extends throughout the γ area. alb, albumin. (From ref. *4*. By permission of the American Society of Microbiology.)

are unnecessary and no point of application is seen. Immunotyping is performed by immunosubtraction, a procedure in which a serum sample is incubated with sepharose beads coupled with anti-γ, α, μ, κ, and λ antisera. After incubation with each of the heavy- and light-chain antisera, the supernates undergo capillary zone electrophoresis to determine which reagents removed the electrophoretic abnormality. Immunosubtraction is technically less demanding and is automated; thus, it is a useful technique for immunotyping M proteins *(3,4)*.

Quantitation of IgG, IgA, and IgM is best performed with a rate nephelometer. Immunodiffusion should not be done to quantify immunoglobulins because it is inaccurate. It must be pointed out that IgM levels determined with nephelometry may be 1000 to 2000 mg/dL higher than the M protein level in the densitometer tracing. The IgG and IgA levels also may be spuriously increased. Consequently, the clinician must use the same technique to measure the M protein on subsequent visits. If the M protein is small, immunoglobulin quantification is more useful than the densitometer tracing.

3. MONOCLONAL GAMMOPATHY
OF UNDETERMINED SIGNIFICANCE

The term *monoclonal gammopathy of undetermined significance* (MGUS) denotes the presence of an M protein in persons without signs or symptoms of multiple myeloma (MM), Waldenström's macroglobulinemia (WM), primary amyloidosis (AL), lymphoproliferative disorders, plasmacytoma, or related disorders. The term *benign monoclonal gammopathy*, which was formerly used, is misleading, because in a proportion of patients MM or related disorders will develop during long-term follow-up periods. It cannot be known at the time of diagnosis whether the process producing an M protein will remain stable and benign or will progress to result in a serious disease.

MGUS is characterized by a serum M protein spike of less than 3 g/dL, fewer than 10% plasma cells in the bone marrow, no or only small amounts of M protein in the urine, absence of lytic bone lesions, no evidence of anemia, hypercalcemia, or renal insufficiency, and no evidence of end-organ damage. The plasma cell proliferation rate (plasma-cell labeling index) is low. Most importantly, M protein levels remain stable and other abnormalities do not develop during long-term follow-up. The finding of an M protein is an unexpected event in the laboratory evaluation of an unrelated disorder, the investigation of increased erythrocyte sedimentation rate (ESR), or in a general health examination. MM, AL, WM, solitary plasmacytoma of bone, extramedullary plasmacytoma, lymphoma, chronic lymphocytic leukemia, and related disorders must be excluded when making the diagnosis of MGUS.

MGUS is found in approx 3% of persons older than 70 yr in Sweden *(5)*, the United States *(6)*, and France *(7)*. The overall rate at which M protein was identified in 6695 persons older than 25 yr in the Swedish study was 1%. In a small Minnesota community with a cluster of MM cases, 15 (1.25%) of 1200 persons 50 yr or older had an M protein, whereas 303 (1.7%) of 17,968 adults 50 yr or older in France had an M protein. In one study, 10% of 111 persons older than 80 yr had an M protein *(8)*. In another, 23% of 439 persons ages 75 to 84 yr had an M protein *(9)*. In our practice during 2002, 629 newly recognized cases of MGUS were identified at the Mayo Clinic in Rochester, Minnesota (Fig. 3).

The incidence of M protein is higher in African-American populations than in whites *(10)*. Cohen and colleagues *(11)* found a prevalence of 8.4% (77 of 916 black persons). Only 29 (3.6%) of 816 non-black persons 70 yr or older had an M protein *(11)*. In contrast, the incidence of gammopathies has been reported to be lower in older Japanese persons *(12)*, although Kurihara and associates *(13)* found that 71 (3.5%) of 2007 inpatients or outpatients in a Japanese University Hospital had an M protein. If the 13 patients with myeloma or macroglobulinemia were excluded, the incidence would be 2.9%.

Because of the considerable prevalence of MGUS and the fact that affected patients are usually seen by physicians in different fields of clinical practice, it is important to know whether the disorder is actually benign or likely to progress to a symptomatic monoclonal gammopathy requiring chemotherapy.

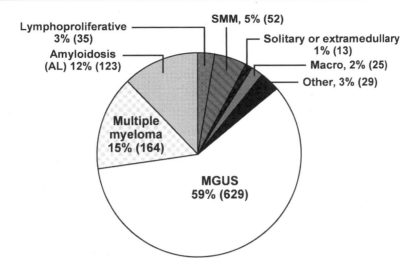

Fig. 3. Monoclonal gammopathies at Mayo Clinic, Rochester, Minnesota, in 2002 ($n = 1070$). Macro, macroglobulinemia; MGUS, monoclonal gammopathy of undetermined significance; SMM, smoldering multiple myeloma.

4. MAYO CLINIC STUDY

A group of 241 patients with MGUS has been followed at Mayo Clinic for 24 to 38 yr, and the data are updated periodically *(14–17)*. No patients have been lost to follow-up. The group consists of 140 men and 101 women with a median age of 64 yr at diagnosis. Only 4% were younger than 40 yr and 33% were 70 yr or older. Hepatomegaly or splenomegaly and laboratory-based diagnoses of such disorders as anemia, thrombocytopenia, hypercalcemia, hypoalbuminemia, and renal insufficiency were the result of unrelated disorders in affected patients. The initial M protein value ranged from 0.3 to 3.2 g/dL (median: 1.7 g/dL). The heavy-chain type was IgG in 73% of patients, IgM in 14%, IgA in 11%, and biclonal in 2%. The light chain was κ in 62% and λ in the remainder. The levels of uninvolved immunoglobulins were reduced in 29% of study participants. Monoclonal light chains were found in urine in 15 patients, but only 3 had more than 1 g/24 h. The percentage of plasma cells ranged from 1 to 10% (median: 3%). Unrelated disorders—e.g., cardiovascular or cerebrovascular disease, connective tissue disorders, inflammatory processes, nonplasma-cell neoplasms, and various other conditions unrelated to the M protein—were found in 76% of participants.

After a 24- to 38-yr follow-up, the patients remaining in the study were categorized as belong to one of four groups (Table 1). Group one consisted of living patients in whom the M protein remained stable and who were identified as having benign disease; this group had decreased to 25 patients (10% of the entire study population alive at follow-up).

Table 1
Course of Disease in 241 Patients With
Monoclonal Gammopathy of Undetermined Significance

Group	Description	At follow-up after 24–38 yr	
		n	%
1	No substantial increase of serum or urine monoclonal protein (benign)	25	10
2	Monoclonal protein 3.0 g/dL, but no myeloma or related disease	26	11
3	Died of unrelated causes	127	53
4	Development of myeloma, macroglobulinemia, amyloidosis, or related disease	63	26
Total		241	100

Modified from ref. *16*. By permission of Mayo Foundation for Medical Education and Research.

The concentration of hemoglobin, amount of serum M protein, type of serum heavy and light chains, decrease in uninvolved immunoglobulins, subclass of IgG heavy chain, and the number and appearance of plasma cells in the bone marrow did not differ substantially from those in the other groups. The M protein disappeared in two patients. The group 1 patients are still at risk for myeloma or related disorders, however, and continue to be followed.

Group 2 is composed of 26 patients in whom the serum M protein value increased to 3 g/dL or more but who did not require chemotherapy for symptomatic MM or macroglobulinemia. The M protein value increased gradually in most persons in this group. Three of these patients are still living. More than half of the total group died of unrelated diseases without developing a malignant plasma cell or lymphoproliferative disorder requiring chemotherapy (group 3—those who died of unrelated causes).

Fifty-five lived at least 10 yr after serum M protein was detected. The most frequent cause of death was cardiovascular or cerebrovascular disease. Fifteen patients died of a nonplasma-cell malignancy.

Group 4 consisted of 63 patients (26%) in whom myeloma, amyloidosis, macroglobulinemia, or a related lymphoproliferative disorder developed. The actuarial rate of development of these diseases was 16% at 10 yr and 40% at 25 yr (Fig. 4). MM developed in 43 (68%) of these 63 patients. The interval from identification of the M protein to the diagnosis of MM ranged from 2 to 29 yr (median: 10 yr). In nine patients, MM was diagnosed more than 20 yr after detection of the serum M protein. The median duration of survival after the diagnosis of MM was 33 mo, which is similar to that in the usual patient with

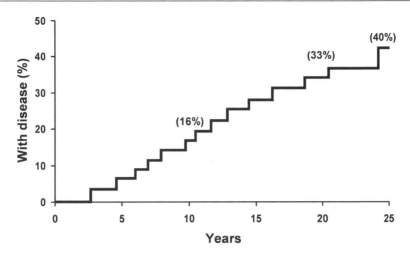

Fig. 4. Incidence of multiple myeloma, macroglobulinemia, amyloidosis, or lymphopro-liferative disease after recognition of monoclonal protein. (From ref. *17a*. By permission of Baillière Tindall.)

myeloma. The development of MM varied from a gradual increase of the M protein to an abrupt increase. AL was found in eight patients 6 to 19 yr after the M protein was identified, and WM developed in seven patients. The median interval from recognition of the M protein to the diagnosis of macroglobulinemia was 8.5 yr. In five patients, a lymphoproliferative disorder (lymphoma in four, chronic lympho-cytic leukemia in one) developed 6 to 22 yr (median, 10.5 yr) after detection of the M protein. The risk of malignant transformation did not differ significantly with the type of M protein. On the basis of the proportional hazards model, the likelihood of developing myeloma or a related disorder was not influenced by the age, gender, class of heavy chain, IgG subclass, type of light chain, presence of hepatomegaly, values for hemoglobin, serum M-protein spike, serum creatinine, or serum albu-min, or the number or appearance of bone marrow plasma cells.

5. LONG-TERM FOLLOW-UP IN 1384 PATIENTS WITH MGUS IN SOUTHEASTERN MINNESOTA

In an effort to confirm the findings of the original Mayo Clinic MGUS series, a population-based study was done of patients from southeastern Minnesota who had been referred to Mayo Clinic. MGUS was identified in 1384 patients who resided in the 11 counties of southeastern Minnesota. The diagnosis was made at Mayo Clinic between January 1, 1960, and December 31, 1994 *(18)*. The group included 753 men (54%) and 631 women (46%) with a median age at diagnosis of 72 yr (compared with 64 yr in the original study group of 241 patients). Only 24 patients (2%) were younger than 40 yr at diagnosis and 810 (59%) were 70 yr

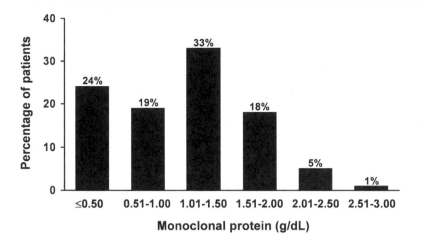

Fig. 5. Initial monoclonal protein values in 1384 residents of southeastern Minnesota in whom monoclonal gammopathy of undetermined significance was diagnosed from 1960 to 1994. (From ref. *18*. By permission of the Massachusetts Medical Society.)

or older. The M protein concentration ranged from immeasurable to 3.0 g/dL (median: 1.2 g/dL) (Fig. 5). In 70% of the patients, the M protein was IgG; in 12%, it was IgA, and in 15%, IgM. Three percent had a biclonal gammopathy. The light chain was κ in 61% of patients and λ in 39%. Reduction of uninvolved (normal or background) immunoglobulin was detected in 38% of the 840 patients for whom immunoglobulin quantification was performed. Electrophoresis, immunoelectrophoresis, and immunofixation of urine samples obtained from 418 of the patients with MGUS indicated that 21% had a monoclonal κ light chain, 10% had a λ light chain, and 69% were negative for monoclonal light chain. Only 17% had a urinary M-protein rate exceeding 150 mg/24 h *(18)*.

The bone marrow of 160 patients (12%) was examined when the M protein was first detected. A median of 3% of the bone marrow consisted of plasma cells (range: 0–10%). The initial hemoglobin values ranged from 5.7 to 18.9 g/dL; the concentration was less than 10 g/dL in 7% of patients and 12.0 g/dL or less in 23%; anemia was associated with causes other than plasma cell proliferation (e.g., iron deficiency, renal insufficiency, or myelodysplasia) in all cases. Renal insufficiency (serum creatinine >2 mg/dL) was identified in 6% of patients at diagnosis and was attributable to conditions such as diabetes, hypertension, and glomerulonephritis. The 1384 patients were followed for 11,009 person-years (median: 15.4 yr; range: 0–35 yr), during which 963 (70%) died. During follow-up, MM, lymphoma with an IgM M protein, AL, macroglobulinemia, chronic lymphocytic leukemia, or plasmacytoma developed in 115 patients (8%) (Table 2). The cumulative probability of progression to one of these disorders was 10% at 10 yr, 21% at 20 yr, and 26% at 25 yr (Fig. 6). The overall risk of progression was

Table 2
Risk of Progression Among 1384 Residents of Southeastern Minnesota
in Whom Monoclonal Gammopathy of Undetermined Significance
Was Diagnosed From 1960 to 1994

Type of progression	Observed no. of patients	Expected no. of patients[a]	Relative risk (95% CI)
Multiple myeloma	75	3.0	25.0 (20–32)
Lymphoma	19[b]	7.8	2.4 (2–4)
Primary amyloidosis	10	1.2	8.4 (4–16)
Macroglobulinemia	7	0.2	46.0 (19–95)
Chronic lymphocytic leukemia	3[c]	3.5	0.9 (0.2–3)
Plasmacytoma	1	0.1	8.5 (0.2–47)
Total group	115	15.8	7.3 (6–9)

[a]Expected numbers of cases were derived from the age- and gender-matched white population of the Surveillance, Epidemiology, and End Results program in Iowa *(19)*, except for primary amyloidosis, for which data are from ref. *20*.

[b]All 19 patients had serum IgM monoclonal protein. If the 30 patients with IgM, IgA, or IgG monoclonal protein and lymphoma were included, the relative risk would be 3.9 (95% CI, 2.6–5.5).

[c]All 3 patients had serum IgM monoclonal protein. If all 6 patients with IgM, IgA, or IgG monoclonal protein and chronic lymphocytic leukemia were included, the relative risk would be 1.7 (95% CI, 0.6–3.7).

From ref. *18*. By permission of the Massachusetts Medical Society.

approx 1% per year, and patients were at risk for progression even after 25 yr or more of stable MGUS. M-protein levels increased to more than 3 g/dL or plasma cell concentrations rose to more than 10% of the bone marrow in an additional 32 patients in whom symptomatic MM or macroglobulinemia did not develop. The cumulative probability of progression to MM or a related disorder and probability of an increase in the concentration of M protein to more than 3 g/dL or an increase in bone marrow plasma cells to more than 10% was 12% at 10 yr, 25% at 20 yr, and 30% at 25 yr (Fig. 6).

The number of patients who progressed to develop a plasma cell disorder ($n = 115$) was 7.3 times the number expected on the basis of incidence rates for those conditions in the Surveillance, Epidemiology, and End Results (SEER) program in Iowa *(19)*. The risk for myeloma increased 25-fold; for WM, 46-fold; and for AL, 8.4-fold *(18)*. The risk for lymphoma increased modestly by 2.4-fold, but the risk is underestimated because only lymphomas associated with an IgM protein counted in the observed numbers, whereas the incidence rates for lymphoma associated with IgG, IgA, and IgM proteins were used to calculate the expected number. The risk for chronic lymphocytic leukemia was only slightly increased when all six cases were included. MM developed in 65% of the 115 patients who progressed to a plasma cell disorder. MM was diagnosed more than

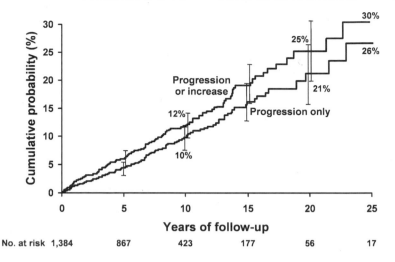

Fig. 6. Probability of progression among 1384 residents of southeastern Minnesota in whom monoclonal gammopathy of undetermined significance (MGUS) was diagnosed from 1960 to 1994. The top curve shows the probability of progression to a plasma cell cancer (115 patients) or of an increase in the monoclonal protein concentration to more than 3 g/dL or the proportion of plasma cells in bone marrow to more than 10% (32 patients). The bottom curve shows only the probability of progression of MGUS to multiple myeloma, IgM lymphoma, primary amyloidosis, macroglobulinemia, chronic lymphocytic leukemia, or plasmacytoma (115 patients). The bars indicate 95% CI. (From ref. *18*. By permission of the Massachusetts Medical Society.)

10 yr after detection of the M protein in 24 patients (32%) and in 5 (7%) after 20 yr of follow-up.

The M protein disappeared during follow-up in 66 patients (5%). Only 17 of the 66 patients had an M-protein value of more than 0.5 g/dL at diagnosis. The M protein disappeared in 39 patients because they were treated for myeloma, lymphoma, or other disorders such as idiopathic thrombocytopenic purpura or vasculitis unrelated to the monoclonal gammopathy. Only 6 of the remaining 27 patients (0.4% of all patients) demonstrated a discrete spike on the densitometer tracing of the initial electrophoretic pattern (median M value: 1.2 g/dL). Thus, spontaneous disappearance of an M protein after the diagnosis of MGUS is rare.

6. IgM MGUS

Little effort has been made to quantitate outcomes of MGUS of the IgM class which progressed to lymphoma or WM, but IgA and IgG MGUS progressed to MM, AL, or a related plasma cell disorder. Of the 213 patients with IgM MGUS from southeastern Minnesota who were followed for 1567 person-years (median: 6.3 yr), lymphoma developed in 17 patients (relative risk [RR]: 14.8), WM in 6

(RR: 262), AL in 3 (RR: 16.3), and chronic lymphocytic leukemia in 3 (RR: 5.7). The relative risk of progression was 16-fold higher in patients with IgM MGUS than in the white population of the SEER Program. The cumulative incidence of progression was 10% at 5 yr, 18% at 10 yr, and 24% at 15 yr. In a multivariate analysis, the concentration of the serum M protein and level of serum albumin at diagnosis were the only risk factors for progression to lymphoma or a related disorder *(21)*.

7. FOLLOW-UP IN OTHER SERIES

In the 20 yr of follow-up of the Swedish series, seven patients (11% of the 64 patients who had an M protein) demonstrated progression of their plasma cell proliferative process. Three of the patients in whom the M-protein value increased and one patient with a large serum IgA κ protein and light-chain proteinuria were still alive without requiring chemotherapy at the time of the report *(22)*. In a series of 20 patients with asymptomatic monoclonal gammopathy, 4 progressed to malignancy during a 3- to 14-yr follow-up *(23)*. In an Italian series of 313 patients with MGUS, 14% of 213 patients followed for 5 to 8 yr and 18% of 100 patients followed for 8 to 13 yr had a malignant transformation *(24)*. The average duration from recognition of the M protein until the development of a serious disease was 63 mo. In another series of 213 patients considered to have MGUS and who had a median follow-up of 38 mo, 10 (4.6%) developed a malignant monoclonal gammopathy after a median of 60 mo *(25)*. In that series, the actuarial risk was 4.5% at 5 yr, 15% at 10 yr, and 26% at 15 y. In another series of 128 patients with MGUS followed for a median of 56 mo, a malignant disease developed in 13 (10.2%). The actuarial probability for development of malignant disease was 8.5% at 5 yr and 19.2% at 10 yr. The median interval from recognition of the M protein to diagnosis of malignant transformation was 42 mo (range: 12–155 mo) *(26)*. In the study by Isaksson et al. *(27)*, a malignant plasma cell dyscrasia developed in 15 (26%) of 57 patients after a median follow-up of 8.4 yr. In a series of 263 cases of MGUS, the actuarial probability of developing a malignancy was 31% at 20 yr *(28)*. Finally, in a group of 335 patients with MGUS, the frequency of progression after a median follow-up of 70 mo was 6.8% *(29)*.

In a series of 1324 patients with MGUS in North Jutland County, Denmark, the standardized mortality ratio was 2.1 *(30)*. In the Danish Cancer Registry, 64 new cases of malignancies (expected: 5.0; RR: 12.9) were found among 1229 patients with MGUS. The risk for MM increased 34.3-fold; for macroglobulinemia, 63.8-fold; and for non-Hodgkin's lymphoma, 5.9-fold. The RR for chronic lymphocytic leukemia did not increase significantly *(31)*. In another series of 88 patients with MGUS, the actuarial risk of progression was 9% at 5 yr and 48% at 20 yr. Those with an M protein value less than 1.0 g/dL and bone marrow with less than 2% plasma cells had a low risk of progression *(32)*. A paraprotein malignancy developed in 51 of 504 patients with MGUS from Iceland after a median follow-up of 6 yr *(33)*. In a group of 1104 patients with MGUS, independent factors influencing the progression of MGUS were a bone marrow plasma cell concentration of more than 5%, Bence Jones proteinuria, polyclonal immunoglobulin reduction, and a high ESR *(34)*. In summary, reported series confirm that the risk for progression from MGUS to myeloma or a related disorder is approx 1% per year and does not disappear even with long-term follow-up.

8. PREDICTORS OF MALIGNANT PROGRESSION

The patient with MGUS is asymptomatic, and the discovery of an M protein is by chance and is unexpected during a routine medical examination. None of the findings at the time of diagnosis of MGUS can be used to distinguish patients whose condition will remain stable from those who will develop a malignant condition.

8.1. Value of M Protein

The value of the M protein is useful for predicting progression, as higher levels are associated with a greater risk for malignancy. A serum M-protein value of more than 3 g/dL usually indicates overt MM, but patients with this M-protein level may have smoldering multiple myeloma (SMM) and remain stable for long periods. Patients with SMM have either an M-protein value of more than 3 g/dL or a bone marrow plasma cell concentration of more than 10%, but no evidence of renal insufficiency, hypercalcemia, lytic lesions, or other clinical manifestations of MM *(35)*. Clinically and biologically, patients with SMM actually have MGUS with a higher M-protein level and greater concentration of plasma cells in the bone marrow. Recognition of these patients is extremely important; they should not be treated with chemotherapy until progression occurs, because they may remain stable for many years.

In our series of 1384 patients with MGUS, the value of the M protein at diagnosis of MGUS was the most important predictor of progression *(18)*. Only the value of the M protein and type of M protein were independent baseline factors for predicting the risk of progression. Age; gender; presence of hepatosplenomegaly; levels of hemoglobin, serum creatinine, and serum albumin; the presence, type, and amount of monoclonal urinary light chain; and the number of bone marrow plasma cells did not predict progression. The presence of a urine M protein (Table 3) and reduction in the concentration of one or more uninvolved immunoglobulins were also not risk factors for progression (Table 4).

The relative risk of progression was related directly to the value of the M protein in the serum at the time of diagnosis of MGUS (Fig. 7). The risk of progression to MM or a related disorder 20 yr after the diagnosis of MGUS was 14% for patients with an initial M-protein level of 0.5 g/dL or less, 16% for a level

Table 3
Rates of Full Progression by Urinary Light Chain Among Residents of Southeastern
Minnesota With Monoclonal Gammopathy of Undetermined Significance

Light chain	Rate of full progression, %			p value
	10 yr	20 yr	25 yr	
κ or λ	12	28	NA	0.12
Negative	11	34	34	

NA, not available.
From ref. *57a*. By permission of Blackwell Publishing.

Table 4
Rates of Full Progression by Reduction of
Uninvolved Immunoglobulins Among Residents of Southeastern Minnesota
With Monoclonal Gammopathy of Undetermined Significance

Uninvolved immunoglobulin reduction, no.	Rate of full progression, %			p value
	10 y	20 y	25 y	
1	12	33	33	0.15
2	22	22	22	0.09
0	8	17	30	

From ref. *58*. By permission of Blackwell Munksgaard.

of 1.0 g/dL, 25% for 1.5 g/dL, 41% for 2.0 g/dL, 49% for 2.5 g/dL, and 64% for 3.0 g/dL (Table 5). The risk of progression with an M-protein level of 1.5 g/dL was almost twice that with an M-protein value of 0.5 g/dL or less, and the risk of progression with an M-protein level of 2.5 g/dL was 4.6 times that with an M-protein value of 0.5 g/dL.

8.2. Type of Immunoglobulin

In the southeastern Minnesota study, patients who had an IgM or IgA M protein had an increased risk of progression compared with those who had an IgG M protein ($p = 0.001$) (Fig. 8). In another study, patients with an IgA M protein had a greater risk of progression than those with IgG or IgM (26).

8.3. Bone Marrow Plasma Cells

The number of plasma cells in the bone marrow may be helpful for predicting progression. In one report, a bone marrow plasma cell concentration of 20% was helpful for distinguishing MGUS from MM (37). In another study,

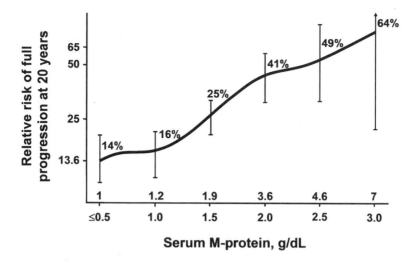

Fig. 7. Actuarial risk of full progression by serum monoclonal protein (M) value at diagnosis of monoclonal gammopathy of undetermined significance in persons from southeastern Minnesota. Numbers above *x*-axis are the relative risks of full progression vs the risk with an M-protein value 0.5g/dL. (From ref. *58*. By permission of Blackwell Munksgaard.)

Table 5
Risk Factors for Progression of Monoclonal Gammopathy of Undetermined Significance to Myeloma or Related Plasma Cell Disorder on Univariate Analysis

Prognostic factor	*Relative risk of progression at 20 yr*	*Absolute risk of progression at 10 yr, %*	*Absolute risk of progression at 20 yr, %*
Monoclonal protein, g/dL *(18)*			
0.5	1	6	14
1.0		7	16
1.5	1.9	11	25
2.0		20	41
2.5	4.6	24	49
3.0	7.0	34	64
Type of immunoglobulin *(18,36)*			
IgG, IgA, and IgM		12	22
IgM		18	29
Bone marrow plasma cell, % *(34)*			
<5	1		
6–9	2.1		

From ref. *58*. By permission of Blackwell Munksgaard.

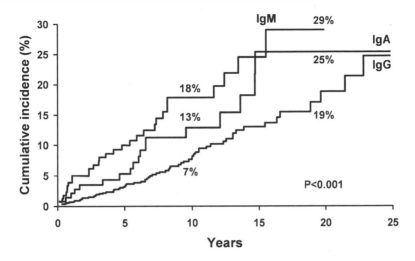

Fig. 8. Monoclonal gammopathy of undetermined significance in residents of south-eastern Minnesota (1960–1994). The risk of full progression is shown by type of monoclonal protein (IgM, IgA, and IgG). (From ref. *57a*. By permission of Blackwell Publishing.)

the transformation rate was 6.8% when the bone marrow plasma cell concentration was less than 10% compared with a transformation rate of 37% in the MGUS group with a bone marrow plasma cell concentration of 10 to 30% *(29)*. In a recent report, a bone marrow plasma cell concentration of more than 5% was considered an independent risk factor for progression to malignancy *(34)*.

8.4. Other Predictors

Cesana and colleagues *(34)* reported that Bence Jones proteinuria and a high ESR were independent factors for progression of the disease to malignancy. In the 263 patients with MGUS reported by Pasqualetti and associates *(38)*, multivariate regression analysis showed that age was the only factor associated significantly with the development of a malignant process.

Magnetic resonance imaging (MRI) may be of some help in differential diagnosis. In a series of 24 patients with newly diagnosed MGUS, MRI results were normal, whereas abnormalities were found in 38 of 44 patients (86%) with MM *(39)*. Histomorphometric studies of bone biopsy specimens reveal normal bone remodeling in patients with MGUS, but increased bone resorption and decreased bone formation in patients with stage III myeloma *(40)*.

Although β_2-microglobulin levels are important for prognosis in MM, they are of little value for distinguishing MGUS from MM owing to a considerable overlap between the two entities. The presence of J chains in malignant plasma cells, increased levels of plasma cell acid phosphatase, a reduced number of CD4 lymphocytes, an increased number of monoclonal idiotype-bearing peripheral blood lymphocytes, and an increased number of immunoglobulin-secreting cells in peripheral blood are all characteristic of MM, but are not reliable for distinguishing them owing to an overlap with MGUS *(41)*. The interleukin (IL)-6 level is more likely to be increased in patients with MM than with MGUS *(42)*. Only 1 of 35 patients with MGUS or SMM had a serum IL-6 level of more than 5 U/mL. However, 35 of 85 patients (41%) with newly diagnosed MM also had normal IL-6 levels *(42)*. An increased IL-6 level probably reflects advanced MM. In another study, 14% of patients with MGUS had increased IL-6 values *(43)*, but the serum IL-6 level cannot be used to distinguish MGUS and MM.

9. DIFFERENTIAL DIAGNOSIS

Distinguishing patients with MGUS from those with MM may be difficult at the time of diagnosis. All clinical and laboratory features—including serum and urine M protein levels; hemoglobin, calcium, and creatinine values; bone marrow plasma cell concentrations, and the presence of lytic bone lesions—are useful. Higher levels of serum M protein are associated with a greater risk for malignancy. A serum M-protein value of more than 3 g/dL usually indicates the presence of MM or WM, although some other conditions, e.g., SMM, also exist *(44)*. Normal or background immunoglobulin levels are not helpful for distinguishing benign and malignant monoclonal gammopathies. Although uninvolved immunoglobulins are also below normal levels in more than 90% of patients with MM, uninvolved immunoglobulins are reduced in almost 40% of patients with MGUS. The presence of a monoclonal light chain in the urine suggests the presence of a malignant gammopathy, but it is not unusual to find small amounts of monoclonal light chain in the urine in patients with MGUS *(45,46)*. Among the 1384 patients with MGUS from southeastern Minnesota in our study, 31% of the 418 tested patients had a monoclonal light chain in the urine, but the amount was small (only 17% had more than 150 mg/24 h). The presence of a monoclonal light chain was not a risk factor for progression. Usually a bone marrow plasma cell concentration of more than 10% suggests MM, but some patients with this extent of plasmacytosis remain stable for long intervals. Patients with a bone marrow plasma concentration of more than 10% are classified as having SMM if no signs or symptoms of MM are present. Generally, the morphologic appearance of the plasma cells is of little help in distinguishing malignant from benign disease. In contrast, Millá and coworkers *(47)* reported that the presence of nucleoli was the most important feature for distinguishing MM from MGUS.

Lytic bone lesions in the skeletal survey strongly suggest a diagnosis of MM. However, if a patient presents with constitutional symptoms, osteolytic lesions, a bone marrow plasma cell concentration less than 10%, and a modest M component, the most likely diagnosis is metastatic carcinoma with an unrelated MGUS.

IL-1β is produced by plasma cells in almost all patients with MM, but is undetectable in most patients with MGUS. IL-1β has strong osteoclast-activating factor activity, increases the expression of adhesion molecules, and induces paracrine IL-6 production. This parallels the development of osteolytic bone lesions, homing of myeloma cells to bone marrow, and IL-6-induced cell growth (48,49).

The presence of normal polyclonal plasma cells expressing CD38 and CD19 but not CD68 with low forward light scatter may be helpful in distinguishing benign from malignant disease. In one study, more than 3% normal polyclonal plasma cells were found in 98% of patients with MGUS but only 1.5% of patients with MM. The monoclonal plasma cell population had a lower CD38 expression rate and a higher forward light scatter and expressed CD56 but not CD19 (50). Expression of CD56/ neural cell adhesion molecules by osteoblasts and plasma cells corresponds with the presence of lytic bone lesions and may be helpful for distinguishing myeloma from benign disease. In 89 patients with myeloma who had lytic lesions, 91% had plasma cells that expressed neural cell adhesion molecules (51).

Conventional cytogenetic studies are not useful for distinguishing MGUS and MM because the number of metaphases available for study in patients with MGUS is too low. The use of fluorescence in situ hybridization (FISH) is of interest. Zandecki and colleagues (52) found trisomy for at least one of chromosomes 3, 7, 9, and 11 in 12% to 72% of bone marrow plasma cells in 12 of 14 hyperdiploid MGUS cases. Drach and colleagues (53) found similar chromosome abnormalities in 19 (53%) of 36 patients with MGUS. We also have seen trisomic clones in patients with MGUS using the three-color FISH procedure (54). Additional FISH studies have shown abnormalities in bone marrow plasma cells in most patients with MGUS (55–57). The genetic changes in MGUS and myeloma were recently reviewed (58).

Vacca and associates (59) demonstrated that bone marrow angiogenesis was increased in MM compared with MGUS. We studied bone marrow angiogenesis in 400 Mayo Clinic patients. Microvessel density was 1.3 in controls, 1.7 in AL, 3 in MGUS, 4 in SMM, 11 in MM, and 20 in relapsed MM. We found an increase in bone marrow angiogenesis among the spectrum of plasma cell disorders, suggesting that angiogenesis may be related to disease progression (60). Vacca and associates (61) reported that 76% of myeloma samples had increased angiogenesis compared with 20% of MGUS samples in an in vitro chick embryo chorioallantoic membrane angiogenesis assay. The role of angiogenesis in MGUS requires more study.

The plasma cell-labeling index is the most useful test for distinguishing MGUS or SMM from overt MM (62). A monoclonal antibody (BU-1) that reacts with 5-bromo-2-deoxyuridine detects cells synthesizing DNA. Because the BU-1 antibody does not require denaturation, monoclonal plasma cells can be identified after staining with κ or λ antisera using immunofluorescence. This test can be performed in 4 to 5 h. An increased plasma cell-labeling index is good evidence that either MM is present or will soon develop. However, approx 40% of patients with active MM have a normal plasma cell-labeling index. There is a good correlation between the peripheral blood and bone marrow labeling index results *(63)*.

The presence of circulating plasma cells of the same isotype in the peripheral blood is a good marker of active disease. Witzig and associates *(64)* demonstrated that monoclonal plasma cells of the same isotype can be detected in the peripheral blood of patients with MM, even though they are not seen in routine peripheral blood smears. In a series of 57 patients with newly diagnosed SMM, 16 had disease progression within 12 mo. Of these 16 patients, 63% had an increased number of peripheral blood plasma cells. In contrast, only 4 of 41 patients who remained stable had an increase in peripheral blood plasma cells *(65)*. Billadeau and coworkers *(66)* demonstrated that clonal circulating cells were present in patients with MGUS, SM, and active myeloma. They used immunofluorescence microscopy with three-color flow cytometry for $CD38^+$, $CD45^-$, and $CD45^{DIM}$ and allele-specific oligonucleotide polymerase chain reaction (PCR), which detected clonal cells in 13 of 16 patients with MGUS, compared with immunofluorescence and flow cytometry, which detected clonal cells in only 4 of the patients with MGUS. Thus, the finding of clonal cells in the peripheral blood of patients with MGUS demonstrates that the clone is present in the circulation early in the disease.

In summary, the diagnosis of MGUS usually is not difficult because the M component is an unexpected finding in the course of evaluation of an unrelated process or in a routine medical examination. However, no single factor can be used to distinguish patients with MGUS from those who will subsequently develop a malignant plasma cell disorder. The patient must be followed at regular intervals to detect the evolution to MM or a related disorder.

10. SURVIVAL AND CAUSE OF DEATH IN PATIENTS WITH MGUS

The survival of 241 patients in whom MGUS was diagnosed before 1971 was 2 yr less than that of an age- and gender-adjusted sample of the US population (13.7 vs 15.7 yr) *(16)*. In contrast, Bladé and colleagues *(26)* found only a trend for shorter survival in patients with MGUS. The median survival of 1384 patients with MGUS was 8.1 yr compared with the 11.8 yr ($p <0.001$) expected for Minnesota residents matched for age and gender (Fig. 9). van de Poel and associates *(67)* reported a slightly shorter survival for 334 patients with MGUS compared with the expected survival of age- and gender-adjusted controls.

It is important to recognize that death from plasma cell disorders occurs much less frequently than from nonplasma-cell disorders. The rate of progression or death at 10 yr in 1384 patients with MGUS was 6% from plasma cell disorders, and 53% from nonplasma-cell disorders (cardiovascular or cerebrovascular diseases and nonplasma-cell malignancies) (Fig. 10). At 20 yr, plasma cell disorders developed in 10%, but 72% had died of nonplasma-cell disorders.

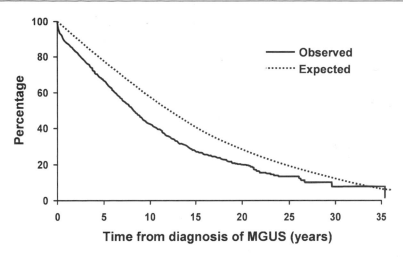

Fig. 9. Survival of 1384 patients with monoclonal gammopathy of undetermined significance (MGUS) from southeastern Minnesota compared with a normal population (8.1 vs 11.8 yr, respectively) (*p* < 0.001). (From ref. *58*. By permission of Blackwell Munksgaard.)

11. MANAGEMENT OF MGUS

MM is distinguished from MGUS by clinical factors such as symptoms, anemia, hypercalcemia, renal insufficiency, and lytic lesions. However, patients with a high plasma cell labeling index need to be monitored more frequently for other evidence of progression. No single factor can be used to distinguish a patient with MGUS from one who will subsequently develop a malignant plasma cell disorder. The serum M-protein value must be measured periodically and clinical evaluation performed to determine whether serious disease has developed.

If the patient has no other features of plasma cell dyscrasia and a serum M spike less than 1.5 g/dL, then serum protein electrophoresis, complete blood count, and measurement of calcium and creatinine levels should be repeated annually. A bone marrow examination, skeletal radiography, and 24-h urine specimen for immunofixation are not necessary in most instances. If the asymptomatic patient has an M-protein value of 1.5 to 2.0 g/dL, additional studies should include collection of a 24-h urine specimen for analysis by electrophoresis and immunofixation. Serum protein electrophoresis, complete blood count, and calcium and creatinine tests should be repeated in 3 to 6 mo. If the results are stable, studies should be repeated annually or sooner if any symptoms or complications develop.

If the serum M spike (IgG or IgA) is more than 2.0 g/dL, there is a greater likelihood of MM. Consequently, a metastatic bone survey—including single views of the humeri and femora—should be done. Aspiration and biopsy of the bone marrow should also be performed. The plasma cell-labeling index and the presence of circulating plasma cell levels in peripheral blood should be

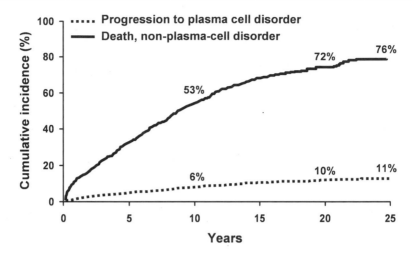

Fig. 10. Rate of death from nonplasma-cell disorders compared with progression to plasma cell disorders in 1384 patients with monoclonal gammopathy of undetermined significance from southeastern Minnesota. (From ref. *58*. By permission of Blackwell Munksgaard.)

determined, and cytogenetic studies should be performed, if available. If the IgM M-protein concentration is more than 2.0 g/dL, computed tomography of the abdomen may be useful for distinguishing lymphadenopathy from macroglobulinemia or a related lymphoproliferative disorder. Additional studies to determine β_2-microglobulin and C-reactive protein levels, for example, should be done. If the results of these studies are satisfactory, serum protein electrophoresis should be repeated in 2 or 3 mo. If the results are stable, it should be repeated in another 3 to 4 mo; if the results are still stable, it should be repeated every 6 to 12 mo. If there is an increase in the value of the serum M protein, the patient should be reevaluated with a complete blood count, serum calcium and creatinine tests, 24-h urine protein, a metastatic bone survey, bone marrow examination, as needed.

12. MONOCLONAL GAMMOPATHIES AND OTHER DISEASES

MGUS frequently occurs as a single abnormality, but is sometimes associated with other diseases, as would be expected in an elderly population. The association of two diseases depends on the frequency with which each occurs independently. Appropriate epidemiologic and statistical studies with a valid control population are essential to evaluate such associations.

12.1. Bone Loss

Previous studies demonstrated enhanced bone resorption activity in the bone marrow in patients with MGUS *(67a)*. A recent study shows increased risk of fractures, especially involving the axial skeleton *(67b)*.

12.2. Lymphoproliferative Disorders

In 1957, Azar and associates *(68)* reported that 13 patients with lymphoma and chronic lymphocytic leukemia had a serum M protein. Three years later, Kyle and colleagues *(69)* described six patients with lymphoma and a serum or urinary M protein detected by a specific electrophoretic pattern. Of 640 patients with diffuse non-Hodgkin's lymphoma or chronic lymphocytic leukemia, 44 had an M-protein component (IgM in 29, IgG in 11), whereas none of 510 patients with nodular lymphoma or Hodgkin's disease had an IgM protein *(70)*.

An M protein is present in serum in approx 5% of patients with chronic lymphocytic leukemia. In a series of 100 patients with chronic lymphocytic leukemia and M protein, the type was IgG in 51, IgM in 38, light chain in only 10, and IgA in one *(71)*. No clinical differences were found between patients who had an IgG vs IgM M protein. M proteins also have been reported in hairy cell leukemia *(72)*, adult T-cell leukemia *(73)*, Sézary syndrome, and mycosis fungoides *(74–76)*.

In a group of 430 patients with an IgM M protein who were evaluated at Mayo Clinic, 242 (56%) were considered to have MGUS. During a median follow-up of 7 yr (1714 patient-years), a lymphoid malignancy developed in 40 (17%) of the 242 patients, macroglobulinemia in 22 patients, malignant lymphoproliferative disease in 9, lymphoma in 6, primary amyloidosis in 2, and chronic lymphocytic leukemia in 1. The median duration from recognition of the M protein to the development of these disorders ranged from 4 to 9 yr. The duration of survival of patients who developed macroglobulinemia after MGUS was diagnosed was identical to that in patients with *de novo* macroglobulinemia *(77)*.

12.3. Other Hematologic Disorders

Chronic neutrophilic leukemia is characterized by persistent leukocytosis consisting of mature neutrophils, a high leukocyte alkaline phosphatase value, and bone marrow granulocytic hyperplasia. In one-third of patients, it is associated with an M protein or myeloma *(78)*. M protein was reported in 6 (13.3%) of 45 patients with refractory anemia *(79)* and 3 of 46 patients with idiopathic myelofibrosis *(80)*. Monoclonal gammopathies have been reported in patients with Gaucher's disease *(81,82)*. A patient with Gaucher's disease and MGUS developed MM developed 12 yr after the diagnosis *(83)*.

Acquired von Willebrand's disease is uncommon, but it often is associated with a monoclonal gammopathy *(84,85)*. In one report, an antibody that inhibited von Willebrand's factor was detected in all five patients who had MGUS and acquired von Willebrand's syndrome. Intravenous immunoglobulin was more effective than von Willebrand's factor concentrates *(86)*. Pernicious anemia, pure red cell aplasia, idiopathic thrombocytopenic purpura, and acute leukemia have all been reported with an M protein, but it is unknown whether the incidence of an M protein is greater in these patients than in a normal population.

12.4. Neurologic Disorders

Peripheral neuropathy has been reported with MGUS *(87)*. Kelly and colleagues *(88)* found 28 patients (10%) with monoclonal gammopathy in a group of 279 patients with a sensorimotor peripheral neuropathy of unknown cause. MGUS was present in 16 patients, AL in 7, MM in 3, and WM and γ heavy-chain type each in 1. The M protein was IgG in 15, IgA in 3, IgM in 4, light chain only in 5, and γ heavy chain in 1. The most common monoclonal gammopathy found in peripheral neuropathy is IgM, followed by IgG and IgA.

The IgM protein binds to the myelin-associated glycoprotein in about half of patients with an IgM protein and peripheral neuropathy *(89,90)*. The neuropathy is mainly sensory and begins in the lower extremities and extends slowly over a period of months to years. Motor involvement is less prominent than sensory. Cranial nerve and autonomic involvement is rare. Clinical and electrodiagnostic features are similar to those in chronic inflammatory demyelinating polyneuropathy. It is important to distinguish MGUS-associated neuropathies from those associated with primary AL. Autonomic features—including postural hypotension, sphincter dysfunction, anhidrosis, and heart or kidney failure—often occur in AL. Autonomic features and organ failure are not part of MGUS neuropathy. Chronic inflammatory demyelinating polyradiculopathy may be confused with MGUS neuropathy. Patients with MGUS have a more indolent course, less severe weakness, and more frequent sensory loss *(91)*. Chronic inflammatory demyelinating polyradiculopathy is likely to occur at a younger age and be characterized by more motor than sensory involvement, a greater tendency for a relapsing course, and an absence of monoclonal gammopathy.

The results of treatment of patients with peripheral neuropathy and monoclonal gammopathy have been disappointing. In a Mayo Clinic study, 39 patients with peripheral neuropathy and MGUS were randomized to plasmapheresis or sham plasmapheresis in a double-blind trial *(92)*. Patients with IgG or IgA gammopathy had a better response to plasma exchange than those with IgM gammopathy. A randomized study comparing intravenous immunoglobulin with placebo followed by a crossover showed minimal benefit. Antibody titers to myelin-associated glycoprotein did not change *(93)*. Rituximab, a monoclonal antibody directed against CD20, was reported to benefit all five patients treated in one study *(94)*. If the patient does not respond, chlorambucil may be useful for patients with an IgM protein or melphalan and prednisone for those with IgG and IgA proteins. Responses have been achieved with chemotherapy, but not enough data are currently available to draw definite conclusions.

Ataxia-telangiectasia is an autosomal recessive disorder characterized by cerebellar ataxia, oculocutaneous telangiectasia, and both T- and B-cell deficiency. Of 86 patients with ataxia-telangiectasia in one study, 5 had a monoclonal gammopathy *(95)*. Other neurologic disorders such as amyotrophic lateral sclerosis and progressive muscular atrophy have been reported with M proteins, but the association may be merely coincidental *(41)*.

12.5. Osteosclerotic Myeloma (POEMS Syndrome)

POEMS syndrome is characterized by polyneuropathy (P), organomegaly (O), endocrinopathy (E), M protein (M), and skin changes (S) *(96,97)*. Affected patients have a chronic inflammatory demyelinating polyneuropathy with more motor involvement than sensory. Sclerotic skeletal lesions are common and provide an important clue to the diagnosis. The cranial nerves are not involved, except for the presence of papilledema. Hepatosplenomegaly and lymphadenopathy may occur. Hyperpigmentation, hypertrichosis, angiomatous lesions, gynecomastia, and testicular atrophy are frequent findings. The most common M protein is IgA, and 90% of patients have a λ light chain. The M protein concentration is almost always less than 3 g/dL, and the bone marrow usually contains fewer than 5% plasma cells. The hemoglobin level is normal or increased, and thrombocytosis is common. The platelet level may correspond to the activity of the disease. Hypercalcemia and renal insufficiency rarely occur. The cause of POEMS syndrome is unknown. Increased levels of IL-1β, tumor necrosis factor-α, IL-6, and vascular endothelial growth factor have been reported. Castleman's disease and POEMS syndrome have been frequently associated. The diagnosis depends on the demonstration of increased numbers of monoclonal plasma cells in a biopsy specimen from the osteosclerotic lesion. The course of POEMS syndrome is chronic, and patients survive for years in contrast with those with MM. In fact, classic MM never occurs. The overall median survival of our 99 patients was 13.7 yr *(98)*. Radiation therapy is effective when the osteosclerotic lesion is localized. More than half of patients improve substantially, but that improvement may not be apparent for 6 mo or longer. Systemic therapy is necessary for patients with widespread osteosclerotic lesions. High-dose melphalan followed by autologous stem cell infusion should be considered for younger patients *(99)*. Melphalan and prednisone comprise the treatment of choice for older patients.

12.6. Dermatologic Diseases

Lichen myxedematosus (scleromyxedema, papular mucinosis) is a rare disease characterized by papules and macules involving the skin. It is usually associated with a cathodal IgGλ M protein *(100)*. The occurrence of pyoderma gangrenosum and monoclonal gammopathy is well established. In one study, 8 of 67 patients with pyoderma gangrenosum had a monoclonal gammopathy *(101)*, and 7 of those 8 patients had an IgA M protein. Necrobiotic xanthogranuloma is frequently associated with an IgG M protein *(102)*. Approximately half of patients with plane xanthomatosis have an M protein *(103)*. Schnitzler's syndrome, which is characterized by chronic urticaria and IgM monoclonal gammopathy, has been reported in several dozen patients *(104)*. Subcorneal pustular dermatosis was reported in 10 patients. IgA M protein was found in three of seven patients who were examined *(105)*. A comprehensive review of monoclonal gammopathies and skin disorders has been published *(106)*.

12.7. Rheumatoid Arthritis and Related Disorders

Rheumatoid arthritis has been associated with monoclonal gammopathies *(107,108)*. Monoclonal gammopathy has also been reported in polymyositis *(109)*. Polymyalgia rheumatica and M proteins have been observed, but both occur in an older population and a significant relationship is unlikely. Myasthenia gravis has also been reported with an M protein *(110)*. Sixteen of 70 patients (23%) with inclusion body myositis had a monoclonal gammopathy; IgG was present in 13 *(111)*. Angioneurotic edema caused by acquired deficiency of C1-esterase inhibitor in monoclonal gammopathies has been reviewed *(103)*. A patient was described with an IgG M-protein value of 4.0 g/dL and severe bleeding. It was found that the purified IgG had formed bonds with thrombin *(112)*.

12.8. Miscellaneous Disorders

Gelfand and colleagues *(113)* described a patient who had angioedema and acquired deficiency of C1-esterase inhibitor and reviewed the reports of 14 other patients in the literature, including 5 with a 7S IgM M protein. In another report, 12 of 19 patients with acquired angioedema type II had MGUS (4 each had IgG, IgA, and IgM) *(114)*. All but one patient had an M protein of the same heavy- and light-chain isotype as the acquired anti-C1 inhibitor antibody. Lofdahl and associates *(115)* reported that eight of nine patients with systemic capillary leak syndrome had an M protein in the serum. In a review of the literature, 21 patients with capillary leak syndrome all had a serum M protein (IgGκ in 12, IgGλ in 7, IgA in 1, and IgG in 1).

The association of MGUS and silicone breast implants is debatable. Karlson and colleagues *(116)* reported MGUS in 5 of 288 women with a silicone breast implant and in 4 of 288 without an implant. An M protein was reported in 11 of 272 patients with chronic active hepatitis *(117)*. M proteins also have been recognized in patients with primary biliary cirrhosis *(118)*. In a series of 102 patients with MM, WM, or MGUS, hepatitis C viral infection was found in 16% but in only 5% of controls *(119)*. In another study, an M protein was found in 11% of 239 patients who were positive for hepatitis C virus but in only 1% of 98 patients who were negative for hepatitis C virus, suggesting an association between M proteins and hepatitis C virus-related liver disease *(120)*.

Corneal crystallin deposits have been found in patients with MGUS *(121,122)*.

12.9. Immunosuppression and Monoclonal Gammopathies

M proteins have been associated with acquired immunodeficiency syndrome (AIDS). Of 341 patients who were positive for human immunodeficiency virus

(HIV), 11 had a serum M protein. After a median follow-up of 50 mo, the M protein disappeared in 7 patients. The presence of an M protein did not appear to influence the course of disease in these patients *(123)*.

Monoclonal gammopathies are common after liver transplantation. In a series of 86 patients, an M protein developed in 26 (30%). Thirteen of the M proteins were transient; the remainder were permanent. A strong correlation between the occurrence of viral infections and persistent M protein was observed, and 3 of the 13 patients with M protein died of posttransplantation lymphoproliferative disorders *(124)*. In another report, an M protein was observed in 57 of 101 patients with a liver transplant, and 5 of 7 (71%) patients with a posttransplantation lymphoproliferative disorder had an M protein. The presence of cytomegalovirus was an important risk factor *(125)*. In a randomized study, the incidence of monoclonal gammopathies was the same for those given tacrolimus (FK506) vs cyclosporine-based immunosuppression *(126)*.

Bone marrow transplantation has also been associated with an increased incidence of monoclonal gammopathies that are usually transient *(127)*. In one report, 12 of 47 patients who had undergone allogeneic bone marrow transplantation had an M protein, and 11 of the 12 developed a cytomegalovirus infection *(128)*. In a report of 550 patients who received an autologous stem cell transplant for MM, abnormal protein bands developed in 55 (10%); 48 additional patients had oligoclonal bands and isotype switch. The authors concluded that the oligoclonal bands and isotype switching were caused by the recovery of immunoglobulin production rather than recurrence of MM *(129)*. Renal transplantation is also associated with an M protein. In one study, an M protein developed after renal transplantation in 18 (13%) of 141 patients; in seven cases, the M proteins were transient *(130)*. In a series of 232 patients who received immunosuppressive therapy during transplantation, 30% had a monoclonal gammopathy; the incidence was higher in older persons *(131)*. In another series of 84 patients who had had a renal transplantation, immunoelectrophoresis revealed an M protein in 21% and Western blotting revealed a monoclonal immunoglobulin in 85.5%. The M proteins were frequently transient *(132)*.

The course of a preexisting MGUS after stem cell transplantation is uncertain. In one report, the M-protein level increased in three of five cases of MGUS after transplantation, and SMM developed in two of those three *(133)*. In another instance, primary AL developed in a patient 10 yr after an IgGκM protein was identified after renal transplantation *(134)*. More data on posttransplantation monoclonal gammopathies are needed.

12.10. Monoclonal Gammopathies With Antibody Activity

M proteins have been reported with specificity against the red blood cell polysaccharide membrane, acid polysaccharides, dextran, antistreptolysin *O*, antistaphylolysin, antinuclear antibody, riboflavin, von Willebrand factor, thyroglobulin, insulin, single- and double-stranded DNA, apolipoprotein, thyroxine, cephalin, lactate dehydrogenase, anti-HIV, platelet glycoprotein III_a, transferrin, α_2-macroglobulin, cardiolipin, chondroitin sulphate, group A streptococci, cytomegalovirus, and antibiotics (41,135).

A patient with MM had xanthoderma-xanthotrichia (yellow discoloration of skin and hair) that was caused by an IgGλ protein with antiriboflavin antibody activity. The xanthoderma disappeared when the IgG level decreased to less than 2 g/dL. Another patient with similar clinical and laboratory features has been reported (136).

The M protein may bind with calcium and produce a high total serum calcium level without symptoms because the ionized calcium level is normal. This possibility should be entertained in asymptomatic patients with hypercalcemia to avoid attempting to reduce their increased calcium levels (137,138). Hypercupremia caused by the binding of copper by an IgGλM protein has been noted (139). In another case, hypercupremia from IgG binding resulted in ocular deposition of copper (140). The binding of an M protein to phosphate and resulting in a high serum phosphorus level has been reported (141). Spurious cases of hyperphosphatemia may result from interference of the M protein with the phosphate chromogenic assay (142).

13. VARIANTS OF MGUS

13.1. Idiopathic Bence Jones Proteinuria

The presence of Bence Jones proteinuria is usually associated with a malignant monoclonal gammopathy. However, cases of patients excreting large amounts of Bence Jones protein with a benign course have been well documented. One patient with a stable serum M protein excreted 0.8 g or more of monoclonal light chain daily for almost 20 yr without developing myeloma or amyloidosis (143). Seven other patients without an M protein in the serum and no evidence of a malignant plasma cell disorder at diagnosis who excreted more than 1 g daily of Bence Jones protein have been described (144). During the follow-up period of 7 to 21 yr, MM developed in three patients, evolving myeloma in one, and asymptomatic myeloma in one. AL developed after 12 yr of follow-up in one patient, and one patient has stable-level Bence Jones proteinuria at 35 yr. Thus, Bence Jones proteinuria may remain stable for years, but in most patients MM or AL develops. These patients must be followed closely.

13.2. Biclonal Gammopathies

Biclonal gammopathies are characterized by the production of two different M proteins that occur in 3 to 4% of patients with monoclonal gammopathies. The presence of 2 M proteins may be the result of the proliferation of two different clones of plasma cells or the production of 2 M proteins by a single clone of plasma cells. The characteristics of 57 patients with biclonal gammopathy have been reviewed *(1)*. Two-thirds had MGUS, and the remainder had MM (16%) or a malignant lymphoproliferative disorder (19%). Thus, the clinical features of patients with biclonal gammopathy are similar to those of patients with monoclonal gammopathy. Serum protein electrophoresis showed only a single band in almost one-third of the cases. The second M protein was not recognized until immunoelectrophoresis or immunofixation was done.

13.3. Triclonal Gammopathies

Triclonal gammopathies have been reported *(145)*. Grosbois and colleagues *(2)* described a patient who had triclonal gammopathy (IgMκ, IgGκ, and IgAκ) and in a review of the literature found 16 cases of triclonal gammopathy that were associated with a malignant immunolymphoproliferative disorder, 5 involving nonhematologic diseases and 3 were of undetermined significance.

13.4. IgD MGUS

The presence of an IgD M protein almost always indicates a malignant plasma cell disorder such as MM or primary amyloidosis. A patient with well-documented MGUS of the IgD type was followed for more than 6 yr, during which time no serious disease developed *(146)*. We described a patient with IgD MGUS who was followed for more than 8 yr and never developed evidence of malignant disease *(147)*.

ACKNOWLEDGMENT

This research was supported in part by research grant CA 62242 from the National Institutes of Health.

REFERENCES

1. Kyle RA, Robinson RA, Katzmann JA. The clinical aspects of biclonal gammopathies: review of 57 cases. Am J Med 1981; 71:999–1008.
2. Grosbois B, Jégo P, de Rosa H, et al. Triclonal gammopathy and malignant immunoproliferative syndrome [French]. Rev Med Interne 1997; 18:470–473.
3. Katzmann JA, Clark R, Sanders E, Landers JP, Kyle RA. Prospective study of serum protein capillary zone electrophoresis and immunotyping of monoclonal proteins by immunosubtraction. Am J Clin Pathol 1998; 110:503–509.
4. Kyle RA, Katzmann JA. Immunochemical characterization of immunoglobulins. In: Rose NR, de Macario EC, Folds JD, Lane HC, Nakamura RM, eds. Manual of Clinical Laboratory Immunology, 5th ed. Washington, DC: ASM Press, 1997:156–176.
5. Axelsson U, Bachmann R, Hallen J. Frequency of pathological proteins (M-components) in 6,995 sera from an adult population. Acta Med Scand 1966; 179:235–247.
6. Kyle RA, Finkelstein S, Elveback LR, Kurland LT. Incidence of monoclonal proteins in a Minnesota community with a cluster of multiple myeloma. Blood 1972; 40:719–724.

7. Saleun JP, Vicariot M, Deroff P, Morin JF. Monoclonal gammopathies in the adult population of Finistere, France. J Clin Pathol 1982; 35:63–68.

8. Crawford J, Eye MK, Cohen HJ. Evaluation of monoclonal gammopathies in the "well" elderly. Am J Med 1987; 82:39–45.

9. Ligthart GJ, Radl J, Corberand JX, et al. Monoclonal gammopathies in human aging: increased occurrence with age and correlation with health status. Mech Ageing Dev 1990; 52:235–243.

10. Shih LY, Dunn P, Leung WM, Chen WJ, Wang PN. Localised plasmacytomas in Taiwan: comparison between extramedullary plasmacytoma and solitary plasmacytoma of bone. Br J Cancer 1995; 71:128–133.

11. Cohen HJ, Crawford J, Rao MK, Pieper CF, Currie MS. Racial differences in the prevalence of monoclonal gammopathy in a community-based sample of the elderly. Am J Med 1998; 104:439–444.

12. Bowden M, Crawford J, Cohen HJ, Noyama O. A comparative study of monoclonal gammopathies and immunoglobulin levels in Japanese and United States elderly. J Am Geriatr Soc 1993; 41:11–14.

13. Kurihara Y, Shiba K, Fukumura Y, Kobayashi I, Kamei S. Occurrence of serum M-protein species in Japanese patients older than 50 years based on relative mobility in cellulose acetate membrane electrophoresis. J Clin Lab Anal 2000; 14:64–69.

14. Kyle RA. Monoclonal gammopathy of undetermined significance: natural history in 241 cases. Am J Med 1978; 64:814–826.

15. Kyle RA. 'Benign' monoclonal gammopathy. A misnomer? JAMA 1984; 251:1849–1854.

16. Kyle RA. "Benign" monoclonal gammopathy—after 20 to 35 years of follow-up. Mayo Clin Proc 1993; 68:26-36.

17. Kyle RA. Monoclonal gammopathy of undetermined significance and solitary plasmacytoma: implications for progression to overt multiple myeloma. Hematol Oncol Clin North Am 1997; 11:71–87.

17a. Kyle RA. Monoclonal gammopathy of undetermined significance [MGUS]. Baillière's Clin Haematol 1995;8:761–781.

18. Kyle RA, Therneau TM, Rajkumar SV, et al. A long-term study of prognosis in monoclonal gammopathy of undetermined significance. N Engl J Med 2002; 346:564–569.

19. Ries LAG, Eisner MP, Kosary CL, et al., eds. SEER Cancer Statistics Review, 1973–1998. Bethesda, Maryland: National Cancer Institute, 2001. http://seer.cancer.gov/Publications/CSR1973_1998/

20. Kyle RA, Linos A, Beard CM, et al. Incidence and natural history of primary systemic amyloidosis in Olmsted County, Minnesota, 1950 through 1989. Blood 1992; 79:1817–1822.

21. Kyle RA, Therneau TM, Rajkumar SV, et al. Long-term follow-up of IgM monoclonal gammopathy of undetermined significance. Blood 2003.

22. Axelsson U. A 20-year follow-up study of 64 subjects with M-components. Acta Med Scand 1986; 219:519–522.

23. Fine JM, Lambin P, Muller JY. The evolution of asymptomatic monoclonal gammopathies: a follow-up of 20 cases over periods of 3–14 years. Acta Med Scand 1979; 205:339–341.

24. Paladini G, Fogher M, Mazzanti G, et al. Idiopathic monoclonal gammopathy: long-term study of 313 cases [Italian]. Recenti Prog Med 1989; 80:123–132.

25. Giraldo MP, Rubio-Félix D, Perella M, Gracia JA, Bergua JM, Giralt M. Monoclonal gammopathies of undetermined significance: clinical course and biological aspects of 397 cases [Spanish]. Sangre (Barc) 1991; 36:377–382.

26. Bladé J, Lopez-Guillermo A, Rozman C, et al. Malignant transformation and life expectancy in monoclonal gammopathy of undetermined significance. Br J Haematol 1992; 81:391–394.

27. Isaksson E, Bjorkholm M, Holm G, et al. Blood clonal B-cell excess in patients with monoclonal gammopathy of undetermined significance (MGUS): association with malignant transformation. Br J Haematol 1996; 92:71–76.

28. Pasqualetti P, Casale R. Risk of malignant transformation in patients with monoclonal gammopathy of undetermined significance. Biomed Pharmacother 1997; 51:74–78.
29. Baldini L, Guffanti A, Cesana BM, et al. Role of different hematologic variables in defining the risk of malignant transformation in monoclonal gammopathy. Blood 1996; 87:912–918.
30. Gregersen H, Salling Ibsen J, Mellemkjær L, Dahlerup JF, Olsen JH, Sørensen HT. Mortality and causes of death in patients with monoclonal gammopathy of undetermined significance. Br J Haematol 2001; 112:353–357.
31. Gregersen H, Mellemkjær L, Salling Ibsen J, et al. Cancer risk in patients with monoclonal gammopathy of undetermined significance. Am J Hematol 2000; 63:1–6.
32. Van De Donk N, De Weerdt O, Eurelings M, Bloem A, Lokhorst H. Malignant transformation of monoclonal gammopathy of undetermined significance: cumulative incidence and prognostic factors. Leuk Lymphoma 2001; 42:609–618.
33. Ögmundsdóttir HM, Haraldsdóttir V, Jóhannesson GM, et al. Monoclonal gammopathy in Iceland: a population-based registry and follow-up. Br J Haematol 2002; 118:166–173.
34. Cesana C, Klersy C, Barbarano L, et al. Prognostic factors for malignant transformation in monoclonal gammopathy of undetermined significance and smoldering multiple myeloma. J Clin Oncol 2002; 20:1625–1634.
35. Kyle RA, Gertz MA, Witzig TE, et al. Review of 1027 patients with newly diagnosed multiple myeloma. Mayo Clin Proc 2003; 78:21–33.
36. Kyle RA, Treon SP, Alexanian R, et al. Prognostic markers and criteria to initiate therapy in Waldenström's macroglobulinemia: consensus panel recommendations from the Second International Workshop on Waldenström's Macroglobulinemia. Semin Oncol 2003; 30:116–120.
37. Ucci G, Riccardi A, Luoni R, Ascari E. Presenting features of monoclonal gammopathies: an analysis of 684 newly diagnosed cases. Cooperative Group for the Study and Treatment of Multiple Myeloma. J Intern Med 1993; 234:165–173.
38. Pasqualetti P, Festuccia V, Collacciani A, Casale R. The natural history of monoclonal gammopathy of undetermined significance: a 5- to 20-year follow-up of 263 cases. Acta Haematol 1997; 97:174–179.
39. Bellaïche I, Laredo JD, Lioté F, et al, and the GRI Study Group. Magnetic resonance appearance of monoclonal gammopathies of unknown significance and multiple myeloma. Spine 1997; 22:2551–2557.
40. Laroche M, Attal M, Dromer C. Bone remodelling in monoclonal gammopathies of uncertain significance, symptomatic and nonsymptomatic myeloma. Clin Rheumatol 1996; 15:347–352.
41. Kyle RA, Lust JA. Myeloma and related disorders: Monoclonal gammopathies of undetermined significance. In: Wiernik PH, Canellos GP, Kyle RA, Schiffer CA, eds. Neoplastic Diseases of the Blood, 2nd ed. New York: Churchill Livingstone, 1991:571–594.
42. Bataille R, Jourdan M, Zhang XG, Klein B. Serum levels of interleukin 6, a potent myeloma cell growth factor, as a reflect of disease severity in plasma cell dyscrasias. J Clin Invest 1989; 84:2008–2011.
43. Filella X, Bladé J, Guillermo AL, Molina R, Rozman C, Ballesta AM. Cytokines (IL-6, TNF-alpha, IL-1alpha) and soluble interleukin-2 receptor as serum tumor markers in multiple myeloma. Cancer Detect Prev 1996; 20:52–56.
44. Kyle RA, Greipp PR. Smoldering multiple myeloma. N Engl J Med 1980; 302:1347–1349.
45. Dammacco F, Waldenström J. Bence Jones proteinuria in benign monoclonal gammapathies: incidence and characteristics. Acta Med Scand 1968; 184:403–409.
46. Lindstrom FD, Dahlstrom U. Multiple myeloma or benign monoclonal gammopathy? A study of differential diagnostic criteria in 44 cases. Clin Immunol Immunopathol 1978; 10:168–174.

47. Millá F, Oriol A, Aguilar J, et al. Usefulness and reproducibility of cytomorphologic evaluations to differentiate myeloma from monoclonal gammopathies of unknown significance. Am J Clin Pathol 2001; 115:127–135.

48. Lust JA, Donovan KA. Biology of the transition of monoclonal gammopathy of undetermined significance (MGUS) to multiple myeloma. Cancer Control 1998; 5:209–217.

49. Lacy MQ, Donovan KA, Heimbach JK, Ahmann GJ, Lust JA. Comparison of interleukin-1 beta expression by in situ hybridization in monoclonal gammopathy of undetermined significance and multiple myeloma. Blood 1999; 93:300–305.

50. Ocqueteau M, Orfao A, Almeida J, et al. Immunophenotypic characterization of plasma cells from monoclonal gammopathy of undetermined significance patients: implications for the differential diagnosis between MGUS and multiple myeloma. Am J Pathol 1998; 152:1655–1665.

51. Ely SA, Knowles DM. Expression of CD56/neural cell adhesion molecule correlates with the presence of lytic bone lesions in multiple myeloma and distinguishes myeloma from monoclonal gammopathy of undetermined significance and lymphomas with plasmacytoid differentiation. Am J Pathol 2002; 160:1293–1299.

52. Zandecki M, Obein V, Bernardi F, et al. Monoclonal gammopathy of undetermined significance: chromosome changes are a common finding within bone marrow plasma cells. Br J Haematol 1995; 90:693–696.

53. Drach J, Angerler J, Schuster J, et al. Interphase fluorescence in situ hybridization identifies chromosomal abnormalities in plasma cells from patients with monoclonal gammopathy of undetermined significance. Blood 1995; 86:3915–3921.

54. Ahmann GJ, Jalal SM, Juneau AL, et al. A novel three-color, clone-specific fluorescence in situ hybridization procedure for monoclonal gammopathies. Cancer Genet Cytogenet 1998; 101:7–11.

55. Avet-Loiseau H, Li JY, Facon T, et al. High incidence of translocations t(11;14)(q13;q32) and t(4;14)(p16;q32) in patients with plasma cell malignancies. Cancer Res 1998; 58:5640–5645.

56. Avet-Loiseau H, Facon T, Daviet A, et al. 14q32 translocations and monosomy 13 observed in monoclonal gammopathy of undetermined significance delineate a multistep process for the oncogenesis of multiple myeloma. Intergroupe Francophone du Myelome. Cancer Res 1999; 59:4546–4550.

57. Fonseca R, Ahmann GJ, Jalal SM, et al. Chromosomal abnormalities in systemic amyloidosis. Br J Haematol 1998; 103:704–710.

57a. Kyle RA, Rajkumar SV. Monoclonal gammopathies of undetermined significance. Rev Clin Exp Hematol 2002;6:225–252.

58. Kyle RA, Rajkumar SV. Monoclonal gammopathies of undetermined significance: a review. Immunol Rev 2003; 194:112–139.

59. Vacca A, Ribatti D, Roncali L, et al. Bone marrow angiogenesis and progression in multiple myeloma. Br J Haematol 1994; 87:503–508.

60. Rajkumar SV, Mesa RA, Fonseca R, et al. Bone marrow angiogenesis in 400 patients with monoclonal gammopathy of undetermined significance, multiple myeloma, and primary amyloidosis. Clin Cancer Res 2002; 8:2210–2216.

61. Vacca A, Ribatti D, Presta M, et al. Bone marrow neovascularization, plasma cell angiogenic potential, and matrix metalloproteinase-2 secretion parallel progression of human multiple myeloma. Blood 1999; 93:3064–3073.

62. Greipp PR, Witzig TE, Gonchoroff NJ, et al. Immunofluorescence labeling indices in myeloma and related monoclonal gammopathies. Mayo Clin Proc 1987; 62:969–977.

63. Witzig TE, Gonchoroff NJ, Katzmann JA, Therneau TM, Kyle RA, Greipp PR. Peripheral blood B cell labeling indices are a measure of disease activity in patients with monoclonal gammopathies. J Clin Oncol 1988; 6:1041–1046.

64. Witzig TE, Kyle RA, Greipp PR. Circulating peripheral blood plasma cells in multiple myeloma. Curr Top Microbiol Immunol 1992; 182:195–199.

65. Witzig TE, Kyle RA, O'Fallon WM, Greipp PR. Detection of peripheral blood plasma cells as a predictor of disease course in patients with smouldering multiple myeloma. Br J Haematol 1994; 87:266–272.

66. Billadeau D, Van Ness B, Kimlinger T, et al. Clonal circulating cells are common in plasma cell proliferative disorders: a comparison of monoclonal gammopathy of undetermined significance, smoldering multiple myeloma, and active myeloma. Blood 1996; 88:289–296.

67. van de Poel MH, Coebergh JW, Hillen HF. Malignant transformation of monoclonal gammopathy of undetermined significance among out-patients of a community hospital in southeastern Netherlands. Br J Haematol 1995; 91:121–125.

67a. Bataille R, Chappard D, Basle M. Quantifiable excess of bone resorption in monoclonal gammopathy is an early symptom of malignancy: a prospective study of 87 biopsies. Blood 1996; 87:4762–4769.

67b. Melton JL, III, Rajkumar SV, Khosla S, Achenbach SJ, Oberg AL, Kyle RA. Fracture risk in monoclonal gammopathy of undetermined significance. J Bone Min Res 2004; 19:1:25–33.

68. Azar HA, Hill WT, Osserman EF. Malignant lymphoma and lymphatic leukemia associated with myeloma-type serum proteins. Am J Med 1957; 23:239–249.

69. Kyle RA, Bayrd ED, McKenzie BF, Heck FJ. Diagnostic criteria for electrophoretic patterns of serum and urinary proteins in multiple myeloma: study of one hundred and sixty-five multiple myeloma patients and of seventy-seven nonmyeloma patients with similar electrophoretic patterns. JAMA 1960; 174:245–251.

70. Alexanian R. Monoclonal gammopathy in lymphoma. Arch Intern Med 1975; 135:62–66.

71. Noel P, Kyle RA. Monoclonal proteins in chronic lymphocytic leukemia. Am J Clin Pathol 1987; 87:385–388.

72. Jansen J, Bolhuis RL, van Nieuwkoop JA, Schuit HR, Kroese WF. Paraproteinaemia plus osteolytic lesions in typical hairy-cell leukaemia. Br J Haematol 1983; 54:531–541.

73. Matsuzaki H, Yamaguchi K, Kagimoto T, Nakai R, Takatsuki K, Oyama W. Monoclonal gammopathies in adult T-cell leukemia. Cancer 1985; 56:1380–1383.

74. Kövary PM, Suter L, Macher E, et al. Monoclonal gammopathies in Sezary syndrome: a report of four new cases and a review of the literature. Cancer 1981; 48:788–792.

75. Venencie PY, Winkelmann RK, Puissant A, Kyle RA. Monoclonal gammopathy in Sezary syndrome: report of three cases and review of the literature. Arch Dermatol 1984; 120:605–608.

76. Venencie PY, Winkelmann RK, Friedman SJ, Kyle RA, Puissant A. Monoclonal gammopathy and mycosis fungoides: report of four cases and review of the literature. J Am Acad Dermatol 1984; 11:576–579.

77. Kyle RA, Garton JP. The spectrum of IgM monoclonal gammopathy in 430 cases. Mayo Clin Proc 1987; 62:719–731.

78. Rovira M, Cervantes F, Nomdedeu B, Rozman C. Chronic neutrophilic leukaemia preceding for seven years the development of multiple myeloma. Acta Haematol 1990; 83:94–95.

79. Economopoulos T, Economidou J, Giannopoulos G, et al. Immune abnormalities in myelodysplastic syndromes. J Clin Pathol 1985; 38:908–911.

80. Dührsen U, Uppenkamp M, Meusers P, König E, Brittinger G. Frequent association of idiopathic myelofibrosis with plasma cell dyscrasias. Blut 1988; 56:97–102.

81. Pratt PW, Kochwa S, Estren S. Immunoglobulin abnormalities in Gaucher's disease: report of 16 cases. Blood 1968; 31:633–640.

82. Shoenfeld Y, Berliner S, Pinkhas J, Beutler E. The association of Gaucher's disease and dysproteinemias. Acta Haematol 1980; 64:241–243.

83. Brady K, Corash L, Bhargava V. Multiple myeloma arising from monoclonal gammopathy of undetermined significance in a patient with Gaucher's disease. Arch Pathol Lab Med 1997; 121:1108–1111.

84. Keren DF. Coagulation disorders in patients with monoclonal gammopathies. Hematol Oncol Clin North Am 1993; 7:1153–1159.

85. Federici AB, Stabile F, Castaman G, Canciani MT, Mannucci PM. Treatment of acquired von Willebrand syndrome in patients with monoclonal gammopathy of uncertain significance: comparison of three different therapeutic approaches. Blood 1998; 92:2707–2711.

86. Lamboley V, Zabraniecki L, Sie P, Pourrat J, Fournie B. Myeloma and monoclonal gammopathy of uncertain significance associated with acquired von Willebrand's syndrome: seven new cases with a literature review. Joint Bone Spine 2002; 69:62–67.

87. Isobe T, Osserman EF. Pathologic conditions associated with plasma cell dyscrasias: a study of 806 cases. Ann N Y Acad Sci 1971; 190:507–518.

88. Kelly JJ, Jr., Kyle RA, O'Brien PC, Dyck PJ. Prevalence of monoclonal protein in peripheral neuropathy. Neurology 1981; 31:1480–1483.

89. Hafler DA, Johnson D, Kelly JJ, Panitch H, Kyle R, Weiner HL. Monoclonal gammopathy and neuropathy: myelin-associated glycoprotein reactivity and clinical characteristics. Neurology 1986; 36:75–78.

90. Kelly JJ, Adelman LS, Berkman E, Bhan I. Polyneuropathies associated with IgM monoclonal gammopathies. Arch Neurol 1988; 45:1355–1359.

91. Simmons Z, Albers JW, Bromberg MB, Feldman EL. Presentation and initial clinical course in patients with chronic inflammatory demyelinating polyradiculoneuropathy: comparison of patients without and with monoclonal gammopathy. Neurology 1993; 43:2202–2209.

92. Dyck PJ, Low PA, Windebank AJ, et al. Plasma exchange in polyneuropathy associated with monoclonal gammopathy of undetermined significance. N Engl J Med 1991; 325:1482–1486.

93. Dalakas MC, Quarles RH, Farrer RG, et al. A controlled study of intravenous immunoglobulin in demyelinating neuropathy with IgM gammopathy. Ann Neurol 1996; 40:792–795.

94. Levine TD, Pestronk A. IgM antibody-related polyneuropathies: B-cell depletion chemotherapy using Rituximab. Neurology 1999; 52:1701–1704.

95. Sadighi Akha AA, Humphrey RL, Winkelstein JA, Loeb DM, Lederman HM. Oligo-/monoclonal gammopathy and hypergammaglobulinemia in ataxia-telangiectasia: a study of 90 patients. Medicine (Baltimore) 1999; 78:370–381.

96. Bardwick PA, Zvaifler NJ, Gill GN, Newman D, Greenway GD, Resnick DL. Plasma cell dyscrasia with polyneuropathy, organomegaly, endocrinopathy, M protein, and skin changes: the POEMS syndrome. Report on two cases and a review of the literature. Medicine (Baltimore) 1980; 59:311–322.

97. Kelly JJ, Jr., Kyle RA, Miles JM, Dyck PJ. Osteosclerotic myeloma and peripheral neuropathy. Neurology 1983; 33:202–210.

98. Dispenzieri A, Kyle RA, Lacy MQ, et al. POEMS syndrome: definitions and long-term outcome. Blood 2003; 101:2496–2506.

99. Jaccard A, Royer B, Bordessoule D, Brouet JC, Fermand JP. High-dose therapy and autologous blood stem cell transplantation in POEMS syndrome. Blood 2002; 99:3057–3059.

100. James K, Fudenberg H, Epstein WL, Shuster J. Studies on a unique diagnostic serum globulin in papular mucinosis (lichen myxedematosus). Clin Exp Immunol 1967; 2:153–166.

101. Powell FC, Schroeter AL, Su WP, Perry HO. Pyoderma gangrenosum and monoclonal gammopathy. Arch Dermatol 1983; 119:468–472.

102. Finan MC, Winkelmann RK. Necrobiotic xanthogranuloma with paraproteinemia: a review of 22 cases. Medicine (Baltimore) 1986; 65:376–388.

103. Pascual M, Mach-Pascual S, Schifferli JA. Paraproteins and complement depletion: pathogenesis and clinical syndromes. Semin Hematol 1997; 34 Suppl 1:40–48.

104. Puddu P, Cianchini G, Girardelli CR, Colonna L, Gatti S, de Pita O. Schnitzler's syndrome: report of a new case and a review of the literature. Clin Exp Rheumatol 1997; 15:91–95.

105. Lutz ME, Daoud MS, McEvoy MT, Gibson LE. Subcorneal pustular dermatosis: a clinical study of ten patients. Cutis 1998; 61:203–208.

106. Daoud MS, Lust JA, Kyle RA, Pittelkow MR. Monoclonal gammopathies and associated skin disorders. J Am Acad Dermatol 1999; 40:507–535.

107. Goldenberg GJ, Paraskevas F, Israels LG. The association of rheumatoid arthritis with plasma cell and lymphocytic neoplasms. Arthritis Rheum 1969; 12:569–579.
108. Zawadzki ZA, Benedek TG. Rheumatoid arthritis, dysproteinemic arthropathy, and paraproteinemia. Arthritis Rheum 1969; 12:555–568.
109. Kiprov DD, Miller RG. Polymyositis associated with monoclonal gammopathy. Lancet 1984; 2:1183–1186.
110. Soppi E, Eskola J, Röyttä M, Veromaa T, Panelius M, Lehtonen A. Thymoma with immunodeficiency (Good's syndrome) associated with myasthenia gravis and benign IgG gammopathy. Arch Intern Med 1985; 145:1704–1707.
111. Dalakas MC, Illa I, Gallardo E, Juarez C. Inclusion body myositis and paraproteinemia: incidence and immunopathologic correlations. Ann Neurol 1997; 41:100–104.
112. Colwell NS, Tollefsen DM, Blinder MA. Identification of a monoclonal thrombin inhibitor associated with multiple myeloma and a severe bleeding disorder. Br J Haematol 1997; 97:219–226.
113. Gelfand JA, Boss GR, Conley CL, Reinhart R, Frank MM. Acquired C1 esterase inhibitor deficiency and angioedema: a review. Medicine (Baltimore) 1979; 58:321–328.
114. Frémeaux-Bacchi V, Guinnepain MT, Cacoub P, et al. Prevalence of monoclonal gammopathy in patients presenting with acquired angioedema type 2. Am J Med 2002; 113:194–199.
115. Lofdahl CG, Solvell L, Laurell AB, Johansson BR. Systemic capillary leak syndrome with monoclonal IgG and complement alterations: a case report on an episodic syndrome. Acta Med Scand 1979; 206:405–412.
116. Karlson EW, Tanasijevic M, Hankinson SE, et al. Monoclonal gammopathy of undetermined significance and exposure to breast implants. Arch Intern Med 2001; 161:864–867.
117. Heer M, Joller-Jemelka H, Fontana A, Seefeld U, Schmid M, Ammann R. Monoclonal gammopathy in chronic active hepatitis. Liver 1984; 4:255–263.
118. Hendrick AM, Mitchison HC, Bird AG, James OF. Paraproteins in primary biliary cirrhosis. Q J Med 1986; 60:681–684.
119. Mangia A, Clemente R, Musto P, et al. Hepatitis C virus infection and monoclonal gammopathies not associated with cryoglobulinemia. Leukemia 1996; 10:1209–1213.
120. Andreone P, Zignego AL, Cursaro C, et al. Prevalence of monoclonal gammopathies in patients with hepatitis C virus infection. Ann Intern Med 1998; 129:294–298.
121. Bourne WM, Kyle RA, Brubaker RF, Greipp PR. Incidence of corneal crystals in the monoclonal gammopathies. Am J Ophthalmol 1989; 107:192–193.
122. Kato T, Nakayasu K, Omata Y, Watanabe Y, Kanai A. Corneal deposits as an alerting sign of monoclonal gammopathy: a case report. Cornea 1999; 18:734–738.
123. Lefrère JJ, Debbia M, Lambin P. Prospective follow-up of monoclonal gammopathies in HIV-infected individuals. Br J Haematol 1993; 84:151–155.
124. Pageaux G-P, Bonnardet A, Picot M-C, et al. Prevalence of monoclonal immunoglobulins after liver transplantation: relationship with posttransplant lymphoproliferative disorders. Transplantation 1998; 65:397–400.
125. Badley AD, Portela DF, Patel R, et al. Development of monoclonal gammopathy precedes the development of Epstein-Barr virus-induced posttransplant lymphoproliferative disorder. Liver Transpl Surg 1996; 2:375–382.
126. Pham H, Lemoine A, Salvucci M, et al. Occurrence of gammopathies and lymphoproliferative disorders in liver transplant recipients randomized to tacrolimus (FK506)- or cyclosporine-based immunosuppression. Liver Transpl Surg 1998; 4:146–151.
127. Hammarström L, Smith CI. Frequent occurrence of monoclonal gammopathies with an imbalanced light-chain ratio following bone marrow transplantation. Transplantation 1987; 43:447–449.
128. Hebart H, Einsele H, Klein R, et al. CMV infection after allogeneic bone marrow transplantation is associated with the occurrence of various autoantibodies and monoclonal gammopathies. Br J Haematol 1996; 95:138–144.

129. Zent CS, Wilson CS, Tricot G, et al. Oligoclonal protein bands and Ig isotype switching in multiple myeloma treated with high-dose therapy and hematopoietic cell transplantation. Blood 1998; 91:3518–3523.

130. Renoult E, Bertrand F, Kessler M. Monoclonal gammopathies in HBsAg-positive patients with renal transplants (letter). N Engl J Med 1988; 318:1205.

131. Radl J, Valentijn RM, Haaijman JJ, Paul LC. Monoclonal gammapathies in patients undergoing immunosuppressive treatment after renal transplantation. Clin Immunol Immunopathol 1985; 37:98–102.

132. Touchard G, Pasdeloup T, Parpeix J, et al. High prevalence and usual persistence of serum monoclonal immunoglobulins evidenced by sensitive methods in renal transplant recipients. Nephrol Dial Transplant 1997; 12:1199–1203.

133. Rostaing L, Modesto A, Abbal M, Durand D. Long-term follow-up of monoclonal gammopathy of undetermined significance in transplant patients. Am J Nephrol 1994; 14:187–191.

134. Dysseleer A, Michaux L, Cosyns JP, Goffin E, Hermans C, Pirson Y. Benign monoclonal gammopathy turning to AL amyloidosis after kidney transplantation. Am J Kidney Dis 1999; 34:166–169.

135. Merlini G, Farhangi M, Osserman EF. Monoclonal immunoglobulins with antibody activity in myeloma, macroglobulinemia and related plasma cell dyscrasias. Semin Oncol 1986; 13:350–365.

136. Merlini G, Bruening R, Kyle RA, Osserman EF. The second riboflavin-binding myeloma IgGλ^{DOT}. I. Biochemical and functional characterization. Mol Immunol 1990; 27:385–394.

137. Annesley TM, Burritt MF, Kyle RA. Artifactual hypercalcemia in multiple myeloma. Mayo Clin Proc 1982; 57:572–575.

138. Merlini G, Fitzpatrick LA, Siris ES, et al. A human myeloma immunoglobulin G binding four moles of calcium associated with asymptomatic hypercalcemia. J Clin Immunol 1984; 4:185–196.

139. Martin NF, Kincaid MC, Stark WJ, et al. Ocular copper deposition associated with pulmonary carcinoma, IgG monoclonal gammopathy and hypercupremia: a clinicopathologic correlation. Ophthalmology 1983; 90:110–116.

140. Probst LE, Hoffman E, Cherian MG, et al. Ocular copper deposition associated with benign monoclonal gammopathy and hypercupremia. Cornea 1996; 15:94–98.

141. Pettersson T, Hortling L, Teppo AM, Totterman KJ, Fyhrquist F. Phosphate binding by a myeloma protein. Acta Med Scand 1987; 222:89–91.

142. Sonnenblick M, Eylath U, Brisk R, Eldad C, Hershko C. Paraprotein interference with colorimetry of phosphate in serum of some patients with multiple myeloma. Clin Chem 1986; 32:1537–1539.

143. Kyle RA, Maldonado JE, Bayrd ED. Idiopathic Bence Jones proteinuria—a distinct entity? Am J Med 1973; 55:222–226.

144. Kyle RA, Greipp PR. "Idiopathic" Bence Jones proteinuria: long-term follow-up in seven patients. N Engl J Med 1982; 306:564–567.

145. Murata T, Fujita H, Harano H, et al. Triclonal gammopathy (IgA kappa, IgG kappa, and IgM kappa) in a patient with plasmacytoid lymphoma derived from a monoclonal origin. Am J Hematol 1993; 42:212–216.

146. O'Connor ML, Rice DT, Buss DH, Muss HB. Immunoglobulin D benign monoclonal gammopathy: a case report. Cancer 1991; 68:611–616.

147. Bladé J, Kyle RA. IgD monoclonal gammopathy with long-term follow-up. Br J Haematol 1994; 88:395–396.

7

Tumor Burden
Staging and Prognostic Factors

Douglas E. Joshua, MBBS, DPhil

Contents

INTRODUCTION
GENETIC CHANGES
SERUM FACTORS
REFERENCES

1. INTRODUCTION

Tumor burden has long been considered a major prognostic indicator in hemato-oncological practice. However, assessment of tumor burden in myeloma differs from that in solid tumors such as lymphoma, where direct assessment of tumor mass is often possible. In myeloma, measures used to quantitate tumor burden are almost all indirect and response to therapy difficult to quantify. The percentage of plasma cells in the bone marrow could be considered a direct measure of tumor mass, but is prone to sampling errors. The paraprotein level in the serum cannot be taken as an absolute indication of tumor mass, because immunoglobulin production per tumor cell varies between patients, although in an individual patient tumor reduction can be equated to paraprotein levels. Traditionally, patients with myeloma have been "staged" by combining a number of prognostic factors. The Durie Salmon *(1)* stage uses indirect measures of tumor bulk and activity such as hemoglobin, calcium, serum and urine M-protein levels, number of bone lesions, and creatinine levels. Combining a series of inaccurate measures of tumor burden has proved to have limitations. In particular, quantification of bone lesions is unreliable, often not an adverse prognostic factor, and falsely classifies patients as having late-stage disease. Although the prognostic validity of this staging system has been confirmed by a number of studies, disease stage has not always been a good predictor of survival, and its predictive value is lost when other important prognostic parameters (e.g., β_2 microglobulin and labeling index) are considered. In a multivariate analysis performed by the Mayo Clinic, no

From: *Current Clinical Oncology: Biology and Management of Multiple Myeloma*
Edited by: J. R. Berenson © Humana Press Inc., Totowa, NJ

other parameters, including stage, added significant prognostic information over that provided by the β_2 microglobulin and labeling index *(2)*.

A number of other staging systems based on relatively simple clinical features and measurements have been proposed, including the Medical Research Council (UK) *(3)* system—which uses hemoglobin, urea, and performance status—and the Grupo Agentino de Tratamiento de la Leucemia Aguda *(4)* and Merlini *(5)* systems. A disadvantage of staging systems is that patients who have high tumor burdens and "indolent" diseases or who present during the plateau phase, and patients who have low tumor burdens with aggressive diseases are often not recognized. None of these systems is clearly superior to the Durie Salmon system, and most have not been widely accepted. The β_2 microglobulin level also represents tumor bulk and is probably secreted directly from the surface of tumor cells. As it is excreted by the kidney, β_2 microglobulin is a direct reflection of renal function, but appears to retain its prognostic significance, even when adjusted for renal failure *(6)*.

A number of newer indices of tumor burden also appear to be valuable. These include the number of circulating monoclonal plasma cells in the blood and their proliferative capacity *(7,8)*. Such cells can be detected by light-chain isotope restriction or by *in situ* hybridization studies *(9)*. A close relationship between the number of tumor cells circulating, the prognosis, and other measures of tumor burden has been reported, and in the majority of patients circulating tumor cells can be documented and both the number and labeling index of these cells are independently prognostically significant *(7,8)*. Additionally, nuclear factor κ B ligand (RANKL):osteoprotegerin (OPG) ratio also correlates with markers of bone resorption, disease activity, and prognosis *(10)*.

Recently, an International Prognostic Index (IPI) has been developed for myeloma based on the β_2 microglobulin and albumin levels alone. This index allows stratification into three groups of patients with differing progresses and has been evaluated internationally *(11)*.

In summary, although measures of tumor burden are useful in identifying low- and high-risk patients, the evaluation of tumor burden is indirect and arbitrary. This often results in the allocation of most patients into late-stage groupings (stage III Durie Salmon), with poor identification of the intermediate-risk group. Although all systems can clearly identify low tumor burden groups, stage 1 disease with a highly proliferative tumor and a poor prognosis cannot easily be identified and results in a variation in the survival of patients with stage 1 disease.

2. GENETIC CHANGES

Genetic alterations include changes in chromosomal structure, oncogene mutations, and abnormalities of oncoprotein expression. Chromosome abnormalities have been difficult to document in myeloma using traditional cytogenetic techniques, because the disease is largely nonproliferative. Overall, in classical banding studies, approx 40% of patients can have clonal chromosomal abnormalities documented *(12)*, but fluorescence *in situ* hybridization (FISH) studies can document abnormalities in almost all patients *(13,14)*. A recent study demonstrated that partial or complete deletions of chromosome 13 or abnormalities involving 11q are associated with poor prognosis. Patients with abnormalities in both 13 and 11 had a particularly poor prognosis, with a medium overall survival of only 1 yr. In this study, there was a significant association between an unfavorable karyotype and other unfavorable prognostic factors, including age and β_2 microglobulin levels. Other karyotypic abnormalities were not shown to be of prognostic significance *(15)*. Recent studies using FISH have confirmed that monosomy 13 is one of the most powerful adverse prognostic indicators *(16,17)*. However, the frequency and prognostic significance of monsomy detected by FISH may differ from that detected by conventional cytogenetics. In two separate studies by FISH, loss of 13q was only of borderline significance *(18,19)*, although such deletions found by conventional cytogenetics confer a significantly worse outcome.

Oncogene abnormalities in myeloma include *ras* and *p53* mutations and deletions *(20–22)* and *Rb* deletions *(23)*, and have been associated with poor prognosis disease. *Ras* mutations in particular appear to represent a late mutagenic event associated with advanced disease, although it is not clear whether they are independent prognostic factors. For example, *ras* mutations are absent in monoclonal gammopathies of undetermined significance (MGUS) and present in 9% of patients with myeloma and approx 30% of patients with plasma cell leukemia, and seem to reflect generally adverse prognostic features, especially heavy bone marrow infiltration and high labeling indices *(22)*. As such, these mutations reflect the genomic instability of the malignant clone and are late molecular lesions generic to the malignancy rather than having a role in tumor initiation. In contrast, abnormalities of the *c-myc* locus are only rarely reported in myeloma, despite the fact that *c-myc* RNA and c-myc oncoproteins are frequently overexpressed in myeloma. Mutations at the *MLV1-4* locus, which maps 20kb 3' of the *c-myc* coding region, are more common, however *(24,25)*.

Studies assessing oncoprotein overexpression show that a wide and disparate range of oncoproteins are overexpressed in multiple myeloma. C-myc is by far the most commonly over expressed oncoprotein, being elevated in approx 40% of cases *(26)*. There is no relationship, however, between the percentage of plasma cells with *c-myc* overexpression and prognosis. Similarly, wild-type *p53* overexpression is not of prognostic significance. The combination of an oncoprotein abnormality and overexpression of a tumor-suppressive gene product is related to progressive rather than stable or plateau-phase disease. These changes are presumably a reflection of progressive genomic instability of the malignant clone *(27)*.

Recent studies have demonstrated that T-cell clones occur in myeloma and their presence is associated with a better prognosis *(22)*. These clones have been detected by molecular techniques, as well as by flow cytometry using monoclonal antibodies to the T-cell receptor V_β regions *(29)*. The prognostic significance of these clones possibly infers an anti-tumor network, but the antigen to which they are directed remains unknown. The phenotype of these clones shows the cells to be mature cytotoxic T cells with little proliferative capacity and mature cytotoxic effector function *(30)*.

2.1. IgH Switch Translocations

During B-cell maturation, the immunoglobulin heavy-chain gene undergoes the process of variable region recombination, followed by isotype switching. Isotype switching is the process by which a given immunoglobulin variable region can be associated with different isotype class conferring different physiological functions. Apart from monsomy 13, switch translocations are the most common cytogenetic abnormality in myeloma. They were initially found by conventional cytogenetics at a frequency of approx 20 to 40%. Using the Southern blot technique to look for illegitimate switch recombinations (ISR) in human myeloma cell lines, it became evident that switch translocation was much more common that previously suspected *(31)*. Approximately 90% of myeloma cell lines have either immunoglobulin heavy-chain or light-chain translocations. Cloning of breakpoints and molecular cytogenetic studies has revealed a large number of chromosomal partners, the most common being chromosomes 11q, 4p, 16q, and 6p, with candidate oncogenes characterized on each partner. Chromosome 11q has been identified as a partner chromosome in 15 to 20% of myeloma with translocation located at 11q13. The finding of cyclin D1 upregulation in myeloma tumors and cell lines bearing (11:14) translocation support cyclin D1 as a candidate oncogene in myeloma. However, studies using interphase FISH have not confirmed a prognostic relationship between cyclin D1 upregulation and aggressive disease *(32)*. In contrast, this translocation is associated with a good prognosis *(32a,32b)*.

Chromosome 4p translocations may lead to an upregulation of the fibroblast growth factor receptor. This is a family of fibroblast growth factor receptor tyrosine kinases that can be dysregulated in myeloma and are overexpressed in several myeloma cell lines *(33)*.

Chromosome 16q is a translocation partner in approx 5 to 10% of myelomas. The candidate oncogene is *c-maf,* which is a basic zipper transcription factor involved in cellular differentiation, proliferation, and interleukin (IL)-6 response *(34)*.

Whether switch translocations represent an early oncogenic change, a late trigger of disease progression, or a nonpathogenic marker of genetic instability is an interesting question with an important implications for our understanding of myeloma pathogenesis. Studies in fresh tissue found that they are only present in approx 50% of primary myeloma samples, and the heterogeneity of chromosomal partners and partner oncogenes would imply that switch translocations cannot be the only oncogenic factor involved in myeloma; therefore, a number of other mechanisms must therefore be considered. Their presence in MGUS suggests that they represent an early factor in the generation of a B-cell clone without necessarily conferring a malignant phenotype *(35)*.

2.2. Other Chromosomal Abnormalities in Myeloma

Molecular cytogenetic studies show that there are a multiple structural abnormalities that do not affect the immunoglobulin locus in myeloma *(36)*. The nonrecurrent nature of such changes makes analysis of their role in the disease difficult, and it is possible they represent a nonspecific phenomenon of genetic instability.

2.2.1. NUMERICAL CHANGES

Numerical changes, such as monosomy and trisomy, are common in myeloma, and hyperdiploidy has been reported in 30 to 45% of abnormal cases *(37,38)*. Similarly, hypodiploidy is a common finding with the loss of chromosome 8, 13, and 14, which is commonly observed using conventional cytogenetics *(39)*. The majority of translocations affecting *c-myc* in myeloma have involved non-immunoglobulin loci, and estimates of the incidence *c-myc* dysregulation vary in primary myeloma tumors. With reported incidences of *c-myc* rearrangement varying from 15 to 50%, it has been considered a representation of late changes in disease progression. The incidence of *c-myc* rearrangements in MGUS and smoldering myeloma is much lower than in active myeloma *(40)*.

2.2.2. OTHER MOLECULAR ABERRATIONS NOT AFFECTING
THE IMMUNOGLOBULIN LOCUS

Other molecular aberrations that do affect the immunoglobulin locus include mutations of N-*ras* and K-*ras* and alterations of *p53*. Mutations of the *ras* oncogene have been reported in approx 40% of patients, but occur rarely in MGUS and are associated with disease progression and resistance to therapy and *ras* mutations are likely to represent late secondary changes in myeloma pathogenesis *(20)*. Aberrations of *p53*—the tumor suppressor gene on chromosome 17p13—have also been postulated to play a role in myeloma progression, with *p53* deletions found to predict poor survival *(41)*.

2.3. Gene Expression Analysis by High-Density
Oligonucleotide Microarray Studies

High-density oligonucleotide microarray technology allows the expression of thousands of genes to be simultaneously screened *(42)*. This technique has been applied to myeloma and the examination of various expression patterns between normal and malignant plasma cells and between myeloma subsets investigated.

Significant differences have been demonstrated between normal and malignant cells in genes covering many important biological functions such as cell cycle control, apoptosis, cellular adhesion and signaling, as well as transcription factors *(43)*.

On the basis of expression patterns derived from microarrays, several subgroups of myeloma could be identified, ranging from those most similar to MGUS to those with expression profiles resembling myeloma cell lines. This categorization was also found to correlate with the clinical indicators, with the cell line-like subgroup more likely to have abnormal karyotypes, higher β_2 microglobulin levels, and deletion of chromosome 13 *(43)*.

Thus, the range of molecular aberrations of myeloma illustrates the extremely complex heterogeneity of this malignancy. Multiple developments in cytogenetics have enabled some elucidation of this spectrum and will have important implications in the investigation of the management and treatment of myeloma in the future. Microarray expression profiles may provide a more accurate and comprehensive assessment of molecular changes in myeloma and thus will become significant tools in prediction of disease behavior and prognosis.

3. SERUM FACTORS

A number of serum markers have been found to be of prognostic value in myeloma. The most important of these is the β_2 microglobulin. The correlation between the serum β_2 microglobulin and survival has been repeatedly documented *(44–46)*. Serum β_2 microglobulin levels can be corrected for renal impairment, although uncorrected values still act as important guides to prognosis because they include important information about renal function.

The prognostic significance of the β_2 microglobulin serum measured at entry and after initial hydration is retained for approx 2 yr *(46)*. A similar 2-yr validity can be found for subsequent determinations. In approx 10% of patients who are considered nonproducers, the β_2 microglobulin does not rise with relapse and thus will not have any prognostic significance *(47)*.

β_2 microglobulin remains a valid prognostic tool, irrespective of chemotherapy protocols, and retains predictive value in patients who are treated with high-dose therapy and autologous transplantation as well as allogeneic transplantation *(48,49)*. It retains its significance in patients who are young (<40 yr) *(50)* and can be used in combination with indices of intrinsic malignancy, e.g., the labeling index, or with bone marrow histology to provide improved prognostic strategies *(51–53)*.

A large number of other serum factors have also been evaluated as prognostic factors in myeloma. These include the serum lactic dehydrogenase (LDH) *(54)* and thymidine kinase (STK) *(55)*. High levels of LDH are associated with plasma cell leukemia, poor responses to chemotherapy, and a reduced median survival. The STK is of prognostic significance, but in multivariant analysis provides no additional prognostic information above the β_2 microglobulin and labeling index *(56)*. In the large Medical Research Council V study, the STK value was only prognostically significant in patients treated with melphalan and not in patients treated with multiagent chemotherapy (ABCM) *(57)*.

An important complex of prognostically significant serum factors are those associated with IL-6, including the soluble IL-6 receptor (IL-6R), IL-6 levels, and C-reactive protein (CRP) levels *(58,59)*. IL-6 is a central growth factor for myeloma cells, and increased levels are seen in advanced disease. CRP production by human hepatocytes in primary culture is directly controlled by IL-6 and appear to be a direct reflection of in vivo IL-6 production. High CRP levels are found in approximately one-third of patients at diagnosis and in almost all patients with terminal progressive disease. The serum soluble IL-6R level acts as an IL-6 agonist and is a powerful prognostic factor *(60,61)*. Serum levels of all these features can be used in combination with β_2 microglobulin to provide a useful staging system. In one study, for example, survival in patients with a high β_2 microglobulin and a high CRP was only 6 mo compared with 54 mo for those patients with a low β_2 microglobulin and a low CRP *(58)* High levels of serum neopterine are associated with disease severity and poor survival. It is not, however, an independent prognostic factor because it is correlated with the level of β_2 microglobulin *(62)*. It has been reported that high levels of serum IL-2 are a favorable prognostic feature, perhaps reflecting T-cell activation and autologous anti-tumor responses *(63)*. Recently, the role of the RANKL:OPG ratio as a marker of prognosis as well as the extent of bone lesions has been confirmed *(10)*.

The determination of a range of prognostic factors allows accurate prognostic information to be developed for individual patients, is useful for assessing treatment strategies and provides us with some insight into the complex therapeutic and immunological interactions responsible for disease progression and survival.

REFERENCES

1. Durie BG, Salmon SE. A clinical staging system for multiple myeloma: correlation of measured myeloma cell mass with presenting clinical features. Cancer 1975; 36:842.
2. Greipp PR Lust JA, O'Fallon WM, Katzmann JA, Witzig TGE, Kyle RA. Plasma cell labelling index and (2-microglobulin predict survival independent of thymidine kinase and C-reactive protein in multiple myeloma. Blood 1993; 81:3382–3387.
3. Medical Research Council's Working Party on Leukaemia in Adults. Prognostic features in the third MRC myelomatosis trial. Br J Cancer 1980; 42:831–840.
4. Corrado C, Santarelli MT, Pavlovsky S, Pizzolato M. Prognostic factors in multiple myeloma: definition of risk groups in 410 previously untreated patients: a Grupo Argentino de Tratamiento de la Leucemia Aguda Study. J Clin Oncol 1989; 7:1839–1844.
5. Merlini GP, Waldenstrom JG, Jayakar SD. A new improved clinical staging system for multiple myeloma based on analysis of 123 treated patients. Blood 1980; 55:1011–1019.
6. Cassuto JP, Krebs BJ, Viot G, Dujardin P, Massejeff R. (2-microglobulin: a tumor marker of lymphoproliferative disorders. Lancet 1978; 11:108–109.

7. Witzig TE, Gertz MA, Lust JA, Kyle RA, O'Fallon WM, Greipp PR. Peripheral blood monoclonal plasma cells as a predictor of survival in patients with multiple myeloma. Blood 1996; 88:1780–1787.

8. Billadeau, D, Ban Ness B, Kimlinger T, et al. Clonal circulating cells are common plasma cell proliferative disorders: a comparison of monoclonal gammopathy of undetermined significance, smoldering multiple myeloma, and active myeloma. Blood 1996; 88:289–296.

9. Brown R, Luo-XF, Gibson J, et al. Idiotypic oligonucleotide probes to detect myeloma cells by mRNA in situ hybridization. Br J Haematol 1995; 90:113–118.

10. Terpos E, Szydlo R, Apperley JF, et al. A soluable receptor activator of nuclear factor Kappa B ligand-osteoprotegrin survival in multiple myeloma: proposal for a novel prognostic index. Blood 2003; 102:1064–1069.

11. Greipp P. The International prognostic index in multiple myeloma IX International Workshop in Myeloma Salamenca 2003. Hematol J 2003;4:S42–S44.

12. Dewald GW, Kyle RA, Hicks GA, Greipp PR. The clinical significance of cytogenetic studies in 100 patients with multiple myeloma, plasma cell leukemia, or amyloidosis. Blood 1985; 66:380–390.

13. Flactif M, Zandecki M, Lai JL, et al. Interphase fluorescence in situ hybridization (FISH) as a powerful tool for the detection of aneuploidy in multiple myeloma. Leukaemia 1995; 9: 2109–2114.

14. Drach J, Schuster J, Nowotny H, et al. Multiple myeloma: high incidence of chromosomal aneuploidy as detected by interphase fluorescence in situ hybridization. Cancer Res 1995; 5517:3854–3859.

15. Tricot G, Barlogie B, Jagannath S, et al. Poor prognosis in multiple myeloma is associated only with partial or complete deletions of chromosome 13 or abnormalities involving 11q and not with other karyotype abnormalities. Blood 1995; 86:4250–4256.

16. Facon T, Avet-Loiseau H, Guillerm G, et al. Chromosome 13 abnormalities identified by FISH analysis and serum (2-microglobulin produce a powerful myeloma staging system for patients receiving high-dose therapy. Blood 2001; 97:1566–1571.

17. Konigsberg R, Zojer N, Ackerman J, et al. Predictive role of interphase cytogenetics for survival of patients with multiple myeloma. J Clin Oncol 2000; 18:804–812.

18. Fonseca R, Harrington D, Blood E, et al. A molecular classification of multiple myeloma based on cytogenic abnormalities detected by interphase FISH is powerful in identifying discrete groups of patients with dissimilar prognosis (Abstract). Blood 2001; 98:734a.

19. Shaughnessy J, Barlogie B, McCoy J, et al. Early relapse after total therapy II for multiple myeloma is significantly associated with cytogenic abnormalities of chromosome 13 but not with interphase FISH-del 13 of plasma cell labeling (Abstract) Blood 2001; 98:734a.

20. Neri A, Murphy JP, Cro L, et al. Ras oncogene mutation in multiple myeloma. J Exp Med 1989; 170:1715–1725.

21. Portier M, Moles JP, Mazars GR, et al. p53 and ras gene mutations in multiple myeloma. Oncogene 1992; 7:2539–2549.

22. Corradini P, Ladetto M, Voena C, et al. Mutational activation of N- and K-ras oncogenes in plasma cell dyscrasias. Blood 1993; 81:2708–2713.

23. Corradini P, Inghirami G, Astolfi M, et al. Inactivation of tumor suppressor genes, p53 and Rb1, in plasma cell dyscrasias. Leukaemia 1994; 8:758–767.

24. Selvanayagam P, Blick M, Narni F, et al. Alteration and abnormal expression of the c-myc oncogene in human multiple myeloma. Blood 1988; 71:30–35.

25. Palumbo AP, Boccadoro M, Battaglio S, et al. Human homologous of Moloney leukaemia virus integration-4 locus (MLVI-4) located 20 kilobases 3' of the c-myc gene is rearranged in multiple myeloma. Cancer Res 1990; 50:6478–6482.

26. Brown RD, Pope B, Luo X-F, Gibson J, Joshua DE. The oncoprotein phenotype of plasma cells from patients with multiple myeloma. Leuk Lymph 1994; 16:147–156.

27. Pope B, Brown R, Luo X-F, Gibson J, Joshua D. Disease progression in patients with multiple myeloma is associated with a concurrent alteration in the expression of both oncogenes and tumor suppressor genes and can be monitored by the oncoprotein phenotype. Leuk Lymph 1997; 25:545–554.

28. Brown R, Yuen Y, Nelson M, Gibson J, Joshua D. The prognostic significance of T cell receptor gene rearrangements and idiotype-reactive T cells in multiple myeloma. Leukemia 1997; 11:1312–1317.

29. Moss P, Gillespie G, Frodsheim P, Bell J, Reyburn H. Clonal populations of CD4+ and CD8+ T cells in patients with multiple myeloma and paraproteinemia. Blood 1996; 87:3297–3306.

30. Sze DM, Giesajtis G, Brown RD, et al. Clonal cytotoxic T cells are expanded in myeloma and reside in the CD8(+) CD57 (+)CD28 (–) compartment. Blood 2001; 98:2817–2827.

31. Bergsagel PL, Chesi M, Nardin E, et al. Promiscuous translocations into immunoglobulin heavy chain switch regions in multiple myeloma. Proc Natl Acad Sci USA 1996; 93: 13931–13936.

32. Avet-Loiseau H, Li J, Facon T, et al. High incidence of translocations t (11;14) (q13;q32) and t(4:14) (p16;q32) in patients with plasma cell malignancies. Canc Res 1998; 58:5640–5645.

32a. Moreau P, Facon T, Leleu X, et al. Recurrent 14q32 translocations determine the prognosis of multiple myeloma, especially in patients receiving intensive chemotherapy. Blood 2002; 100:1579–1583.

32b. Soverini S, Cavo M, Cellini C, et al. Cyclin D1 overexpression is a favorable prognostic variable for newly diagnosed multiple myeloma patients treated with high-dose chemotherapy and single or double autologous transplantation. Blood 2003; 102:1588–1593.

33. Chesi M, Brents LA, Ely SA, et al. Activated fibroblast growth factor receptor 3 is an oncogene that contributes to tumor progression in multiple myeloma. Blood 2001; 97:729–736.

34. Kataoka K, Nishizawa M, Kawai S. Structure–function analysis of the maf oncogene product, a member of the b-Zip protein family. J Virol 1993; 67:2133–2141.

35. Ho PJ. Brown Rd, Pelka G et al. Illegitimate switch recombinations are present in approx half of primary myeloma tumors, but do not relate to known prognostic indicators or survival. Blood 2001; 97:490–495.

36. Sawyer JR, Lukacs JL, Munshi N, et al. Identification of new nonrandom translocation in multiple myeloma with multicolor spectral karyotyping. Blood 1998; 92:5269–5278.

37. Calasanz MJ, Cigudosa JC, Odero MD, et al. Cytogenetic analysis of 280 patients with multiple myeloma and related disorders: primary breakpoints and clinical correlations. Genes Chrom Cancer 1997; 18:84–93.

38. Sawyer JR, Waldron JA, Jagannath S, et al. Cytogenetic findings in 200 patients with multiple myeloma. Canc Genet Cytogene 1995; 82:41–49.

39. Smadja NV, Bastard C, Brigaudeau C, et al. Hypodiploidy is a major prognostic factor in multiple myeloma. Blood 2001; 98:2229–2238.

40. Avet-Loiseau H, Gerson F, Magrangeas F, et al. Rearrangements of the c-myc oncogene are present in 15% of primary human multiple myeloma tumors. Blood 2001; 98:3082–3086.

41. Drach J, Ackermann J, Fritz E, et al. Presence of a p53 gene deletion in patient with multiple myeloma predicts for short survival after conventional-dose chemotherapy. Blood 1998; 92:802–809.

42. Lipshutz RJ, Fodor SP, Gingeras TR, et al. High density synthetic oligonucleotide arrays. Nature Genet 1999; 21:20–24.

43. Zhan F, Hardin J, Kordsmeier B, et al. Global gene expression profiling of multiple myeloma, monoclonal gammopathy of undetermined significance, and normal bone marrow plasma cells. Blood 2003; 99:1745–1757.

44. Child JA, Crawford SM, Norfolk DR, O'Quinley JH, Struthers LPL. Evaluation of serum (2-microglobulin as a prognostic indicator in myelomatosis. Br J Cancer 1993; 178:1091–1096.

45. Durie BGM, Stock-Novack D, Salmon SE, et al. Prognostic value of pretreatment serum (2-microglobulin in myeloma: a Southwest Oncology Group Study. Blood 1990; 75:823–830.

46. Cuzick J, De Stavola BL, Cooper EH, Chapman C, MacLennan, ICM. Long-term prognostic value of serum (2-microglobulin in myelomatosis. Br J Haematol, 1990; 75:506–510.

47. Bataille R, Granier J, Sany J. Unexpected normal serum (-microglobulin levels in multiple myeloma. Anticancer Res 1987; 7:513–515.

48. Bjorkstrand B, Ljungman P, Bird JM, et al. Autologous stem cell transplantation in multiple myeloma: results of the European Group for Bone Marrow Transplantation. Stem-Cells-Dayt 1995; 13:140–146.

49. Gahrton G, Tura S, Ljungman P, et al. An update of prognostic factors for allogeneic bone marrow transplantation in multiple myeloma using matched sibling donors. European Group for Blood and Marrow Transplantation. Stem-Cells-Dayt 1995; 13:122–125.

50. Blade J, Kyle RA, Greipp PR. Presenting features and prognosis in 72 patients with multiple myeloma who were younger than 40 years. Br J Haematol 1996; 93:345–351.

51. Greipp PR, Katzmann JA, O'Fallon WM, Kyle RA. Value of beta 2-microglobulin level and plasma cell labelling indices as prognostic factors in patients with newly diagnosed myeloma. Blood 1988; 72:219–223.

52. Pasqualetti P, Casale R, Collacciani A, Colantonio D. Prognostic factors in multiple myeloma: a new staging system based on clinical and morphological features. Eur J Cancer 1991; 27: 1123–1126.

53. Schambeck CM, Bartl R, Hochtlen-Vollmar W, Wick M, Lamerz R, Fateh-Moghadam A. Characterization of myeloma cells by means of labelling index, bone marrow histology, and serum beta 2-microglobulin. Am J Clin Pathol 1996; 106:64–68.

54. Barlogie B, Smallwood L, Smith T, Alexanian R. High serum levels of lactic dehydrogenase identify a high-grade lymphoma-like myeloma. Ann Int Med, 1989; 110:521–525.

55. Simonsson B, Kallander CFR, Brenning G, Killander A, Ahre A, Gronowitz JS. Evaluation of serum deoxythymidine kinase as a marker in multiple myeloma. Br J Haematol 1985;61:215–224.

56. Greipp PR, Lust JA, O'Fallon WM, et al. Plasma cell labelling index and (2- microglobulin predict survival independent of thymidine kinase and C-reactive protein in multiple myeloma. Blood 1993; 81:3382–2287.

57. Brown RD, Joshua DE, Nelson M, Gibson J, Dunn J, MacLennan ICM. Serum thymidine kinase as a prognostic indicator for patients with multiple myeloma; results from the MRC (UK) V Trial. Br J Haematol 1993; 84:238–241.

58. Bataille R, Boccadoro M, Klein B, Durie BGM, Pileri A. C-reactive protein and serum (2-microglobulin produce a simple and powerful myeloma staging system. Blood 1992; 80:733–737.

59. Pelliniemi TT, Irjala K, Mattila K, et al. Immunoreactive interleukin-6 and acute phase proteins as prognostic factors in multiple myeloma. Finnish Leukemia Group. Blood 1995; 85:765–771.

60. Pulkki K, Pelliniemi TT, Rajamaki A, Tienhaara A, Laakso M, Lahtinen R. Soluble interleukin-6 receptor as a prognostic factor in multiple myeloma. Finnish Leukemia Group. Br J Hematol 1996; 92:370–374.

61. Ohtani K, Ninomiya H, Hasegawa Y, et al. Clinical significance of elevated soluble interleukin-6 receptor levels in the sera of patients with plasma cell dyscrasias. Br J Haematol 1995; 91:116–120.

62. Boccadoro M, Battaglio S, Omede P, et al. Increased serum neopterin concentration as indicator of disease severity and poor survival in multiple myeloma. Eur J Hematol, 1991; 47:305–309.

63. Nucci GD, Magliocca V, Petrucci MT, Poyi G, Sgadari C. High serum IL-2 levels are predictive of prolonged survival in multiple myeloma. Br J Haematol 1990; 75:373–377.

8 Treatment of Multiple Myeloma

Meletios A. Dimopoulos, MD, and Robert A. Kyle, MD

1. INTRODUCTION

Multiple myeloma (MM) is a relatively common hematologic neoplasia with an annual incidence in the United States of approx 13,000 newly diagnosed patients and responsible for 1% of all cancer deaths. Some patients are diagnosed by chance and should not be treated unless there is evidence of an imminent complication or demonstration of progressive disease. However, most patients present with a variety of symptoms and signs that require immediate treatment. At present, the disease is considered incurable with conventional treatment and the realistic goals of treatment are relief of symptoms and prolongation of a good quality of life for as long as possible. The treatment of MM should focus on the management of the complications of the disease, along with attempts to reduce the growth of malignant plasma cells.

The role of high-dose therapy supported by stem cell transplantation (SCT) in the management of myeloma is being defined, and there is evidence that many patients benefit from this procedure. Each physician who treats patients with MM who are younger than 70 yr and do not have significant concomitant medical problems should discuss with the patient the possibility of autologous blood SCT. This procedure may not be applicable in older patients. We will thus discuss

From: *Current Clinical Oncology: Biology and Management of Multiple Myeloma*
Edited by: J. R. Berenson © Humana Press Inc., Totowa, NJ

the conventional treatment of myeloma in terms of whether the patient is a candidate for autologous SCT.

2. TREATMENT OF MYELOMA

2.1. Primary Therapy in Patients Without the Option of Stem Cell Transplantation

Most patients with MM present with painful bone lesions. Mild or moderate pain can usually be managed with analgesics, a corset with plastic stays, and a rolling walker, along with systemic anti-myeloma therapy. Physical activity must be encouraged. For severe pain resulting from a well-defined focal process that does not respond to chemotherapy, radiotherapy in a dose of 30 Gy administered over 10 d is very effective. Femoral or humeral fractures require prompt fixation with an intramedullary rod.

Chemotherapy and glucocorticoids is the preferred initial treatment for elderly patients with symptomatic MM, for patients who have significant medical problems that are unrelated to the underlying myeloma, or for those who decline or are ineligible for high-dose therapy. Intermittent courses of melphalan and prednisone have been the standard chemotherapy for patients with MM over the last 30 yr (1). Melphalan is usually administered at a dosage of 8 mg/m twice daily and prednisone at a dose of 60 mg/m twice daily by mouth for four consecutive days. Melphalan can also be administered orally at a dosage of 0.15 mg/kg/d for 7 d and prednisone at a dosage of 20 mg three times daily orally for the same 7 d. Melphalan should be given before breakfast because food reduces its absorption by approx 50% (2). If renal failure is present, the initial dose of oral melphalan should be reduced by 25% to avoid significant myelosuppression. Because gastrointestinal absorption of melphalan is unpredictable, mild cytopenia (neutrophils: 1.0–1.5 µL; or platelets: 100,000/µL) should be confirmed 3 wk after administration of the drug so that the subsequent dose of melphalan can be adjusted. Treatment should be repeated at intervals of 4 to 6 wk, and unless the disease progresses rapidly despite an adequate dose of melphalan, at least three courses of melphalan and prednisone should be given before resistance is confirmed. With this regimen, an objective response may not be obtained for 6 to 12 mo, even longer in some patients. Furthermore, a significant and early reduction in monoclonal protein levels after the first or second course may be a sign of a poor prognosis, because high chemosensitivity may reflect a high proliferative rate for myeloma cells, which can subsequently result in early relapse and reduced survival (3). The oral administration of melphalan and prednisone produces an objective response, defined by a 50% or more reduction in serum or urine myeloma protein levels and a reduction in bone marrow plasmatocytosis without evidence of new bone lesions in approx 50% of patients. A complete response—

which is indicated by the disappearance of serum and urine monoclonal protein with immunofixation and a normal bone marrow biopsy—occurs in fewer than 5% of patients treated with melphalan and prednisone. The median duration of response is approx 2 yr and the median survival of patients is approx 3 yr; 5% of patients are alive after 10 yr of treatment.

Because of the limitations of melphalan and prednisone therapy, several combinations of multiple alkylating agents—administered with or without the addition of a vinca alkaloid, an athracycline, or a nitrosourea—have been used. The combination of vincristine, bleomycin and carmustine (BCNU), melphalan, cyclophosphamide, and prednisone (collectively known as VBMCP) has induced objective responses in approx 70% of patients, but the median duration of survival is not significantly different from that obtained with melphalan and prednisone *(4)*. The VCMP–vincristine, carmustine, doxorubicin, and prednisone (VBAP) alternating chemotherapy has been prospectively compared with melphalan and prednisone. The Southwest Oncology Group reported a response and a survival advantage for the alternating combination *(5)*, but other randomized studies failed to confirm these data *(6,7)*. The Medical Research Council compared the combination of adriamycin, BCNU, cyclophosphamide, and melphalan (ABCM) with melphalan monotherapy and concluded that the combination was associated with a longer survival *(8)*. Most investigators, however, consider that melphalan alone was a suboptimal standard arm. A meta-analysis of 18 published trials involving almost 4000 patients randomized to melphalan–prednisone (MP) or various combinations of chemotherapy for primary treatment revealed that these treatments were equivalent in efficacy. The authors observed that the median survival varied widely in the MP control groups and they noted an improved outcome for combination chemotherapy in those studies characterized by a worse-than-expected survival in the MP arm *(9)*. Another overview by the Myeloma Trialist's Collaborative Group, which included data on 6623 patients enrolled in 27 trials worldwide, also showed that MP and combination therapy were comparable in effectiveness *(10)*. Furthermore, both publications failed to confirm the long-held impression that multiagent chemotherapy conferred a survival advantage in high-risk patients *(9,10)*. A recent randomized trial compared standard doses of VCMP/ VBAP with increased doses of cyclophosphamide and doxorubicin. With the increased dose intensity, a higher response rate was noted at the expense of an increased early death rate. No significant differences in response duration and survival were found *(11)*.

Chemotherapy should be continued until the patient achieves a plateau phase, which is defined by serum and urine monoclonal protein levels that remain stable for at least 4 to 6 mo and no evidence of disease progression or symptoms. Chemotherapy should be discontinued in such patients, because there is no evidence that maintenance chemotherapy prolongs patient survival *(12)*, although a recently randomized Southwest Oncology Group study shows oral prednisone alone (50 mg qod) is effective as maintenance therapy *(12a)*. In contrast, continued chemotherapy containing alkylating agents or nitrosoureas may be associated with a higher frequency of myelodysplastic syndrome or acute leukemia *(13,14)*. Likewise, the administration of systemic radiotherapy using double hemibody irradiation as a consolidation treatment does not prolong survival *(15)*.

The VAD regimen combines vincristine 0.4 mg/d and doxorubicin 9 mg/m twice a day administered by continuous infusion for 4 d with oral dexamethasone 20 mg/m twice daily for days 1 through 4, 9 through 12, and 17 through 20. This regimen, which is active in many patients with disease that is resistant to alkylating agents, has been administered in previously untreated patients. The response rate is approx 60%, and it offers no obvious survival benefits compared with standard alkylating agent-based therapies *(16–18)*. The time required to reduce the monoclonal protein level by half is less with VAD than with other regimens that do not include high-dose steroids. Therefore, the VAD regimen may be preferable for patients in whom a rapid onset of response is desirable, e.g., patients with hypercalcemia, renal failure, or widespread painful bone lesions. Furthermore, VAD appears to be indicated for patients with renal failure, because none of its components is excreted by the kidneys and, thus, dose adjustments are not required. The occasional patient who presents with plasma cell leukemia should also be treated with VAD because standard alkylating agents are ineffective in these patients *(19)*. No more than three courses of VAD are usually needed to confirm a response or resistance to this regimen *(17)*. To avoid the inconvenience of the continuous 4-d intravenous infusion, VAD has been also administered on an outpatient basis using a 4-d schedule of intravenous bolus injections. Responses have been observed in 67% of patients *(20)*. Doxorubicin has recently been encapsulated in "stealth" liposomes. Liposomal doxorubicin, because of its longer half-life, can be administered once in each treatment cycle and is considered less toxic than doxorubicin, especially as far as cardiotoxicity is concerned. A phase II study of VAD using liposomal doxorubicin as the primary outpatient treatment in patients with MM resulted in objective responses in 88% of patients, including a complete response in 12% *(21)*. The previously mentioned "VAD-like" regimens were prospectively compared as primary treatment for patients with myeloma. With either bolus VAD or VAD with liposomal doxorubicin, an objective response was noted in 61% of patients, including a complete response in 12% *(22)*. In a recent study comparing MP alone or alternating VAD/MP or alternating vincristine, mitoxantrone, dexamethasone (VND)/MP therapy, the alternating regimens were associated with more severe granulocytopenia and infections, but did not increase the objective response rate and survival over those observed with MP alone *(23)*.

High-dose intermittent oral dexamethasone is also an active primary therapy in patients with myeloma, with response and survival rates similar to those achieved with other standard regimens *(24)*. Because dexamethasone is not associated with myelosuppression, it is indicated for patients who require radiotherapy for the treatment of painful bone lesions. Dexamethasone may be the primary treatment of choice in the occasional patient who presents with pancytopenia if the pancytopenia is thought to be secondary to causes other than florid myeloma.

The addition of interferon (IFN)-α to standard chemotherapy has been considered because this agent has some activity (15%) in previously untreated patients and because INF may have a different mechanism of action than that of classical chemotherapeutic agents *(25)*. The combination of VBMCP and INF-α was associated with a modest increase in the complete response rate *(26)*. However, in three large prospective studies, the addition of INF-α to MP *(27,28)* or to VBMCP *(29)* did not result in any survival advantage when compared with MP or VBMCP alone. The comparison of an INF–dexamethasone combination with dexamethasone alone in previously untreated patients indicated similar response and survival rates *(30)*. Furthermore, the addition of interferon to VAD did not improve the response and survival rates *(31)*. Within the context of a prospective randomized study, INF-α was added to both MP and to VBMPC induction treatment in patients with MM and a good prognosis. Response rate, duration of response, and survival were similar *(32)*.

The introduction of oral idarubicin provided the opportunity to combine this anthracyline with high-dose dexamethasone. This oral combination induced objective responses in 80% of previously untreated patients, including a complete response in 7%. Responses appeared as rapidly as those observed with VAD. However, no data are available indicating the long-term outcome with this regimen and caution is required in patients with renal impairment *(33)*.

While patients are on initial treatment, they should be seen every 1–2 mo for evaluation, including M-protein measurements, chemistries, blood counts, and physical examination. During the plateau phase, the patient should be followed every 3 or 4 mo with a physical examination, blood counts, renal function tests, and calcium levels, along with serum and urine electrophoretic studies. Evaluation of bone marrow and bones should also be carried out, as indicated. It should be remembered that a relapse can occur, characterized by am increase in size and/or number of bone lesions without a corresponding increase of monoclonal protein levels.

2.2. Primary Therapy in Candidates for Stem Cell Transplantation

There is cumulative evidence (described in detail in other chapters of this book) that high-dose therapy supported by autologous blood SCT is beneficial for many patients with MM *(34,35)*. This procedure is usually applied in patients younger than 70 yr who lack significant comorbid conditions. Patients who are potential candidates for high-dose therapy during some phase of their disease should not be exposed to standard melphalan- or other alkylating agent-containing combinations in order to avoid damaging hematopoietic stem cells *(36,37)*.

Radiotherapy also reduces the yield in blood stem cell collection and should be restricted to patients with an absolute indication, e.g., spinal cord compression. A rapid response is desirable; for this reason, primary therapy with the VAD regimen is recommended because it causes less damage to bone marrow progenitor cells. Nonrandomized studies have indicated that the addition of weekly cyclophosphamide to the VAMP (vincristine, doxorubicin, methylprednisolone) regimen enhances responses in previously untreated patients without compromising subsequent stem cell collection (38). Collection and cryopreservation of blood stem cells should be carried out as soon as the best response is observed. One may proceed with a SCT even if the patient does not respond to VAD. In some studies, the sequential administration of VAD followed by high-dose cyclophosphamide followed by the combination of etoposide, dexamethasone, cytarabine and cisplatin increased the complete response rate and allowed the collection of enough blood stem cells to support two autologous transplants (39).

Recent data indicate that age exceeding 65 yr and renal impairment are not significant adverse factors for high-dose therapy with SCT (40,41). Thus, the number of patients for whom primary therapy will have to be selected carefully because of the possible need for high-dose therapy in the future is increasing.

3. TREATMENT OF REFRACTORY MULTIPLE MYELOMA

Before a second-line treatment can be selected for a patient with MM, the disease phase should be clearly defined. Primary refractory disease is defined by the absence of response to primary treatment. Some patients with primary refractory disease have nonprogressive disease without significant symptoms, whereas other patients have rapidly evolving myeloma. Refractory relapse is characterized by a response to primary therapy as well as disease progression despite the continuation of previously effective treatment. Finally, some patients undergo a relapse associated with an unmaintained response or INF maintenance.

A patient who experiences a relapse when no treatment is taken has a 50% chance of responding again to the original treatment. MP therapy is effective in approx 30% of patients who experience a relapse while maintained on INF (30). High-dose oral dexamethasone or high-dose IV methylprednisolone has induced responses in approximately one-third of patients with primary disease that is refractory to standard alkylating agents, the VAD regimen, or high-dose steroids (42–44). Patients experiencing a relapse to refractory disease are more likely to benefit from the VAD regimen, which induces a response in 40 to 50% of such patients, which is sustained for a median duration of approx 1 yr (42,45). The addition of INF-α to VAD was not associated with an improved outcome (46). The greater efficacy associated with VAD compared with dexamethasone in relapsing patients has been attributed to the greater sensitivity of proliferating tumor cells to the cycle-active drugs vincristine and doxorubicin. The combina-

tion of bolus intravenous vincristine, BCNU, and doxorubicin with oral prednisone (VBAP) has been effective in 30% of patients *(47)*.

For patients who fail to respond to or relapse after exposure to VAD or to a
high-dose corticosteroid regimen, alternative nonmyeloablative options are limited. Attempts to reverse the expression of the multidrug resistance gene *(MDR)*
initially focused on the addition of high-dose verapamil to VAD. This imprac-
tical regimen, which necessitates close cardiac monitoring, appeared to be effective for a short period in approx 20% of patients with VAD-resistant myeloma
(48). A randomized trial of VAD vs VAD plus oral verapamil in alkylating agent-
resistant MM revealed similar response and survival rates *(49)*. Quinine has also
been shown to inhibit expression of *MDR*, but showed no efficacy when added
to a VAD-like regimen in a large, randomized clinical trial conducted by the
Southwest Oncology Group *(12a)*. Initial reports of the role of cyclosporine as
an agent with clinically evident inhibition of *MDR* indicated that the VAD–
cyclosporine combination induced responses in 40% of VAD-resistant patients
(50). A lower response rate and higher toxicity grades were subsequently reported
(51). Cyclosporine-*A* combined with VAD was prospectively compared with
VAD in patients who were refractory to or relapsing after treatment with alkylating agents. The objective response rate, median time to progression, and
median survival were similar in both arms *(52)*.

High-dose alkylating agents without stem cell support have also been
administered in patients with VAD-refractory myeloma. High-dose melphalan at doses up to 100 mg/m twice daily appeared to be active in approximately one-third of patients, but with a significant treatment-related
mortality of 15% *(53)*. The addition of growth factor support reduced the
toxic death rate *(54)*. Other combinations—e.g., etoposide, dexamethasone, cytarabine and cisplatin *(55)*, high-dose cyclophosphamide alone *(56)*
or with the addition of etoposide *(57)*, and hyperfractionated cyclophosphamide added to VAD *(58)*—have been administered within the context
of phase II studies. No more than one-third of patients seem to benefit for
periods of approx 6 mo. Patients with relapsing myeloma or those with
elevated levels of lactate dehydrogenase and β_2 microglobulin are less likely
to benefit from these salvage treatments. The combination of dexamethasone, cyclophosphamide, etoposide, and cisplatin (DCEP) resulted in a
complete response rate of 10% and partial response rate of 41% in patients
who relapsed after autologous SCT *(59)*. It is unlikely that most of these
phase II studies can be easily reproduced because of differences in methods
of assessing resistance to previous treatments used among these studies and
because of patient selection bias.

Over the last 10 yr, several new agents have been administered to patients
with MM. Most of these were inactive and a few have shown limited activity.
All-*trans* retinoic acid inhibits the growth of some human myeloma cell lines,

presumably through the down-regulation of interleukin (IL)-6 receptor. However, phase II trials of this agent did not demonstrate activity in either refractory or previously untreated patients *(60,61)*. Three purine analogues—fludarabine, pentostatin, and cladribine—have been administered to patients with previously treated myeloma. Despite the significant activity of these agents against other chronic lymphoproliferative disorders, their effect against myeloma was disappointing *(62–64)*. Paclitaxel has been evaluated both in previously treated and in newly diagnosed patients with MM. Despite significant hematologic toxicity, the activity of this agent in MM was limited *(65)*. Docetaxel was inactive in patients with refractory or relapsing myeloma *(66)*. Gemcitabine, a cytosine arabinoside analog, did not induce objective responses *(67)*. Of 17 patients with refractory myeloma, 2 had an objective reduction in tumor mass after treatment with IL-2 *(68)*. Vinorelbine, a new vinca alkaloid, has been administered to pretreated patients with myeloma and 15% of patients responded *(69)*. Topotecan, a topoisomerase I inhibitor, was administered at a twice daily dose of 1.25 mg/m for five consecutive days, with growth factor support, to patients with relapsing or refractory MM. The major toxicity was myelosuppression and the response rate was 16% *(70)*. Idarubicin is an anthracycline, which can be administered orally. Its administration was associated with activity in approx 20% of patients with advanced myeloma and in 2 of 14 patients with prior exposure to doxorubicin *(71)*.

3.1. Thalidomide and Its Derivatives

Thalidomide is an oral drug with anti-angiogenic and immunomodulatory properties that has been recently shown to possess significant activity in MM. Singhal and colleagues first reported that thalidomide induced partial or complete responses in approx 30% of patients with refractory myeloma, most of whom had failed high-dose therapy *(72)*. Several other studies have confirmed these results *(73)*. This agent was originally administered daily at bedtime with a starting dose of 200 mg and an increase of dose in 200-mg increments every 2 wk to a maximum dose of 800 mg. The administration of thalidomide is associated with a variety of side effects such as constipation, weakness, somnolence, mood changes, skin rash, tremor, edema, deep vein thrombosis, and peripheral neuropathy. Some of these side effects are age- and dose-related. Nearly half of the patients who take it are unable to take the maximum 800-mg dose *(72)*. Nevertheless, some studies have indicated that there is a dose–response effect *(74,75)*. Other studies reported similar activity with lower doses *(76)*; thus, the optimal dose of thalidomide has not been established. Outside the context of a clinical study, thalidomide therapy should be individualized to a dose that achieves a response and is well tolerated. The median survival of thalidomide-treated patients exceeds 1 yr. Prognostic factors associated with a longer survival include low serum β_2 microglobulin, absence of abnormal chromosome 13, younger age, and low plasma cell-labeling index *(74)*.

The activity of thalidomide as a single agent in advanced myeloma, along with in vitro evidence of synergism with dexamethasone, provided the rationale for investigating the combination of thalidomide and dexamethasone. Several reports have indicated that this combination was active in approx 50% of patients with refractory or relapsing myeloma. Moreover, the addition of dexamethasone to thalidomide reduced the median time to response to 1 mo or even less *(77,78)*. Nevertheless, it is not clear that the combination of thalidomide and dexamethasone improves event-free or overall survival compared with thalidomide monotherapy. From a practical point of view, the thalidomide–dexamethasone regimen could be administered to patients with myeloma resistant to chemotherapy, especially when rapid disease control is required. For patients who have a relatively asymptomatic relapse, thalidomide monotherapy may be appropriate; dexamethasone can be added if there is no evidence of response to thalidomide monotherapy. It is important to recognize that the optimal dose of steroids in this combination is unknown. Certainly, efficacy of this combination has been observed with lower doses of dexamethasone and other weaker steroids in anecdotal reports.

Thalidomide and dexamethasone have also been combined with chemotherapy for the treatment of patients with refractory myeloma. Several series have added cytotoxic drugs such as cyclophosphamide, etoposide, doxorubicin, and cisplatin. Objective responses have been documented in at least two-thirds of patients and the median duration of survival exceeds 18 mo *(79)*. However, it is not clear whether the addition of chemotherapy to thalidomide therapy actually improves patient survival. Furthermore, the side effects of these regimens include not only thalidomide-related complications but also myelosuppression and infections.

In view of the significant activity of thalidomide in refractory and relapsing myeloma, this agent—alone or in combination with other drugs—has been administered to previously untreated patients with multiple myeloma. Two phase II trials have administered single-agent thalidomide to patients with smoldering or asymptomatic myeloma and observed partial responses in one-third of them *(80,81)*. In the Mayo Clinic series, the 2-yr progression-free survival was 63 vs 47% for thalidomide-treated patients vs similar patients who were followed in previous years without any treatment *(80)*. Patients with smoldering or asymptomatic myeloma should not be treated with thalidomide outside the context of a clinical trial, however. Prospective randomized studies are needed to define the role of thalidomide in patients with early myeloma. The combination of thalidomide with dexamethasone has been administered to newly diagnosed patients with symptomatic myeloma. Sixty to 70% of patients have achieved objective responses, the median time to response was less than 1 mo, and an adequate number of blood stem cells was collected from patients eligible for subsequent high-dose therapy *(81,82)*. This oral and nonmyelosuppresive regimen may be used as primary treatment for MM when blood stem cell collection is planned if there is evidence of neutropenia or thrombocytopenia or when concomitant administration of radiotherapy is required. No more than 4 mo of treatment with high-dose dexamethasone and no more than 400 mg/d of thalidomide are recommended. There are preliminary reports on the addition of cytotoxic drugs to thalidomide–dexamethasone in previously untreated patients with MM. The largest randomized study is being conducted at the University of Arkansas as of this writing. Patients are treated with sequential chemotherapy and tandem autotransplants with or without thalidomide, which is being administered at a daily dose of 400 mg. Response and survival data are not yet available, but a high incidence of vein thrombosis has been reported among patients receiving thalidomide (28 vs 4%) *(83)*. The risk of thrombosis is increased by the addition of steroids or anthracyclines *(83a,83b)* to thalidomide.

Owing to encouraging activity of thalidomide in myeloma, new analogs of this drug are being developed. Among these, the immunomodulatory drug CC-5013 has been tested in phase II studies. Approximately one-third of patients with refractory myeloma responded to this agent, including patients who had previously failed thalidomide therapy. In contrast to thalidomide, no significant somnolence, constipation, or neuropathy was noted in either study *(84)*.

3.1.1. BORTEZOMIB

Recent data indicate that bortezomib, a selective proteasome inhibitor, has significant activity in patients with refractory MM. The proteasome is a multi-enzyme complex that causes proteolysis of the endogenous inhibitor of the nuclear factor-KB (NF-KB), IkB. Proteasomal degradation of IkB activates NF-KB, which induces the transcription of proteins that promote survival, stimulate growth, and reduce susceptibility to apoptosis in myeloma cells. NF-KB also modulates the secretion of IL-6 by bone marrow stomal cells *(85)*.

In a multicenter phase II trial, 202 patients with advanced myeloma refractory to the treatment they had received most recently were treated with IV bortezomib at a dose of 1.3 mg/m^2 twice weekly for 2 wk, followed by 1 wk without treatment. Up to eight cycles of bortezomib were administered; in patients with a suboptimal response, oral dexamethasone was added. Of these patients, 27% achieved at least a 50% reduction in monoclonal protein levels to bortezomid alone, including 4% of patients who were rated as complete responders using negative immunofixation. The median duration of the response was 12 mo. Response to this agent was not affected by the number or types of previous treatments received, including thalidomide *(86)*. Since NF-KB activity is associated with the development of chemotherapy resistance, bortezomib has been used and shown to overcome resistance to both melphalan and doxorabicin *(78a)*. Because of this, the drug has recently been combined with liposomal doxoubicin *(78b)* or oral melphalan *(78c)* in clinical studies with early encouraging results.

3.1.2. ARSENIC TRIOXIDE

Arsenic trioxide is a novel anti-cancer agent with established activity in acute promyelocytic leukemia. In vitro data have shown that human myeloma cell lines and freshly isolated myeloma cells are particularly sensitive to arsenic trioxide at clinically relevant concentrations. Recent data suggest that arsenic trioxide exerts its anti-myeloma effect by inducing apoptosis, integrin modulation, caspase activation, and overexpression of CD38 and its ligand on plasma cells and lymphokine-activated killer cells, respectively (87). In addition, the drug reduces NF-KB activity by inhibiting the degradation of the inhibitor complex IKB (87a). Preliminary clinical data show that arsenic trioxide administered daily has activity in approx 20% of patients with refractory MM (88). Another recently completed study using single-agent arsenic trioxide showed responses (M-protein reduction of 25%) in nearly half of heavily pretreated patients (88a). Because arsenic trioxide's ability to kill tumor cells is related to oxygen radical formation, intracellular molecules such as glutathione that reduce oxygen radical levels inhibit arsenic trioxide efficacy. Thus, the use of agents such as ascorbic acid that reduce glutathione levels enhance the anti-MM effects of arsenic trioxide (88b). Because in vitro studies had shown the ability of arsenic trioxide to overcome chemotherapy resistance (87a), a small pilot study was initiated combining arsenic trioxide with low doses of melphalan and ascorbic acid (88b). Responses were observed in these patients, including five patients with renal failure. Because of these promising early results, a large multicenter study is being conducted. Ongoing studies are evaluating the combination of arsenic trioxide with dexamethasone in resistant disease.

4. MANAGEMENT OF THE COMPLICATIONS

4.1. Hypercalcemia

Hypercalcemia is found in approx 25% of patients at diagnosis and is identified much more commonly during disease progression. The presence of hypercalcemia should be suspected in patients with myeloma who report nausea, fatigue, weight loss, confusion, polyuria, or constipation. The most effective treatment for hypercalcemia consists of high doses of a glucocorticoid and hydration with isotonic saline. Bisphosphonates are potent inhibitors of bone resorption and have been used successfully in the treatment of hypercalcemia. Zoledronic acid is a new, more potent bisphosphonate in vitro. It is administered intravenously at a dose of 4 mg and requires only a 15-min infusion. It has been shown to be more effective than pamidronate in the treatment of hypercalcemia (89). However, the widespread use of chronic bisphosphonates in patients with MM has reduced the risk of this complication.

4.2. Renal Failure

Approximately 20% of patients with myeloma present with renal insufficiency; this incidence rate increases during the course of the disease. Hypercalcemia, Bence-Jones proteinuria, or a combination of both conditions causes renal impairment in more than 95% of patients *(90)*. Other causes and contributing factors include hyperuricemia, amyloidosis, immunoglobulin deposition disease, pyelonephritis, nephrotoxic drugs, and unrelated medical disorders *(91)*. Maintenance of a high fluid intake to produce 3 L of urine daily is important to prevent renal failure in patients with Bence-Jones proteinuria.

In approx 50% of untreated patients, renal insufficiency can be reversed, especially when it is recognized and treated promptly. For most patients with mild and moderate renal failure, the combination of chemotherapy, hydration, and allopurinol (to treat hyperuricemia) is effective. Patients should receive intravenous fluid to achieve a urine flow exceeding 3 L daily; bicarbonate may be added to achieve a urine pH above 7.0. Infection should be treated promptly with intravenous antibiotics. The preferred chemotherapy consists of VAD, which does not require dosage adjustments for renal failure and provides the best chance for rapid disease control. Recent studies suggest that thalidomide, bortezomib, or arsenic trioxide may also be effective, particularly when chemotherapy is added. Dexamethasone monotherapy is also an option. Plasmapheresis has been proposed by some, but controlled studies have not shown that this approach yields any improvement in survival *(92)*. Other patients who present with severe renal failure may require temporary hemodialysis along with chemotherapy. Long-term hemodialysis or peritoneal dialysis is an option for some patients in whom myeloma has responded to chemotherapy.

4.3. Anemia

Anemia is present in 60% of patients with myeloma at the time of diagnosis, and almost every patient eventually becomes anemic. The anemia is primarily caused by decreased production of red blood cells (RBC) secondary to suppression of marrow erythroporesis by the presence of malignant plasma cells. Patients with renal failure also have decreased production of erythropoietin (EPO), which may worsen the degree of anemia. A mild shortening of red cell survival, as well as iron deficiency, may also contribute to the anemia. The plasma volume is often expanded in patients with high levels of immunoglobulin (Ig)A or IgG, so that the hematocrit level may be as much as 6% less than the value expected based on the measured RBC volume *(93)*. This factor must be considered before ordering red cell transfusions for anemic patients.

Moderate anemia is usually well tolerated, unless there is significant coronary artery disease or cerebrovascular insufficiency. Severe anemia is usually reversed with the control of myeloma by chemotherapy and with improvement in renal function. Administration of recombinant EPO can increase hemoglobin levels in patients with myeloma; this may be a useful therapeutic approach when a patient with anemia reaches a therapeutic plateau *(94,95)*. Prerequisites for benefit seem to be a serum EPO level that is inappropriately low for the hematocrit level and an adequate iron supply.

Several placebo-controlled trials of EPO in anemic patients with myeloma receiving chemotherapy have been reported. Osterborg and colleagues found an improvement in hemoglobin level and elimination of transfusion requirement in 60% of patients taking EPO compared with 24% of the control group *(96)*. Dammacco and colleagues also observed that hemoglobin levels increased by a mean of 1.8 g/dL in patients receiving EPO and 28% required transfusion during the first 3 mo of treatment compared with no rise in hemoglobin levels and a 47% incidence of transfusion requirement in patients receiving placebo *(97)*. With appropriate dosages of EPO, at least 80% of patients show a hemoglobin increment of more than 1 g/dL after 4 wk of treatment, and an improved quality of life is documented in responding patients *(98)*.

Darbepoietin-α is a novel erythropoiesis-stimulating protein with a prolonged half-life and the potential to be administered less frequently than EPO. Once-weekly administration of darbepoietin-α to anemic patients with either lymphoma or myeloma who are receiving chemotherapy was associated with a hemoglobin response in 50% of patients. As of this writing, ongoing trials are evaluating the efficacy of darbepoietin administered once every 2 or 3 wk *(99)*.

5. NEUROLOGICAL EFFECTS

It is unusual for the nervous system to be involved in patients with myeloma, other than through spinal cord or nerve compression by plasma cell tumors. Peripheral neuropathy can occur in occasional patients with myeloma, but is particularly common in amyloidosis or osteosclerotic myeloma. In many patients, there are associated endocrine abnormalities that can result in organomegaly, anasarca, hyperpigmentation, hypertichosis, gynecomastia, or hirsutism. The occurrence of polyneuropathy with organomegaly, endocrinopathy, myeloma and skin changes has been named the POEMS syndrome *(100)*.

When neuropathy is seen in myeloma, it is typically distal, symmetrical, and slowly progressive. Pathological studies show axonal degeneration and demyelination *(101)*. Treatment consisting of plasma exchange and chemotherapy may improve the neuropathy *(102)*.

5.1. Serum Immunoglobulin Effects

Features of hyperviscosity syndrome may occur when the IgG or IgA myeloma levels exceed 5 g/dL. A serum viscosity measurement at least four times that of normal is usually required to produce symptoms, which include fatigue, blurred vision, confusion, tinnitus, and an increased bleeding tendency. Myeloma proteins of IgA or IgG3 type are more likely to produce hyperviscosity because of their increased tendency to polymerize *(103)*. Prompt plasmapheresis using a continuous flow blood cell separator, combined with chemotherapy will rapidly reduce the monoclonal protein level *(104)*.

Bleeding diathesis is an unusual feature in myeloma. The coating of platelets by myeloma proteins may result in a prolonged bleeding time and abnormal platelet adhesiveness *(105)*. Inhibitors of coagulation factors, thrombocytopenia associated with marrow infiltration or chemotherapy, and the production of anticoagulants by neoplastic plasma cells may also cause bleeding *(106)*.

The monoclonal protein may have the properties of a cryoglobulin. Type I cryoglobulinemia is asymptomatic in most instances, whereas type II and occasionally type III cryoglobulinemia are associated with Raynaud's phenomenon, vascular purpura, and vasculitis *(107)*.

5.2. Infection

Frequent bacterial infections are a common cause of morbidity and result from both neutropenia, as well as from the marked reduction of normal immunoglobulin production and the inability to mount an adequate response to antigenic challenges. In mouse plasmacytomas, a protein produced by the tumor cells (PC factor) induces normal macrophages to secrete a second humoral substance—plasmacytoma-induced macrophage substance—which suppresses antibody production and B-cell proliferation *(108)*. In humans, the mechanism involved in immunosuppression is less clear, although a circulating phagocytic mononuclear cell from myeloma patients that suppresses the secretion of mitogen-stimulated normal human B cells in culture has been described *(109)*. Neutropenia may result most commonly from chemotherapy and less commonly from marrow infiltration with tumor cells. There is also evidence of impaired granulocyte and complement function *(110,111)*.

The incidence of bacterial infections in patients with myeloma is significantly higher than in healthy people. Pneumonia is the most common infection, followed by urinary tract infections. The pattern of infection is biphasic, with episodes caused by *Pneumococcus* and *Hemophilus* predominating early in the course of the disease, whereas Gram-negative bacilli and *Staphylococcus aureus* predominate later in the course of the illness *(112)*. Further risk of infection is imposed on myeloma patients by chemotherapy-induced neutropenia, as well as by anemia and uremia. The risk is greater during the first 2 mo after initiation of therapy and during relapse *(113)*. Prophylactic trimethoprim–sulfamethoxazole may be useful during the first 2 mo of therapy *(114)*. In addition, the risk of infection is particularly high during high-dose chemotherapy. Localized herpes zoster infections occur commonly in patients with MM and should be treated with immediate appropriate anti-viral therapy to avoid systemic infection and symptomatic post-herpetic neuralgia.

Febrile patients, especially those who are neutropenic, need immediate hospitalization and empirical therapy using broad-spectrum antibiotics after appropriate cultures have been made. Pneumococcal and influenza vaccines should be administered prophylactically, even though the antibody response is defective in most patients. Recent evidence suggests that intravenously administered immunoglobulin therapy may be helpful for patients with recurrent infections, especially when serum levels of uninvolved immunoglobulins are low *(115)*. This treatment is too expensive for long-term therapy, however.

ACKNOWLEDGMENTS

We wish to thank Konstantina Kakoyiannis and Asimina Petropoulou for their excellent secretarial assistance.

REFERENCES

1. Alexanian R, Haut A, Khan AU, et al. Treatment for multiple myeloma: combination chemotherapy with different melphalan dose regimens. JAMA 1969; 208:1680–1685.
2. Alberts DS, Chang SY, Chen HS, Evans TL, Moon TE. Oral melphalan kinetics. Clin Pharmacol Ther 1979; 26:737–745.
3. Boccadoro M, Marmont F, Tribalto M, et al. Early responder myeloma: kinetic studies identify a patient subgroup characterized by a very poor prognosis. J Clin Oncol 1989; 7:119–125.
4. Oken MM, Harrington DP, Abramson N, et al. Comparison of melphalan and prednisone with vincristine, carmustine, melphalan, cyclophosphamide, and prednisone in the treatment of multiple myeloma. Results of Eastern Cooperative Oncology Group study E2479. Cancer 1997; 79:1561–1567.
5. Salmon SE, Haut A, Bonnet JD, et al. Alternating combination chemotherapy and levamisole improves survival in multiple myeloma: a Southwest Oncology Group study. J Clin Oncol 1983; 1:453–461.
6. Cooper MR, McIntyre OR, Propert KJ, et al. Single, sequential, and multiple alkylating agent therapy for multiple myeloma: a CALGB study. J Clin Oncol 1986; 4:1331–1339.
7. Boccadoro M, Marmont F, Tribalto M, et al. Multiple myeloma: VMPC/VBAP alternating combination chemotherapy is not superior to melphalan and prednisone even in high-risk patients. J Clin Oncol 1991; 9:444–448.
8. MacLennan IC, Chapman C, Dunn J et al. Combined chemotherapy with ABCM versus melphalan for treatment of myelomatosis. Lancet 1992; 339:200–205.
9. Gregory WM, Richards MA, Malpas JS. Combination chemotherapy versus melphalan and prednisone in the treatment of multiple myeloma: an over-view of published trials. J Clin Oncol 1992; 10:334–342.
10. Myeloma Trialists' Collaborative Group. Combination chemotherapy versus melphalan plus prednisone as treatment for multiple myeloma: an overview of 6633 patients from 27 randomized trials. J Clin Oncol 1998; 16:3832–3842.
11. Blade J, San Miguel JF, Fontanillas M, et al. Increased conventional chemotherapy does not improve survival in multiple myeloma: long-term results of two PETHEMA trials including 914 patients. Hematol J 2001; 2:272–278.
12. Alexanian R, Gehan E, Haut A, Saiki J, Weick J. Unmaintained remissions in multiple myeloma. Blood 1978; 51:1005–1011.

12a. Berenson JR, Crowley JJ, Grogan TM, et al. Maintenance therapy with alternate-day prednisone improves survival in multiple myeloma patients. Blood 2002; 99:3163–3168.

13. Bersagel DE, Bailey AJ, Langley GR, MacDonald RN, White DF, Miller AB. The chemotherapy of plasma-cell myeloma and the incidence of acute leukemia. N Engl J Med 1979; 301:743–748.

14. Rowley JD, Golomb HM, Vardiman JW. Nonrandom chromosome abnormalities in acute leukemia and dysmyelopoietic syndromes in patients with previously treated malignant disease. Blood 1981; 58:759–767.

15. Mackenzie MR, Wold H, George C, et al. Consolidation hemibody radiotherapy following induction combination chemotherapy in high-tumor burden multiple myeloma. J Clin Oncol 1992; 10:1769–1774.

16. Samson D, Gaminara E, Newland A, et al. Infusion of vincristine and doxorubicin with oral dexamethasone as first-line therapy for multiple myeloma. Lancet 1989; 2:882–885.

17. Alexanian R, Barlogie B, Tucker S. VAD-based regimens as primary treatment for multiple myeloma. Am J Hematol 1990; 33:86–89.

18. Monconduit M, Menard JF, Michaux JL, et al. VAD or VMBCP in severe multiple myeloma: the Groupe d'Etudes et de Recherche sur le Myelome (GERM). Br J Haematol 1992; 80: 199–204.

19. Dimopoulos MA, Palumbo A, Delasalle KB, Alexanian R. Primary plasma cell leukemia. Br J Haematol 1994; 88:754–759.

20. Segeren CM, Sonneveld P, Van der Holt, et al. Vincristine, doxorubicin and dexamethasone (VAD) administered as rapid intravenous infusion for first line treatment in untreated multiple myeloma. Br J Haematol 1999; 105:127–130.

21. Hussein MA, Wood L, His E, et al. A phase II trial of pegylated liposomal doxorubicin, vincristine, and reduced-dose dexamethasone combination therapy in newly diagnosed multiple myeloma patients. Cancer 2002; 95:2160–2168.

22. Dimopoulos MA, Pouli A, Zervas K, et al. Prospective randomized comparison of vincristine, doxorubicin and dexamethasone (VAD) administered as intravenous bolus injection and VAD with liposomal doxorubicin as first-line treatment in multiple myeloma. Ann Oncol 2003; 14:1039–1044.

23. Caro M, Benni M, Ronconi S, et al. Melphalan-prednisone versus alternating combination VAD/MP or VIVD/MP as primary treatment for multiple myeloma, final analysis of a randomized clinical study. Haematologica 2002; 87:934–942.

24. Alexanian R, Dimopoulos MA, Dellasalle K, Barlogie B. Primary dexamethasone treatment of multiple myeloma. Blood 1992; 80:887–890.

25. Quesada JR, Alexanian R, Hawkins M, et al. Treatment of multiple myeloma with recombinant alpha-interferon. Blood 1986; 67:275–278.

26. Oken MM, Kyle RA, Greipp PR, et al. Complete remission induction with combined VBMCP chemotherapy and interferon in patients with multiple myeloma. Leukemia and Lymphoma 1996; 20:447–451.

27. Cooper MR, Dear K, McIntyre OR, et al. A randomized clinical trial comparing melphalan/prednisone with or without interferon alfa-2b in newly diagnosed patients with multiple myeloma: a Cancer and Leukemia Group B study. J Clin Oncol 1993; 11:155–160.

28. Osterborg A, Bjorkholm M, Bjoreman M, et al. Natural interferon-a in combination with melphalan/prednisone versus melphalan/prednisone in the treatment of multiple myeloma stages II and III: a randomized study from the Myeloma Group of Central Sweden. Blood; 81:1428–1434.

29. Oken MM, Leong T, Kay NE, et al. The effect of adding interferon or high-dose cyclophosphamide to VBMCP to treat multiple myeloma: results from an ECOG phase III trial. Blood 1995; 86(suppl 1):441 a.

30. Dimopoulos MA, Weber D, Delasalle KB, Alexanian R. Combination therapy with Interferon-dexamethasone for newly diagnosed patients with multiple myeloma. Cancer 1993; 72:2589–2592.
31. Abrahamson GM, Bird JM, Newland AC, et al. A randomized study of VAD therapy with either concurrent or maintenance interferon in patients with newly diagnosed multiple myeloma. Br J Haematol 1996; 94:659–664.
32. Zervas K, Pouli A, Grigoraki B, et al. Comparison of vincristine, carmustine, melphalan, cyclophosphamide, prednisone (VBMCP) and interferon-alpha with melphalan and prednisone (MP) and interferon-alpha in patients with good-prognosis multiple myeloma: a prospective randomized study. Greek Myeloma Study Group. Eur J Haematol 2001; 66:18–23.
33. Cook G, Sharp RA, Tansey P, et al. A phase I/II trial of 2-Dex (oral idarubicin and dexamethasone), an oral equivalent of VAD, as initial treatment or progression in multiple myeloma. Br J Haematol 1996; 93:931–934.
34. Attal M, Harousseau JL, Stoppa AM, et al. A prospective randomized trial of autologous bone marrow transplantation and chemotherapy in multiple myeloma. N Engl J Med 1996; 335:91–97.
35. Child JA, Morgan GJ, Davies FE, et al. High-dose chemotherapy with hematopoietic stem-cell rescue for multiple myeloma. N Engl J Med 2003; 348:1857–1883.
36. Tricot G, Jagannath S, Vesole D, et al. Peripheral blood stem cell transplants for multiple myeloma: Identification of favorable variables for rapid engraftment in 225 patients. Blood 1995; 85:588–596.
37. Boccadoro M, Palumbo A, Bringhen S, et al. Oral melphalan at diagnosis hampers adequate collection of peripheral blood progenitor cells in multiple myeloma. Haematologica 2002; 87:846–850.
38. Raje N, Powles R, Kulkarni S, et al. A comparison of vincristine and doxorubicin infusional chemotherapy with methylprednisolone (VAMP) with the addition of weekly cyclophosphamide (C-VAMP) as induction treatment followed by autografting in previously untreated myeloma. Br Haematol 1997; 97:153–160.
39. Barlogie B Jagannath S, Vesole DH, et al . Superiority of tandem autologous transplantation over standard therapy for previously untreated multiple myeloma. Blood 1997; 89:789–793.
40. Singhal DS, Desikan KR, Mehta J, et al. Age is not a prognostic variable with autotransplants for multiple myeloma. Blood 1999; 93:51–54.
41. Tricot G, Alberts DS, Johnson C, et al. Safety of autotransplants with high dose melphalan in renal failure: a pharmacokinetic and toxicity study. Clin Cancer Res 1996; 2:947–952.
42. Barlogie B, Smith L, Alexanian R. Effective treatment of advanced multiple myeloma refractory to alkylating agents. N Engl J Med 1984; 310:1353–1356.
43. Alexanian R, Barlogie B, Dixon D. High-dose glucocorticoid treatment of resistant myeloma. Ann Intern Med 1986; 105:8–11.
44. Gertz MA, Garton JP, Greipp PR, et al. A phase II study of high-dose methylprednisolone in refractory or relapsed multiple myeloma. Leukemia 1995; 9:2115–2118.
45. Lokhorst HM, Menwissen OJ, Bast EJ, Dekker AW: VAD chemotherapy for refractory multiple myeloma. Br J Haematol 1989; 71:25–30.
46. Alexanian R, Barlogie B, Gutterman J. Alpha-interferon combination therapy of resistant myeloma. Am J Clin Oncol 1991; 14:188–192.
47. Blade J, San Miguel, Sanz MA, et al. Treatment of melphalan-resistant multiple myeloma with vincristine, BCNU, doxorubicin, and high dose dexamethasone (VBAD). Eur J Cancer 1992; 29A:57–62.
48. Salmon SE, Dalton WS, Grogan TM, et al. Multidrug resistant myeloma: Laboratory and clinical effects of verapamil as a chemosensitizer. Blood 1991; 78:44–50.
49. Dalton WS, Crowley J, Salmon SS, et al. A phase III randomized study of oral verapamil as a chemosensitizer to reverse drug resistance in patients with refractory myeloma. A Southwest Oncology Group Study. Cancer 1995; 75:815–820.

50. Sonneveld P, Durie BG, Lokhorst HM, et al. Modulation of multidrug-resistant multiple myeloma by cyclosporine: the Leukaemia Group of the EORTC and the HOVON. Lancet 1992; 340:255–259.

51. Weber D, Dimopoulos M, Sinicrope F, Alexanian R. VAD-cyclosporine for VAD-resistant myeloma. Leuk Lymphoma 1995; 19:159–163.

52. Sonneveld P, Suciu S, Weijermans P, et al. Cyclosporine-A combined with vincristine, doxorubicin and dexamethasone (VAD) vs VAD in patients with advanced refractory multiple myeloma: An EORTC-HOVOIY randomized phase III study. Br J Haematol 2001; 115:895–902 .

53. Barlogie B, Alexanian R, Smallwood L, et al. Prognostic factors with high-dose melphalan for refractory multiple myeloma. Blood 1988; 72:2015–2019.

54. Barlogie B, Jagannath S, Dixon DO, et al. High-dose melphalan and granulocyte-macrophage colony-stimulating factor for refractory multiple myeloma. Blood 1990; 76:677–680.

55. Barlogie B, Velasquez WS, Alexanian R, Cabanillas F. Etoposide, dexamethasone, cytarabine, and cisplatin in vincristine, doxorubicin and dexamethasone-refractory myeloma. J Clin Oncol 1989; 7:1514–1517.

56. Lenhard RE, Daniels MJ, Oken MM, et al. An aggressive high dose cyclophosphamide and prednisone regimen for advanced multiple myeloma. Leuk Lymphoma 1944; 16:589–592.

57. Dimopoulos MA, Delassalle KB, Champlin R, Alexanian R. Cyclophosphamide and etoposide therapy with GM-CSF for VAD-resistant multiple myeloma. Br J Haematol 1993; 83:240–244.

58. Dimopoulos MA, Weber D, Kantarjian H, et al. HyperCVAD for VAD-resistant multiple myeloma. Am J Haematol 1996; 52:77–81.

59. Munshi NC, Desikan KR, Jagannath S, et al. Dexamethasone, cyclophosphamide, etoposide and cisplatinum (DCEP), an effective regimen for relapse after high-dose chemotherapy and autologous transplantation. Blood 1995; 88(Suppl1):586a.

60. Siegel D, Niesvisky R, Miller J et al. All-trans retinoic acid and interferon synergistically inhibit myeloma cell growth and induce retinoic acid receptor expression. Blood; 1992(:suppl 1):12/a.

61. Weber DM, Bseiso A, Wood A, Gavino M, Alexanian R. All-trans retinoic acid for multiple myeloma. Blood (suppl 1):357a.

62. Belch AR, Henderson JF, Brox LW. Treatment of multiple myeloma with deoxycoformycin. Cancer Chemother Pharmacol 1985; 14:49–52.

63. Lichtman SM, Mittelman A, Budman DR, et al. Phase II trial of fludarabine phosphate in multiple myeloma using a loading dose and continues infusion schedule. Leukemia and Lymphoma 1991; 6:61–63.

64. Dimopoulos MA, Kantarjian H, Estey EH, Alexanian R. 2-Chlorodeoxyadenosine in the treatment of multiple myeloma. Blood 1992; 80:1626.

65. Dimopoulos MA, Arbuck S, Huber M, et al. Primary therapy of multiple myeloma with paclitaxel. Ann Oncol 1994; 5:757–759.

66. Friedenberg WR, Graham D, Greipp P, et al. The treatment of multiple myeloma with docetaxel (an ECOG study). Leuk Res 2003; 27:751–754.

67. Weick JK, Crowley JJ, Hussein MA, et al. The evaluation of gemcitabine in resistant or relapsing multiple myeloma, phase II: a South-West Oncology Group Study. Invest New Drugs 2002; 20:117–121.

68. Peest D, Leo R, Bloche S, et al. Low-dose recombinant interleukin-2 therapy in advanced multiple myeloma. Br J Haematol 1995; 89:328–337.

69. Harousseau JL, Maloisel F, Sotto JJ et al. Vinorelbine in patients with recurrent multiple myeloma: a phase II study. Proc Am Soc Clin Oncol 1997; 16:11a.

70. Kraut EH, Crowley JJ, Wade JL, et al. Evaluation of topotecan in resistant and relapsing multiple myeloma: A Southwest Oncology Group Study. J Clin Oncol 1998; 16:589–592.

71. Chisesi T, Capnist G, De Dominicis E, Din E. A phase II study of idarubicin in advanced myeloma. Eur J Cancer Clin Oncol 1988; 24:681–684.

72. Singhal S, Mehta J, Desikan R, et al. Anti-tumor activity of thalidomide in refractory multiple myeloma. N Engl J Med 1999; 341:1565–1571.

73. Richardson P, Hideshima T and Anderson K: Thalidomide: emerging role in cancer medicine. Annu Rev Med 2002; 53:629–657.

74. Barlogie B, Desikan R, Eddlemon P, et al. Extended survival in advanced and refractory multiple myeloma after single-agent thalidomide: identification of prognostic factors in a phase 2 study of 169 patients. Blood 2001; 98:492–494.

75. Neben K, Moehler T, Benner A, et al. Dose-dependent effect of thalidomide on overall survival in relapsed multiple myeloma. Clin Cancer Res 2002; 8:3377–3382.

76. Durie BGM: Low-dose thalidomide in myeloma: Efficacy and biologic significance. Semin Oncol 2002; 29(Suppl 17):34–38.

77. Dimopoulos MA, Zervas K, Kouvatseas G, et al. Thalidomide and dexamethasone combination for refractory multiple myeloma. Ann Oncol 2001; 12:991–995.

78. Anagnostopoulos A, Weber D, Rankin K, et al. Thalidomide and dexamethasone for resistant multiple myeloma. Br J Haematol 2003; 121:768–769.

78a. Ma MH, Yang HH, Parker K, et al. The proteasome inhibitor PS-341 markedly enhances sensitivity of multiple myeloma tumor cells to chemotherapeutic agents. Clin Cancer Res 2003; 9:1136–1144.

78b. Orlowski RZ, Voorhees PM, Garcia RA, et al. Phase I study of the proteasome inhibitore bortezomib in combination with pegylated liposomal doxorubicin in patients with refractory hematologic malignancies. Blood 2003; 102:abstract 1639.

78c. Yang HH, Yan X, Chen H, Berenson JR. Differential synergistic anti-myeloma effects of the COX-2 inhibitor NS398 and bortezomib on doxorubicin-sensitive and resistant myeloma cells. Blood 2003; 102:abstract 3488.

79. Cavanaugh JD, Oakervee H: Thalidomide in multiple myeloma: current status and future prospects. Br J Haematol 2003; 18–26.

80. Rajkumar SV, Gertz MA, Lacy MQ, et al. Thalidomide as initial therapy for early-stage myeloma. Leukemia 2003; 17:775–779.

81. Weber D, Rankin K, Gavino M, et al. Thalidomide alone or with dexamethasone for previously untreated multiple myeloma. J Clin Oncol 2003; 21:16–19.

82. Rajkumar SV, Hayman S, Gertz MA, et al. Combination therapy with thalidomide plus dexamethasone for newly diagnosed myeloma. J Clin Oncol 2002; 20:4319–4323.

83. Zangari MA, Annaissie E, Barlogie B, et al. Increased risk of deep-vein thrombosis in patients with multiple myeloma receiving thalidomide and chemotherapy. Blood 2001; 98:1614–1615.

83a. Dimopoulos MA, Anagnostopoulos A, Weber D. Treatment of plasma cell dyscrasias with thalidomide and its derivatives. J Clin Oncol 2003; 21:23:4444–4454.

83b. Zangari M, Siegel E, Barlogie B, et al. Thrombogenic acitivity of doxorubicin in myeloma patients receiving thalidomide: Implications for therapy. Blood 2002; 100:1158–1171.

84. Richardson PG, Schlossman RL, Weller E, et al. Immunomodulatory drug CC-5013 overcomes drug resistance and is well tolerated in patients with relapsed multiple myeloma. Blood 2002; 100:3063–3067.

85. Mitsiades N, Mitsiades CS, Poulaki V, et al. Biologic sequelae of nuclear factor-kappa B blockade in multiple myeloma: therapeutic implications. Blood 2002; 99:4079–4086.

86. Richardson PG, Barlogie B, Berenson J, et al. A phase 2 study of bortezomib in relapsed, refractory myeloma. N Engl J Med 2003; 348:2609–2617.

87. Hayashi T, Hideshima T, Akiyama M, et al. Arsenic trioxide inhibits growth of human multiple myeloma cells in the bone marrow microenvironment. Mol Cancer Ther 2002; 1:851–860.

87a. Friedman JM, Ma MH, Manyak SJ, et al. Arsenic trioxide causes apoptosis, growth inhibition and increased sensitivity to chemotherapeutic agents in multiple myeloma cells through inhibition of nuclear factor (NF)-κB activity. Proc Am Assoc Cancer Res 2002; Abstract 4585.

88. Munshi NC, Tricot G, Desikan R, et al. Clinical activity of arsenic trioxide for the treatment of multiple myeloma. Leukemia 2002; 16:1835–1837.

88a. Hussein MA, Paradise C, Carozza R, et al. Arsenic trioxide in patients with relapsed or refractory multiple myeloma: Final report of a phase II clinical study. Blood 2002; 100: abstract 5138.

88b. Grad JM, Bahlis NJ, Reis I, Oshiro MM, Dalton WS, Boise LH. Ascorbic acid enhances arsenic trioxide-induced cytotoxicity in multiple myeloma cells. Blood 2001; 98:3: 805–813.

88c. Borad M, Swift RA, Sadler K, Yang H, Berenson JR. Melphalan, arsenic trioxide and ascorbic acid (MAC) is effective in the treatment of refractory and relapsed multiple myeloma (MM). Blood 2003; 102:abstract 827.

89. Major P, Lortholary A, Hon J, et al. Zoledronic acid is superior to pamidronate in the treatment of hypercalcemia of malignancy: a pooled analysis of two randomized, controlled clinical trials. J Clin Oncol 2001; 19:558–567.

90. Alexanian R, Barlogie B and Dixon D. Renal failure in multiple myeloma. Arch Intern Med 1990; 150:1693–1695.

91. Clark AD, Shetty A, Soutar R. Renal failure and multiple myeloma: pathogenesis and treatment of renal failure and management of underlying myeloma. Blood Rev 1999; 13:79–90.

92. Johnson WJ, Kyle RA, Pineda AA et al. Treatment of renal failure associated with multiple myeloma: plasmapheresis, hemodialysis and chemotherapy. Arch Intern Med 1990; 150:863–869.

93. Alexanian R. Blood volume in monoclonal gammopathy. Blood 1997; 49:301–304.

94. Ludwig H, Fritz E, Kotzmann H et al. Erythropoietin treatment of anemia associated with multiple myeloma. N Engl J Med 1990; 322:1693–1699.

95. Garton JP, Gertz MA, Witzig TE, et al. Epoetin alpha for the treatment of the anemia of multiple myeloma. A prospective, randomized, placebo-controlled, double-blind trial. Arch Inter Med 1995; 155:2069–2074.

96. Osterborg A, Boogaerts MA, Gimino R, et al. Recombinant human erythropoietin in transfusion-dependent anemic patients with multiple myeloma and non-Hodgkin's lymphoma. Blood 1996; 87:2675–2682.

97. Dammacco F, Castoldi G, Rogers S. Efficacy of epoetin alfa in the treatment of anemia of multiple myeloma. Br Haematol 2001; 106:172–179.

98. Demetri G, Kris M, Wade J, et al. Quality of life benefit in chemotherapy patients treated with epoietin alfa is independent of disease response or tumor type: results from a prospective community oncology study. J Clin Oncol 1998; 16:3413–3425.

99. Smith R. Applications of Darbepoietin, a novel erythropoiesis-stimulating protein in Oncology. Curr Opin Hematol 2002; 9:228–233.

100. Dispenzieri A, Kyle RA, Lacy MQ, et al. POEMS syndrome: definitions and long-term outcome. Blood 2003; 101:2496–1506.

101. Ohi T, Kyle RA & Dyck PJ. Axonal attenuation and secondary segmental demyelination in myeloma neuropathies. Ann Neurol 1985; 17:255–261.

102. Dyck PJ, Low PA, Windebank AJ et al. Plasma exchange in polyneuropathy associated with monoclonal gammopathy of undetermined significance. N Engl J Med 1991; 325:1482–1486.

103. Capra JD & Kunkel JG. Aggregation of IG3 proteins: relevance to the hyperviscosity syndrome. J Clin Invest 1970; 49:610–621.

104. Beck JR, Quinn BM, Meier FA, Rawnsley HM. Hyperviscosity syndrome in paraproteinemia managed by plasma exchange. Transfusion 1982; 22:51–53.

105. Perkins HA, Mackenzie MR, Fudenberg HH. Hemostatic defects in dysproteinemias. Blood 1970; 35:695–707.

106. Kaufman PA, Gockerman JP, Greenberg CS. Production of a novel anticoagulant by neoplastic plasma cells: report of a case and review to the literature. Am J Med 1989; 86:612–616.
107. Brouet JC, Clauvel JP, Danon F, et al. Biologic and clinical significance of cryoglobulins. Am J Med 1974; 57:775–790.
108. Kolb JP, Arrian S, Zolla-Pazner S. Suppression of the humoral immune response by plasmacytoma. J of Immunol 1977; 18:702–709.
109. Broder S, Humphrey R, Durm M, et al. Impaired synthesis of polyclonal immunoglobulins by circulating lymphocytes from patients with multiple myeloma. N Engl J Med 1975; 293:887–892.
110. Mc Gregor RR, Negendank WG, Schreiber AD. Impaired granulocyte adherence in multiple myeloma: relationship to complement system, granulocytic delivery and infection. Blood 1978; 51:591–599.
111. Cheson BD, Walker HS, Heath ME, et al. Defective binding of the third component of complement to Streptococcus pneumoniae in multiple myeloma. Blood 1984; 63:949–957.
112. Savage DG, Lindenbaum K, Garrett TJ. Biphasic pattern of bacterial infection in multiple myeloma. Ann Intern Med 1982; 96:47–50.
113. Perri RT, Hebbel RP, Oken MM. Influence of treatment and response status on infection risk in multiple myeloma. Am J Med 1981; 293:887–892.
114. Oken MM, Pomeroy C, Weisdorf D, Bennett JM. Prophylactic antibiotics for the prevention of early infection in multiple myeloma. Am J Med 1996; 100:624–628.
115. Chapel H, Lee M, Hargreaves R. Randomized trial of intravenous immunoglobulin as prophylaxis against infections in plateau phase myeloma. Lancet 1994; 343:1059–1063.

9
Dose-Intensive Therapy With Autologous Stem Cell Transplantation for Patients With Multiple Myeloma

Jean-Luc Harousseau, MD, Michel Attal, MD, and Gary J. Schiller, MD

1. INTRODUCTION

Despite their sensitivity to alkylator-based chemotherapy, dose-intensive regimens with a source of hematopoietic support have only recently been exploited for the treatment of patients with multiple myeloma (MM) *(1–6)*. The concept of dose-intensification as a means of inducing prolonged remission did not appear to be relevant in myeloma, a disease in which conventional chemotherapy may effect a response but has little or no impact on progression-free survival *(7–10)*. Furthermore, allogeneic bone marrow transplantation (BMT), the historic form of hematopoietic support for patients receiving dose-intensive chemotherapy, is usually reserved for younger patients with a human lymphocyte antigen (HLA)-identical sibling. Because of both advanced age at presentation and subsequent

From: *Current Clinical Oncology: Biology and Management of Multiple Myeloma*
Edited by: J. R. Berenson © Humana Press Inc., Totowa, NJ

high treatment-related mortality, allogeneic transplantation has been reserved for a relatively small number of patients with MM *(11–13)*. Barlogie and colleagues introduced the concept of high-dose chemotherapy followed by autologous stem cell transplantation in the 1980s *(3,4)* and rapidly several large trials were performed in patients with MM *(14–19)*.

2. AUTOLOGOUS STEM CELL TRANSPLANTATION IN RESISTANT MYELOMA

Dose-intensification was first used in patients with poor-risk MM. After the pioneering work by McElwain and colleagues in 1983 *(2)*, studies began using high-dose intravenous phenylalanine melphalan without hematopoietic cell support *(20–23)*.

Dose-intensive chemotherapy was associated with severe myelosuppression, with a median time to granulocyte and platelet recovery of nearly 1 mo and a high risk of toxic death, even with hematopoietic growth factors administered following dose-intensive chemotherapy *(20–23)*. Support from hematopoietic stem cells from autologous bone marrow, peripheral blood progenitor cells, or syngeneic bone marrow—ameliorates the myelosuppressive effect of high-dose chemotherapy and allows the additional use of total body irradiation (TBI) *(4)*. This strategy proved effective in shortening the duration of neutropenia and thrombocytopenia, and, at least to some degree, decreased the risk of infectious complications. More importantly, a proof of principle was confirmed, i.e., that high-dose cytotoxic chemotherapy could induce a response, even in patients whose disease was resistant to conventional agents. The rate of response (>75% reduction in myeloma protein production and the disappearance of Bence-Jones proteinuria) ranged from 39 to 100% with a median relapse-free survival of 4 to 12 mo (Table 1) *(3,19,24–26)*. The addition of autologous bone marrow support did not affect response duration, but permitted further dose escalation. Several regimens were proposed, including high-dose melphalan with TBI, and dose-intensive busulfan and cyclophosphamide. They all resulted in a significant anti-tumor response in patients with highly resistant disease, but the response duration was typically measured in months.

These early studies confirmed that dose-intensification therapy in patients with MM resistant to conventional chemotherapy could be used to achieve an impressive anti-tumor response (indicated by a decrease in monoclonal paraprotein and bone marrow plasmacytosis), but the response duration was relatively short and there was no evidence of a sustained progression-free survival. The dissociation between response and progression-free survival could be considered a result of incomplete response criteria or patient eligibility. When dose-intensive conditioning is applied to a similar group of resistant patients with acute leukemia or non-Hodgkin's lymphoma, a response is also relatively easy

Table 1

Results of Early Studies of Dose-Intensive Therapy for Resistant Multiple Myeloma

Author (reference)	No. of Patients	Preparative Regimen[a]	Stem Cell Support[b]	Response	Survival
Barlogie (3)	23	HDM 80–140 mg/m^2	None	60%	progression-free: 4 mo overall: 4 mo
Bensinger (19)	41 (of 63)	Busulfan (14–16 mg/kg) Cy (120–174 mg/kg) ± TBI	BM ± PSC	65%	progression-free <12 mo
Fermand (24)	8	HDM, VP16, NU + TBI	PSC	100%	11 mo
Dimopoulos (25)	17	Cy (3g/m^2) + VP16 (900/m^2)	PSC	59%	progression-free: 12 mo
Mansi (26)	15	Busulfan (16 mg/kg)	BM	46%	8 mo

[a]HDM, high-dose melphalan; Cy, cyclophosphamide; VP16, etoposide; NU, nitrosourea; TBI, total body irradiation.
[b]BM, bone marrow; PSC, peripheral stem cells.

to achieve and progression-free survival is also rare *(27)*. For this reason, the next generation of studies concentrated on high-dose therapy for patients with newly diagnosed MM.

3. AUTOLOGOUS STEM CELL TRANSPLANTATION IN NEWLY DIAGNOSED PATIENTS

3.1. AutoSCT vs Conventional Chemotherapy

In the absence of significant improvement in survival with a variety of conventional chemotherapy regimes, high-dose therapy with autologous (auto)SCT has been used with increased frequency during the past 15 years as part of frontline treatment *(28)*. Nonrandomized studies have shown that autoSCT is a safe (5% toxic deaths) and effective consolidation therapy *(29–32)* in patients who had not progressed from initial induction of conventional doses of chemotherapy. Most importantly, some studies have suggested that a 30 to 50% complete remission could be achieved using this approach in patients with newly diagnosed MM and that this more important tumor burden reduction could be converted into a prolonged remission and survival *(29)*. However, these pilot studies are difficult to analyze because the recruitment of patients was subject to selection bias regarding age, performance status, renal function, and response to initial chemotherapy. Blade and colleagues studied the outcome of a subgroup of patients who were potential candidates for high-dose therapy but were treated only with conventional chemotherapy *(33)*. Their median survival was 60 mo and 52 mo from the time when high-dose therapy would be considered. Thus, they stated that survival duration for these patients was similar to that reported in selected series of patients given high-dose therapy early during the course of their disease. In three other historical comparisons, however, high-dose therapy appeared to be superior to conventional chemotherapy (Table 2) *(34–36)*.

Therefore, assessing the actual impact of dose-intensive strategies on event-free survival and overall survival required further evaluation. The Intergroupe Français du Myélome (IFM) was the first to conduct a randomized multicenter trial showing the superiority of high-dose therapy in patients aged 65 yr or less *(37)*. An intent-to-treat analysis of 200 patients with newly diagnosed MM indicated that autologous BMT improved the response rate significantly, because 38% of patients enrolled in the high-dose therapy arm achieved complete remission or very good partial remission (>90% reduction of the M component) compared with 14% of patients enrolled in the conventional chemotherapy arm ($p < 0.001$). An updated analysis of this study confirms the published results and shows that with a median follow-up period of 7 yr, high-dose therapy significantly improves event free survival (median: 28 vs 18 mo; 7-yr event-free survival: 16% vs 8%, $p = 0.01$) and overall survival (median: 57 vs 44 mo; 7-yr overall survival: 43% vs 25%, $p = 0.03$).

Table 2
Conventional Chemotherapy vs High-Dose Therapy: Historical Comparisons

Author (reference)	No. of patients		Type of HDT	Age	Median survival (months)		p value
	HDT	CC			CC	HDT	
Barlogie (34)	123	116[a]	Tandem transplantation	<70	48	62+	0.01
Lenhoff (35)	274	274[b]	HDM 200mg/m^2+ ASCT	<60	44	NR	0.001
Palumbo (36)	71	71[c]	HDM 100 mg/m^2 + ASCT (2–3 courses)	55–75	48	56+	< 0.01

[a]matched for age, β_2 microglobulin, creatinine
[b]fulfilling eligibility criteria for HDT
[c]matched for age and β_2 microglobuline
CC, conventional chemotherapy; HDT, high-dose therapy; HDM, high-dose melphalan; ASCT, autologous stem cell transplantation.

In other randomized studies comparing conventional chemotherapy and autologous transplant, inclusion criteria and treatment details were variable (Table 3) (38–41). However, in all of these studies, high-dose therapy with an autologous transplant resulted in a significantly improved rate of complete remission. The median progression-free survival was prolonged in the transplant arm in each study (5–13 mo), and that difference was significant in four out of five trials. The median overall survival was also prolonged in the transplant arm in four of five studies, although the difference was significant only in the IFM90 (37) and in the Medical Research Council (MRC)7 trials (41). However, the survival benefit associated with autoSCT up front could be underestimated, because in recently conducted trials, a significant number of patients allocated to the conventional chemotherapy arm underwent transplant following relapse. This strategy was supported by the results of another randomized study showing no significant survival benefit for an early transplant compared with transplant for disease progression after conventional chemotherapy (62). However, a recently completed study comparing autologous transplant to the use of this treatment at the time of relapse showed no difference in outcome (62a).

In conclusion, the MRC7 recently confirmed the IFM90 trial results by showing that high-dose therapy significantly increased rate of complete remission, event-free survival, and overall survival on a larger number of patients compared with conventional chemotherapy (41). As a consequence of these two trials, high-dose therapy plus autologous stem cell support is now considered the standard of care for patients with newly diagnosed MM up to the age of 65.

Table 3
Conventional chemotherapy vs High-Dose Therapy: Results of Randomized Studies

Group/Trial (reference)	No. of patients	Age	Median follow-up	CR rate (%) CC	CR rate (%) HDT	Median EFS (mo) CC	Median EFS (mo) HDT	Median OS (mo) CC	Median OS (mo) HDT
IFM90 (37)	200	<65 yr	7 yr	5[a]	22[a]	18[a]	28[a]	44[a]	57[a]
MAG91 (38)	190	55–65 yr	56 mo	NA	NA	19[a]	24[a]	50	55
Pethema (39)	164	Median 56 yr	44 mo	11[a]	30[a]	33	43	56	62
Italian MMSG (40)	195	<70 yr	2 yr	6[a]	28[a]	21[a]	34[a]	NR	NR
MRC7 (41)	407	<65 yr	42 mo	8	44	19[a]	31[a]	42[a]	54[a]

[a]significant difference.
EFS, event-free survival; NA, not available; CC, conventional chemotherapy; OS, overall survival; NR, not reached; CR, complete remission; HDT, high-dose therapy.

3.2. Source of Hematopoietic Stem Cells

The use of peripheral blood progenitor cells (PBPC) as the source of stem cells for hematopoietic rescue after myeloablative therapy for MM was introduced during the late 1980s *(24,43)*.

Hematopoietic progenitors were first collected from the blood during hematopoietic recovery after moderately intensive forms of chemotherapy, e.g., high-dose cyclophosphamide or high-dose therapy with cyclophosphamide, hydroxydaunomycin, vincristine, and prednisone (CHOP therapy) *(24,43,44)*. The introduction of hematopoietic growth factors profoundly modified the practice of stem cell autografting. Gianni and colleagues first used granulocyte-macrophage colony-stimulating factor (GM-CSF) after chemotherapy to increase the number of hematopoietic progenitors in the cytapheresis product *(45)*. Other investigators used GM-CSF or granulocyte colony-stimulating factor (G-CSF) after high-dose cyclophosphamide therapy *(44,46)*. Currently, PBPCs are collected either after priming by chemotherapy (usually high-dose cyclophosphamide therapy) with G-CSF or only by G-CSF. As in other hematological malignancies, the benefit of PBPC compared to bone marrow are a more rapid hematopoietic reconstitution and an earlier accessibility. The actual effect of autologous PBPC transplantation on overall survival in MM cannot be assessed based on early studies because of variable inclusion criteria, the conditioning regimens, and the response criteria. The β_2 microglobulin level, the duration of chemotherapy prior to transplant, the number of regimens and treatment cycles, and the response to initial cytotoxic chemotherapy were the most important prognostic factors. In a series of 225 patients treated for newly diagnosed or refractory MM, Tricot and colleagues retrospectively analyzed variables affecting PBPC mobilization and the speed of engraftment *(47)* and found a highly significant correlation between the number of CD34-positive cells infused and a prompt recovery of both granulocytes and platelets. Prior exposure to chemotherapy, especially with alkylating agents, significantly delayed the posttransplant hematopoietic recovery. The threshold CD34-positive cell dose necessary for prompt engraftment was less than or equal to 2×10^6/kg for patients with no more than 24 mo of chemotherapy; in contrast, more than 5×10^6/kg CD34-positive cells were required for a rapid recovery in patients with longer exposure. Rapid platelet recovery (before day 14) was almost invariably seen (94%) when more than 5×10^6/kg were infused, irrespective of the duration of prior therapy. In the absence of CD34-positive measurements, rapid platelet recovery after priming with high-dose cyclophosphamide and fewer than 12 mo of prior chemotherapy were the best predictors of early engraftment. In another study in 116 patients, Marit and colleagues found that the number of granulocyte-macrophage colony-forming unit (CFU-GM) cells infused (25×10^4/kg) was the most important parameter for rapid and complete hematological recovery after autologous PBPC transplantation *(48)*. Previous use of alkylating agents, response to previous chemotherapy,

and the interval between diagnosis and priming chemotherapy were also significant factors. In a series of 103 patients treated with 7 g/m^2 cyclophosphamide plus
G-CSF, Goldschmidt and colleagues found that the most significant predictor of
impaired PBPC collection was the duration of previous melphalan therapy *(49)*.

Other smaller studies confirm that either the duration of melphalan therapy or
bone marrow plasma cell infiltration can be used to predict the CFU-GM yield
and speed of engraftment *(46,50)*. As a consequence, melphalan should not be
administered in patients scheduled for an autologous PBPC transplantation procedure. Alternatively, PBPCs should be collected early in the course of the
disease.

The optimal dose of cyclophosphamide for priming PBPCs in MM has yet to
be determined and, most probably, will never be studied. There is an apparent
dose–response relationship. In comparative studies, higher doses of cyclophosphamide (7 g/m^2) were more efficient and associated with an increased number
of harvested PBPCs compared with lower doses (4 g/m ^{2}) *(49,51)*. Moreover,
higher doses could reduce both graft contamination by malignant plasma cells
and tumor cell mass *(49,52)*. However, the administration of cyclophosphamide
at a dosage of 7 g/m^2 is associated with increased toxicity. Significant morbidity as
well as several toxic deaths have been recorded with this dosage, mostly in pretreated patients *(46,48,51,52)*. Although the number of CD34-positive cells collected appears to be superior after priming with high-dose cyclophosphamide
followed by G-CSF compared with G-CSF alone, collection after G-CSF alone in
a steady state should also be considered, at least in newly diagnosed patients. The
CD34-positive cell yield achieved with G-CSF alone is greater than 2.5×10^6/kg
in most cases and allows for safe and rapid hematopoietic reconstitution *(53)*.
The major advantage of collecting PBPC after priming with G-CSF alone is the
reduced risk and cost of the procedure, owing to the avoidance of hospitalization
(54). However, the risk of mobilizing clonal myeloma cells associated with the
process of priming with growth factors without chemotherapy has been suggested by some case reports *(55,56)*.

Combinations of hematopoietic growth factors could further enhance the
amount of PBPCs collected. Preliminary results of the use of a combination of
stem cell factor (SCF) and G-CSF have been encouraging *(57,58)*. In heavily
pretreated patients, this combination allows for the collection of an adequate
number of CD34-positive cells in more patients *(42)*, whereas in newly diagnosed patients, the optimal yield of 5×10^6 CD34/kg is obtained a in a fewer
number of cytaphereses *(58)*. The impact of hematopoietic growth factors
administered after autologous PBPC transplantation is not completely clear.
Although the use of growth factors could reduce the time to platelet recovery
in patients who receive low amounts of CD34-positive cells, there are no dis-
cernible effects in patients who receive more than 5×10^6 CD34-positive
cells/kg *(59)*.

3.3. Selection of Patients

Usually, autologous transplant is offered only to patients aged 65 yr or younger with a performance status of grade 0 to 2 and normal renal function, which are the eligibility criteria for most of the studies described. The issue of age is important because the median age of patients with MM is more than 65 yr and because age is a well-known prognostic factor. The introduction of hematopoietic growth factors and the use of PBPC instead of bone marrow have significantly modified the practice of autoSCT. This form of hematopoietic support, collected after priming with G-CSF, seems to have made transplantation safer, such that it is now offered to older patients. The Arkansas group compared the outcome of autologous transplantation in 49 patients aged 65 yr and older with that in 49 younger matched patients selected from a cohort of 550 patients *(60)*. Because progression-free and overall survival were comparable, the authors concluded that age is not a biologically adverse parameter for patients treated with high-dose therapy and progenitor-cell support, and should not constitute an exclusion criteria for participation in studies of what appears to be superior therapy. The same group published the results of autologous PBPC transplantation in 70 patients aged more than 70 yr. Although transplant appeared to be feasible in this age group, the use of higher dose melphalan (200 mg/m^2) produced excessive toxicity *(61)*. Palumbo and colleagues showed that two to three courses of melphalan 100 mg/m^2 supported by PBPC is feasible on an outpatient basis in patients aged 75 yr or less. They compared 71 patients treated with this approach to 71 matched patients treated with conventional chemotherapy and concluded that intensive therapy was superior in terms of the rate of complete remission and event-free and overall survival *(53)*. However, the issue of selection bias can be raised in all studies of dose-intensive therapy given to elderly patients. The benefit of autologous transplantation and the optimal conditioning regimen for this patient population needs further evaluation in the setting of randomized trials.

Because of concerns regarding excessive toxicity, patients with severe renal failure are typically excluded from dose-intensive therapy and autologous transplantation. A retrospective study of the Spanish Registry showed high transplant-related mortality in patients who had renal failure at the time of high-dose therapy *(62)*. However, in a study of 81 patients with renal failure at the time of autologous transplant, the Arkansas Group stated that renal failure had no impact on the quality of stem cell collection and did not affect engraftment *(63)*. Transplantation was feasible, even in patients on dialysis. However, extrahematologic toxicity was more severe and occurred more frequently after melphalan 200 mg/m^2 than after melphalan 140 mg/m^2. Although compromised renal function at presentation should not exclude patients from high-dose therapy, the impact of renal failure at the time of autologous transplantation requires further study.

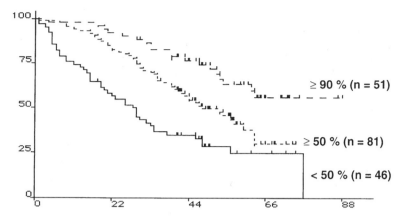

Fig. 1. IFM90 trial: impact of response on survival.

4. POSSIBLE METHODS OF IMPROVING THE RESULTS OF AUTOLOGOUS TRANSPLANTATION

In the IFM90 trial, the 7-yr event-free survival for patients enrolled in the high-dose therapy arm was only 16% with autologous transplantation, and there was no evidence of a plateau in the survival curve. Thus, strategies for improving these results were clearly warranted. Because the achievement of complete remission or a very good partial remission was significantly associated with prolonged survival in this trial (Fig. 1), the aim of subsequent studies was to increase the complete remission rate as a surrogate for improved progression-free and overall survival.

4.1. Conditioning Regimen

Improving the conditioning regimen has been determined to be a means of improving the response rate. The optimal preparative conditioning regimen has not yet been determined. Since its introduction in 1987 (4), TBI has been used in many nonrandomized studies. The combination of TBI plus high-dose melphalan (140 mg/m^2) therapy yields complete remission rates that range from 20 to 50%, depending on the disease status at transplantation and the criteria used to define remission. This conditioning regimen was used in the IFM90 trial and could, therefore, be considered standard. However, in newly diagnosed patients, the Royal Marsden Group reported an impressive 70% rate of complete remission with high-dose melphalan (200 mg/m^2), with minimal extramedullary toxicity (64).

In 1995, the IFM initiated a randomized study comparing single-agent high-dose melphalan (200 mg/m^2) with melphalan (140 mg/m^2) plus TBI in 282 patients newly diagnosed with MM (65). In this study, single-agent melphalan

Table 4
IFM9502 Study

	HDM 140 mg/m^2 + TBI N = 140	HDM 200 mg/m^2 N = 142	p Value
Duration neutropenia (median)	4–34 (10)	4–34 (8)	<0.001
Duration thrombocytopenia (median)	0–110 (7)	0–30 (7)	<0.001
Number of platelet transfusion (median)	0–30 (2)	0-18 (1)	<0.001
Mucositis grade 3–4 (%)	51	30	<0.001
CR + VGPR (%)	43	55	0.06
Toxic death	5	4	0.07
Median event-free survival (mo)	21	20.5	0.6
4-yr survival (%)	45.5	66	0.05

HDM, high-dose melphalan; CR, complete remission; VGPR, very good partial remission.

200 mg/m^2 therapy was significantly less toxic (i.e., resulted in a shorter duration of neutropenia and thrombocytopenia, lower incidence of grade-3 mucositis, no toxic death, compared with five deaths in the TBI group). Although the response rate and the event-free survival were identical in these two groups, overall survival was superior in the melphalan 200 mg/m^2 group, apparently because of a better likelihood of salvage after relapse (Table 4). In two other nonrandomized studies, investigators also failed to show a survival benefit for TBI-containing regimens (66,67). In fact, European Bone Marrow Transplant registry data showed a worse outcome for patients placed on regimens containing TBI. Therefore, 200 mg/m^2 melphalan should be preferred over regimens containing 140 mg/m^2 melphalan plus TBI. Knowing the tolerability of 200 mg/m^2 melphalan, higher doses of melphalan alone or in combination with an anti-interleukin-6 antibody have been explored, with encouraging results (68–69). To further improve the efficacy of conditioning regimens, current studies use radioconjugates (Holmium, Samarium) that localize preferentially in bone (70). Other combinations have been explored, including busulfan–cyclophosphamide or busulfan–melphalan. Both the University of California at Los Angeles group and the Seattle group have utilized preparative regimens containing busulfan 0.8 mg/kg and cyclophosphamide (19). In a large retrospective analysis of 821 Spanish Registry patients showed that busulfan–melphalan combination therapy yielded significantly better response rates compared with other regimens and suggested that event-free survival and overall survival could be longer as well (71). Because this was not a randomized study, however, 200 mg/m^2 melphalan

is still considered the standard conditioning regimen to which all others should be prospectively compared.

4.2. Purging the Graft

As in other malignant conditions, progenitor cells procured from the peripheral blood have almost completely replaced bone marrow in autologous transplantation for MM. The main reasons for this choice are easier accessibility and availability and faster hematopoietic recovery, although bone marrow mobilized with G-CSF may provide the same degree of rapid recovery. Tumor-cell contamination is lower in blood-derived progenitor-cell harvests than in bone marrow, but the superiority of PBPC autologous transplantation in terms of clinical outcome has not been demonstrated by a randomized trial. Sensitive polymerase chain reaction (PCR)-based techniques have demonstrated that virtually all peripheral blood-derived cell harvests are contaminated with malignant cells (72–75). Although the prognostic significance of malignant cells detected with such sensitive methods is still unknown, reducing tumor-cell contamination of the grafts has long been a concern.

No single antigen has been identified as specific for the malignant plasma cell. Consequently, negative selection of tumor cells by means of antibody purging requires a panel of monoclonal antibodies (MAbs) to be successful and may still fail to identify all malignant cells (76). The low rate of plasma cell replication makes it difficult to eliminate malignant cells in the autograft by exposing it to cytotoxic agents. Furthermore, extensive exposure to previous chemotherapy may render any form of chemotherapeutic purging hazardous because of a well-recognized risk of delayed engraftment. Prolonged pancytopenia has been noted with the use of 4-hydroperoxycyclophosphamide-purged autografts (77). In studies using MAb purging, the median time to neutrophil engraftment is 19 to 25 d (76,78). Therefore, the inherent methodologic risks involved in antibody purging and in vitro exposure to cytotoxic agents have made these forms of autologous transplant less desirable, and they have not been extensively pursued. Selection of CD34-positive progenitors appeared to be a promising alternative with a 2.5- to 4.5-log depletion of plasma cells (79,80). Several studies have confirmed the feasibility and safety of autologous transplants with CD34-positive-selected blood-derived cells in MM (81–83). In a multicenter, randomized, phase III trial comparing selected and unselected peripheral blood cell-derived grafts in 131 patients with myeloma, successful neutrophil engraftment was achieved in all patients by day 15 and there was no significant difference between the two groups regarding platelet engraftment (85). However, a recent analysis of this trial failed to show improvement in progression-free survival or overall survival with CD34-positive cell selection, although the study may not have had sufficient power to detect such differences (85). The results of two other randomized studies have not been published yet, but preliminary results do not show any benefit for using CD34-positive-selected progenitor cells. Moreover, in both studies, the incidence of opportunistic infection appears greater in the CD34-positive -selected PBPC arm *(86–87)*.

Sensitive PCR techniques using patient-specific oligonucleotide primers show the persistence of myeloma cells in the CD34-positive cell fractions in some patients, whereas highly purified CD34-positive lin-thy 1-positive stem cells do no appear to contain clonal myeloma cells *(88)*. Thus, an additional purging step might be necessary to obtain tumor-free grafts. This approach could induce delayed hematopoietic and immunologic recovery, however, and would have uncertain effects on progression-free survival *(89)*.

Encouraging results have been obtained with negative selection using mono-clonal magnetic microbeads against CD19, CD56, and CD138 *(90)*. This approach warrants further evaluation. Currently, unselected PBPCs remain the standard source of stem cells for autologous transplant.

4.3. Single vs Double Transplant

One way to increase the rate of complete remission and, by inference, progres-sion-free survival could be to repeat intensive treatments. The IFM group was the first to explore this strategy. Unfortunately, the hematopoietic toxicity of the first course of dose-intensive therapy was severe in the absence of any hematopoietic support *(6)*. Thanks to autologous PBPC transplantation and hematopoietic growth factors, the use of two sequential courses of dose-intensive conditioning has become more feasible and appears to increase the rate of complete remission *(91,92)* and even induce molecular remission *(93)*.

The largest experience in this setting comes from the University of Arkansas *(94)*. Out of 495 patients enrolled to undergo 2 transplants, including 315 pre-treated patients, 95% completed the first course of 200 mg/m- of melphalan with blood SCT and 73% completed both courses of melphalan and both transplant procedures. The rate of complete remission increased from 24% after the first transplant to 43% after the second transplant. This experience has now been extended to more than 1000 patients *(95)*. However, the impact of tandem trans-plantations on progression-free and overall survival needs to be compared with the effects of less aggressive strategies.

In 1994, the IFM initiated such a randomized trial (IFM94) comparing one vs two autologous transplant procedures carried out between October 1994 and March 1997. The results of this trial have recently been published *(96)*. In this trial, 403 untreated patients aged less than 60 yr were enrolled by 45 centers *(97)*. At diagnosis, they were randomized to a single autologous transplant with melphalan 140 mg/m^2 and TBI (8 Gy) or a double transplant—the first prepared with melphalan 140 mg/m^2 and the second prepared with melphalan 140 mg/m^2 and TBI (8 Gy). After the initial cytoreduction with dexamethasone and infusional vincristine and doxorubicin (VAD), 343 patients who were eligible

Table 5
Single vs Double Autologous Stem Cell Transplantation
Results of the IFM94 Trial

	Single ASCT N = 199	p Value	Double ASCT N = 200
CR rate (%)	34		35
CR + VGPR rate (%)	42		50
Median EFS (mo)	25	0.03[a]	30
7-yr EFS (%)	10*		20
Median OS (mo)	48	0.02[a]	58
7-yr OS (%)	21		42

[a]log-rank test.

ASCT, autologus stem cell transplantation; CR, complete emission; VGPR, very good partial remission; EFS, event-free survival; OS, overall survival.

for a transplantation underwent a second randomization to PBPC vs bone marrow to support high-dose melphalan (140 mg/m^2) plus TBI. Because there was no difference in the outcome between the use of PBPC vs bone marrow, the results were pooled for comparison.

Overall, 399 patients were evaluable. Of the 199 patients assigned to the single autologous transplant arm, 177 (85%) received the planned transplant and 3 experienced a toxic death. Of the 200 patients randomized in the double transplant arm, 156 (78%) received two transplants and 5 experienced a toxic death.

There is no significant difference in the rate of complete remission between single and double autologous transplant (Table 5). However, with a median follow-up period of 6 yr, the median event-free survival and overall survival were superior in the double-transplant arm (Figs. 2 and 3). Further analysis showed the most benefit among patients who did not achieve a CR or very good partial response (>90% reduction in M-protein) from the first high-dose treatment.

Three other randomized trials have been conducted to compare the efficacy of one vs two autologous transplants (Table 6). With a median follow-up period of 53 mo, the French MAG95 group failed to observe any significant survival benefit with the double transplant (86). The Bologna group enrolled 358 patients and currently 220 patients are evaluable (97). The rate of complete remission was 39% in the double-transplant arm vs 30% in the single-transplant arm. With a median follow-up period of 38 mo, there was no difference in overall survival but a significant increase in median event-free survival in the double-transplant arm compared with the single-transplant arm (34 vs 25 mo). The Dutch group, which recruited 378 patients, observed a significant increase in 4-yr event-free survival (29 vs 15%) following a median 40-mo follow-up period, but no difference in overall survival (98). However, it should be noted that the survival curves in the

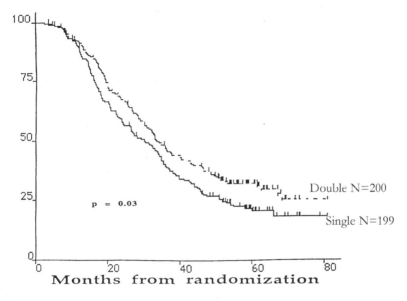

Fig. 2. IFM94 trial: Comparison of single vs double autotransplantation (intent-to-treat analysis)—event-free survival.

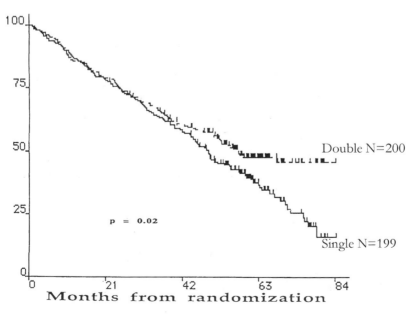

Fig. 3. IFM94 trial: Comparison of single vs double autotransplantation (intent-to-treat analysis)—overall survival.

Table 6
Single vs Double ASCT: Results of Multicenter Randomized Studies

Group/trial (reference)	No. of patients	Median follow-up	Results
IFM94 (96)	399	75 mo	Better EFS and OS[a]
Hovon (98)[b]	378	40 mo	Higher CR rate[a] and better EFS[a]
Bologna (97)[c]	220	38 mo	Better EFS[a]
MAG95 (86)[d]	227	53 mo	No significant difference

[a]in favor of the more intensive treatment arm
[b]2 × 70 mg/m melphalan + CTX-TBI/PBSCT
[c]200 mg/m melphalan/PBSCT + Bu-Mel/PBSCT
[d]VAD + HD chemo + TBI/PBSCT vs 140 mg/m Mel/PBSCT + HD chemo + TBI/PBSCT
EFS, event-free survival; OS, overall survival; CR, complete remission.

IFM94 trial separate only after 4 yr. Therefore, the median follow-up time of at least two of the studies is still short; a longer observation period is needed before any definite conclusion can be drawn.

From the only randomized study with mature data, we can conclude that double autologous transplant is:

1. Feasible in younger patients with newly diagnosed myeloma (78% of patients actually received two transplants).
2. Safe (only 3% of participants had a toxic death).
3. Significantly superior to single transplant in terms of event-free survival and overall survival.

However, improvement remains insufficient because the median survival in this series is only 58 mo and the 7-yr event-free survival is only 21%. The Royal Marsden Hospital group recently reported a 5.7-yr median survival in a large series of patients treated with a single autologous transplant prepared by 200 g/m- melphalan, with a second transplant at relapse in approx 25% of patients (99). They stated that this approach could yield results equal to those achieved with a double transplant, although their results may have been biased, which is suggested by the fact that 18% of patients were already in complete remission at the time of the transplant.

A key issue is to determine which patients will benefit more from a double transplant. The group at the University of Arkansas analyzed prognostic factors in a large series of patients treated with a double transplant and found several initial parameters to be associated with a poor outcome: high β_2-microglobulin or lactate dehydrogenase (LDH) levels, low albumin levels, hypodiploidy characterized by a chromosome-13 abnormality (detected by conventional cytogenetics) (95,100).

Survival

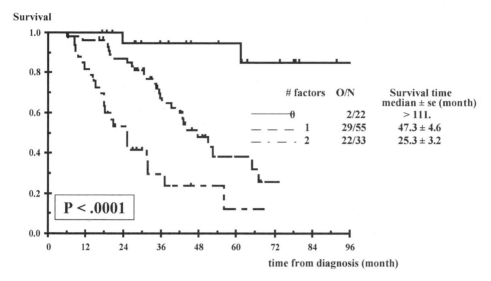

Fig. 4. Prognostic impact of (β_2 microglobulin level and chromosome 13 abnormalities (detected by FISH analysis)—overall survival. FISH, fluorescence *in situ* hybridization.

When these factors are combined, a subgroup of patients with a very poor prognosis can be identified *(100,101)*. Patients with high β_2-microglobulin (or low albumin) and with a chromosome-13 deletion have a short survival, even with tandem transplants (Fig. 4) *(102)*. For these patients, new therapies are clearly needed, e.g., the introduction of novel agents (e.g., thalidomide, bortezomib or CC-5013) for frontline therapy. On the other hand, patients with none of these unfavorable prognostic factors may achieve prolonged event-free survival and overall survival after a double autologous transplant with a potential curve plateau for 45% patients *(101,103)*.

In the IFM94 trial, the response to a single transplant was found to be of prognostic significance. In patients who achieved at least a very good partial remission, there was no apparent benefit to performing a second transplant. However, in patients with less than 90% of the M component remaining after the first transplant, survival was significantly longer in patients who received two transplants (Figs. 5 and 6).

The search for a better type of transplant continues. The availability of allogeneic transplantation as an option to treat patients with MM is limited in this patient population because of recipient age and the limited availability of histocompatible donors. Although registry studies continue to show a poor outcome from allogeneic transplants (i.e., a high risk for treatment-related complications) *(104)*, a variety of allogeneic strategies are currently under investigation, including allogeneic transplantation after a nonmyeloablative preparative regimen during the immediate post-autotransplant period *(105,106)*. Other options

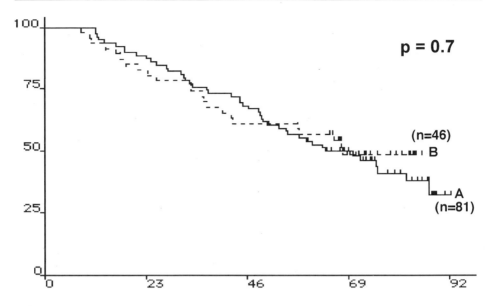

Fig. 5. IFM94 trial: overall survival if response to one autograft is at least 90%. (A) single transplant; (B) double transplant.

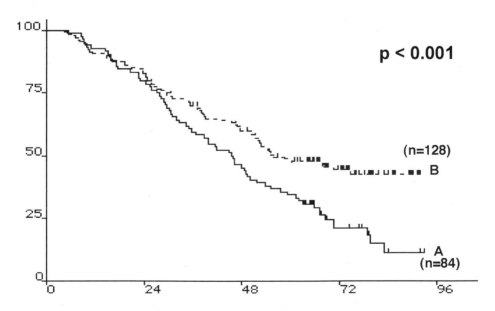

Fig. 6. IFM94 trial: overall survival if response to one autograft is less than 90%. (A) single transplant; (B) double transplant.

include maintenance therapy after autotransplant with an immunomodulatory agent, bisphosphonate, or some other agent. Given the high response rate and the likelihood of prolonged progression-free survival with relatively low treatment-related mortality, high-dose chemotherapy with some type of autograft support should be considered for patients with symptomatic MM who are aged 65 yr or younger.

REFERENCES

1. Buckner CD, Fefer A, Bensinger WI, et al. Marrow transplantation for malignant plasma cell disorders: summary of the Seattle experience. Eur J Haematol 1989; 51:185 190.
2. McElwain TJ, Powles RL. High-dose intravenous melphalan for plasma-cell leukaemia and myeloma. Lancet 1993; 822–824.
3. Barlogie B, Hall R, Zander A, et al. High-dose melphalan with autologous bone marrow transplantation for multiple myeloma. Blood 1986; 67:1298–1301.
4. Barlogie B, Alexanian R, Dicke K, et al. High-dose chemoradiotherapy and autologous bone marrow transplantation for resistant multiple myeloma. Blood 1987; 70:869–872.
5. Copeland EA, Tutschka PJ. Marrow transplantation following busulfan and cyclophosphamide in multiple myeloma. Bone Marrow Transplant 1988; 3:363–365.
6. Harousseau JL, Milpied N, Laporte JP, et al. Double-intensive therapy in high-risk multiple myeloma. Blood 1992; 79:2827–2833.
7. Gregory WM, Richards MA, Malpas JS. Combination chemotherapy versus melphalan and prednisolone in the treatment of multiple myeloma: an overview of published trials. J Clin Oncol 1992; 10:334–342.
8. Hjorth M, Hellquist L, Holmberg E, et al. Initial treatment in multiple myeloma: no advantage of multidrug chemotherapy over melphalan–prednisone. Br J Haematol 1990; 74:185–191.
9. Bladé J, San Miguel, Alcalá A, et al. Alternating combination VCMP/VBAP chemotherapy versus melphalan/prednisone in the treatment of multiple myeloma: a randomized multicentric study of 487 patients. J Clin Oncol 1993; 11:1165–1171.
10. Nimer S. Use a gentle approach for refractory myeloma patients. J Clin Oncol 1988; 6:757–758.
11. Gahrton G, Tura S, Ljungman P, et al for the European Group for Bone Marrow Transplantation. Allogeneic bone marrow transplantation in multiple myeloma. New Engl J Med 1991; 325:1267–1273.
12. Bjorkstrand BB, Ljungman P, Svensson H, et al. Allogeneic bone marrow transplantation vs. Autologous stem cell transplantation in multiple myeloma: a retrospective case-matched study from the European Group for Blood and Marrow Transplantation. Blood 1996; 88:4711–4718.
13. Bensinger WI, Buckner CD, Anasetti C, et al. Allogeneic marrow transplantation for multiple myeloma: an analysis of risk factors on outcome. Blood 88:2787–2793, 1996.
14. Attal M, Huguet F, Schlaifer D, et al. Intensive combined therapy for previously untreated aggressive myeloma. Blood 1992; 79:1130.
15. Jagannath S, Barlogie B, Dicke K, et al. Autologous bone marrow transplantation in multiple myeloma: identification of prognostic factors. Blood 1990; 76:1860–1866.
16. Fermand JP, Chevret S, Ravaud P, et al. High-dose chemoradiotherapy and autologous blood stem cell transplantation in multiple myeloma: results of a phase II trial involving 63 patients. Blood 1993; 82:2005–2009.
17. Schiller G, Vescio R, Freytes C, et al. Autologous CD34-selected peripheral blood progenitor cell transplantation for patients with advanced multiple myeloma. Bone Marrow Transplantation 1998; 21:141–145.

18. Marit G, Faberes C, Pico JL, et al. Autologous peripheral-blood progenitor-cell support following high-dose chemotherapy or chemoradiotherapy in patients with high-risk multiple myeloma. J Clin Oncol 1996; 14:1306–1313.

19. Bensinger WI, Rowley SD, Demirer T, et al. High-dose therapy followed by autologous hematopoietic stem-cell infusion for patients with multiple myeloma. J Clin Oncol 1996; 14:1447–1456.

20. Barlogie B, Jagannath S, Dixon DO, et al. High-dose melphalan and granulocyte-macrophage colony-stimulating factor for refractory multiple myeloma. Blood 1990; 76:677–680.

21. Nimer SD. High-dose melphalan for refractory myeloma—the M.D. Anderson experience. Hematol Oncol 1988; 6:167–172.

22. Buzaid AC, Durie BGM. Management of refractory myeloma: a review. J Clin Oncol 1988; 6:889–905.

23. Moreau P, Fiere D, Bezwoda WR, et al. Prospective randomized placebo-controlled study of granulocyte-macrophage colony-stimulating factor without stem-cell transplantation after high-dose melphalan in patients with multiple myeloma. J Clin Oncol 1997; 15:660–666.

24. Fermand JP, Levy Y, Gerota J, et al. Treatment of aggressive multiple myeloma by high-dose chemotherapy and total body irradiation followed by blood stem cells autologous graft. Blood 1989; 73:20–23. Bensinger WI, Buckner CD, Clift RA, et al. Phase I study of busulfan and cyclophosphamide in preparation for allogeneic marrow transplant for patients with multiple myeloma. J Clin Oncol 1992; 10:1492–1497.

25. Dimopoulos MA, Hester J, Huh Y, Champlin R, Alexanian R. Intensive chemotherapy with blood progenitor transplantation for primary resistant multiple myeloma. Br J Haematol 1994; 87:730–734.

26. Mansi J, da Costa F, Viner C, Judson I, Gore M, Cunningham D. High-dose busulfan in patients with myeloma. J Clin Oncol 1992; 10:1569–1573.

27. Surbone A, Armitage JO, Gale RP. Autotransplantation in lymphoma: better therapy or healthier patients? Ann Internal Med 1991; 114:1059–1060.

28. Bataille R, Harousseau JL. Multiple Myeloma [review]. New Engl J Med 1997; 36:1657–1664.

29. Harousseau JL, Attal M. The role of autologous hematopoietic stem cell transplantation in multiple myeloma. Semin Hematol 1997; 34 (suppl 1):61–66.

39. Harousseau JL, Attal M, Divine M, et al. Autologous stem cell transplantation after first remission induction treatment in multiple myeloma: a report of the French registry on autologous transplantation in multiple myeloma. Blood 1995; 85:3077–3085.

31. Gore ME, Viner C, Meldrum M, et al. Intensive treatment of multiple myeloma and criteria for complete remission. Lancet 1989; 879–881.

32. Alexanian R, Dimopoulos MA, Hester J, Delasalle K, Champlin R. Early myeloablative therapy for multiple myeloma. Blood 1994; 84:4278–4282.

33. Blade J, San Miguel JF, Fontanillas M, Alcala A, Maldonado J, Garcia-Conde J, et al. Survival of multiple myeloma patients who are potential candidates for early high-dose therapy intensification/autotransplantation and who were conventionally treated. J Clin Oncol 1996; 14:2167–2173.

34. Barlogie B, Jagannath S, Vesole D, Naucke S, Cheson B, Mattox S, et al. Superiority of tandem autologous transplantation over standard therapy for previously untreated multiple myeloma. Blood 1997; 89:789–793.

35. Lenhoff S, Hjorth M, Holmberg E, Turesson I, Westin J, Nielsen JL, et al. Impact of survival of high-dose therapy with autologous stem cell support in patients younger than 60 years with newly diagnosed multiple myeloma. Blood 2000; 95:7–11.

36. Palumbo A, Triolo S, Argentino C, et al. Dose intensive melphalan with stem-cell support is superior to standard treatment in elderly myeloma patients. Blood 1999; 94:1248–1253.

37. Attal M, Harousseau JL, Stoppa AM, et al. A prospective, randomized trial of autologous bone marrow transplantation and chemotherapy in multiple myeloma. N Engl J Med 1996; 335:91–97.
38. Fermand JP, Ravaud P, Katsahian S, et al. High dose therapy and autologous blood stem cell transplantation versus conventional treatment in multiple myeloma: results of a randomized trial in 190 patients 55 to 65 years of age [abstract]. Blood 1999; 94(suppl 1):396 a.
39. Blade J, Sureda A, Ribera JM, et al. High-dose therapy autotransplantation/intensification vs continued conventional chemotherapy in multiple myeloma in patients responding to initial treatment chemotherapy: results of a prospective randomized trial from the Spanish Cooperative Group PETHEMA [abstract]. Blood 2001; 98:815a.
40. Palumbo A, Bringhen S, Rus C, et al. A prospective randomized trial of intermediate dose melphalan (100 mg/m-) vs oral melphalan/prednisone: an interim analysis [abstract]. Blood 2001; 98:849a.
41. Child JA, Morgan GJ, Davies FE, et al. High dose chemotherapy with hematopoietic stem-cell rescue for multiple myeloma. N Engl J Med 2003; 348:1875–1883.
42. Fermand JP, Ravaud P, Chevret S, et al. High-dose therapy and autologous peripheral blood stem cell transplantation in multiple myeloma: up-front or resume treatment? Results of a multicenter sequential randomized clinical trial. Blood 1998; 92:3131–3136.
43. Reiffers J, Marit G, Boiron JM. Autologous blood stem cell transplantation in high risk multiple myeloma. Br J Haematol 1989; 72:296.
44. Jagannath S, Vesole DH, Glenn L, Crowley J, Barlogie B. Low-risk intensive therapy for multiple myeloma with combined autologous bone marrow and blood stem cell support. Blood 1992; 80:1666–1672.
45. Gianni AM, Sienna S, Bregni M, et al. Granulocyte-macrophage colony-stimulating factor to harvest circulating haematopoietic stem cells for autotransplantation. Lancet 1989; 8863:580.
46. Tarella C, Boccadoro M, Omede P, et al. Role of chemotherapy and GM-CSF on hemopoietic progenitor cell mobilization in multiple myeloma. Bone Marrow Transplantation 1993; 11:271–277.
47. Tricot G, Jagannath S, Vesole D, Nelson J, et al. Peripheral blood stem cell transplants for multiple myeloma: identification of favorable variables for rapid engraftment in 225 patients. Blood 1995; 85:588–596.
48. Marit G, Thiessard F, Faberes F, et al. Factors affecting both peripheral blood progenitor cell mobilization and hematopoietic recovery following autologous blood progenitor cell transplantation in patients with multiple myeloma: monocentric study. Leukemia 1998; 12:1447–1456.
49. Goldschmidt H, Hegenbart U, Haas R, et al. Mobilization of peripheral blood progenitor cells with high-dose cyclophosphamide (4 or 7 g/m2) and granulocyte colony stimulating factor in patients with multiple myeloma. Bone Marrow Transplantation 1996; 17:691–697.
50. Prince HM, Imrie K, Sutherland DR, et al. Peripheral blood progenitor cell collections in multiple myeloma: predictors and management of inadequate collections. Br J Haematol 1996; 93:142–145.
51. Kotasek D, Shepherd KM, Sage RE, et al. Factors affecting blood stem cell collections following high-dose cyclophosphamide mobilization in lymphoma, myeloma and solid tumors. Bone Marrow Transplantation 1992; 9:11–17.
52. Goldschmidt H, Hegenbart U, Wallmeier M, et al. Factors influencing collection of peripheral blood progenitor cells following high-dose cyclophosphamide and granulocyte-colony stimulating factor. Br J Haematol 1997; 98:736–744.
53. Mahé B, Milpied N, Hermouet S, et al. G-CSF alone mobilizes sufficient blood CD34+ cells for positive selection in newly diagnosed patients with myeloma and lymphoma. Br J Haematol 1996; 92:263–268.

54. Alegre A, Tomas JF, Martinez-Chamorro C, et al. Comparison of peripheral blood progenitor cell mobilization in patients with multiple myeloma : high-dose cyclophosphamide plus GM-CSF vs G-CSF alone. Bone Marrow Transplantation 1997; 20:211–221.

55. Celsing F, Hast R, Stenke L, Hansson H, Pisa P. Extramedullary progression of multiple myeloma following GM-CSF treatment: grounds for caution? Eur J Haematol 1992; 49:108.

56. Vora AJ, Cheng HT, Peel J, Greaves M. Use of granulocyte colony-stimulating factor G-CSF for mobilizing peripheral blood stem cells: risk of mobilizing clonal myeloma cells in patients with bone marrow infiltration. Br J Haematol 1994; 86:180–182.

57. Tricot G, Jagannath S, Desikan KR, et al. Superior mobilization of peripheral blood progenitors with r-metHuSCF and r-metHuG-CSF in heavily pretreated multiple myeloma patients [abstract]. Blood 1996; 83:388a.

58. Facon T, Harousseau JL, Maloisel F et al. Stem cell factor in combination with filgrastim after chemotherapy improves peripheral blood progenitor cell yield and reduces apheresis requirements in multiple myeloma: a randomized, controlled trial. Blood 1999; 94:1218–1225.

59. Bensinger W, Appelbaum F, Rowley S, et al. Factors that influence collection and engraftment of autologous peripheral blood stem cells. J Clin Oncol 1995; 10:2547–2555.

60. Siegel DS, Desikan KR, Nehta J, et al. Age is not a prognostic variable with autotransplants for multiple myeloma. Blood 1999; 93:51–54.

61. Badros A, Barlogie B, Siegel E, et al. Autologous stem cell transplantation in elderly multiple myeloma patients over the age of 70 years. Br J Haematol 2001; 114:600–607.

62. San Miguel J, Lahuerta JJ, Garcia-Sanz R, et al. Are myeloma patients with renal failure candidate for autologous stem cell transplantation. Hematol J 2000; 1:28–36.

62a. Barlogie B, Kyle R, Anderson K, et al. Comparable survival in multiple myeloma (MM) with high dose therapy (HDT) employing MEL 140 mg/m^2 + TBI 12 Gy autotransplants versus standard dose therapy with VBMCP and no benefit from interferon (IFN) maintenance: Results of Intergroup Trial S9321. Blood 2003; 102:abstract 135.

63. Badros A, Barlogie B, Siegel E, et al. Results of autologous stem cell transplant in multiple myeloma patients with renal failure. Br J Haematol 2001; 114:822–829.

64. Cunningham D, Paz-Ares L, Milan S, et al. High dose Melphalan and autologous bone marrow transplantation as consolidation in previously untreated myeloma. J Clin Oncol 1994; 12:759–763.

65. Moreau P, Facon T, Attal M, et al. Comparison of 200 mg/m^2 melphalan and 8 Gy total body irradiation plus 140 mg/m^2 as conditioning regimens for peripheral blood stem cell transplantation in patients with newly diagnosed multiple myeloma: final analysis of the IFM 95-02 randomized trial. Blood 2002; 99:731–735.

66. Goldschmidt H, Hegenbart U, Wallmeier M, et al. High-dose therapy with peripheral blood progenitor cell transplantation in multiple myeloma. Ann Oncol 1997; 8:243–246.

67. Bjorkstrand B, Svensson H, Goldschmidt H, et al. 5489 autotransplants in multiple myeloma: A registry from the EBMT [abstract]. Blood 1999; 94(suppl 1):714a.

68. Moreau P, Milpied N, Mahé B, et al. Melphalan 220 mg/m^2 followed by peripheral blood stem cell transplantation in 27 patients with advanced multiple myeloma. Bone Marrow Transplant 1999; 23:1000–1006.

69. Moreau P, Harousseau JL, Wijdenes J, Morineau N, Milpied N, Bataille R. A combination of anti-interleukin 6 murine monoclonal antibody with dexamethasone and high-dose melphalan induces high complete response rate in advanced multiple myeloma. Br J Haematol 2000; 109:661–664.

70. Giralt S, Bensinger W, Goodman M, et al. Ho-DOTMP plus melphalan by peripheral blood stem cell transplantation in patients with multiple myeloma: results of two phase I/II trials. Blood 2003; 102:2684–2691.

71. Lahuerta JJ, Grande C, Blade J, et al. Myeloablative treatments for multiple myeloma: update of comparative study of different regimens used in patients from the Spanish Registry for Transplantation in Multiple Myeloma. Leuk Lymph 2002; 43:67–74.
72. Billadeau O, Quam L, Thomas W, et al. Detection and quantification of malignant cells in the peripheral blood of multiple myeloma patients. Blood 1992; 80:1818–1824.
73. Bird JM, Bloxham D, Samson D. Molecular detection of clonally rearranged cells in peripheral blood progenitor cell harvests from multiple myeloma patients. Br J Haematol 1994; 88:110–116.
74. Corradini P, Voena C, Astolfi M, et al. High-dose sequential chemotherapy in multiple myeloma: residual tumor cells are detectable in bone marrow and peripheral blood cell harvests and after autografting. Blood 1995; 85:1596–1602.
75. Dreyfus F, Ribrag V, Leblond V, et al. Detection of malignant B cells in peripheral blood stem cell collections after chemotherapy in patients with multiple myeloma. Bone Marrow Transplant 1995; 15:707–711.
76. Anderson KC, Barut BA, Ritz J, et al. Monoclonal antibody-purged autologous bone marrow transplantation therapy for multiple myeloma. Blood 1991; 77:712–720.
77. Reece DE, Barnett MJ, Connors JM. Treatment of multiple myeloma with intensive chemotherapy followed by autologous BMT using marrow purged with 4-hydroxyperoxy cyclophosphamide. Bone Marrow Transplant 1993; 11:139–146.
78. Gobbi M, Cavo M, Tazzari PL, et al. Autologous bone marrow transplantation with immunotoxin-purged marrow for advanced multiple myeloma. Eur J Haematol 1989; 51:176–181.
79. Schiller G, Vescio R, Freytes C, et al. Transplantation of CD 34+ peripheral blood progenitor cell after high-dose chemotherapy for patients with advanced multiple myeloma. Blood 1995; 86:390–397.
80. Lemoli RM, Fortuna A, Motta MR, et al. Concomitant mobilization of plasma cells and hematopoietic progenitors into peripheral blood of multiple myeloma patients: positive selection and transplantation of enriched CD 34+ cells to remove circulating tumor cells. Blood 1996; 87:1625–1634.
81. Schiller G, Vesico R, Freytes C, et al. Autologous CD34- selected blood progenitor cell transplants for patients with multiple myeloma. Bonne Marrow Transplant 1998; 21:141–147.
82. Morineau N, Tang XW, Moreau P, et al. Lack of benefit of CD34+ cell selected over non-selected peripheral blood stem cell transplantation in multiple myeloma: results of a single center study. Leukemia 2000; 14:1815–1820.
83. Lemoli R, Martinelli G, Zamagni E, et al. Engraftment, clinical and molecular follow-up of patients with multiple myeloma who were reinfused with highly purified CD34+ cells to support single or tandem high-dose chemotherapy. Blood 2000; 95:2234–2239.
84. Vescio RA, Schiller G, Stewart K, et al. Multicenter phase III trial to evaluate CD 34+ selected versus unselected autologous peripheral blood progenitor cell transplantation in multiple myeloma. Blood 1999; 93:1858–1868.
85. Stewart AK, Vescio K, Schiller G, et al. Purging of autologous peripheral blood stem cells using CD34 selection does not improve overall or progression free survival after high-dose therapy for multiple myeloma: results of a multicenter randomized controlled trial. J Clin Oncol 2001; 198:3771–3779.
86. Fermand JP, Marolleau JP, Alberti C, et al. Single versus tandem high dose therapy supported with autologous stem cell transplantation using unselected or CD 34 enriched ABSC: preliminary results of a two by two designed randomized trial in 23 young patients with multiple myeloma [abstract]. Blood 2001; 98:815a.
87. Goldschmidt H, Bouko Y, Bourhis JH, et al. CD 34+ selected PBPCT results in an increased infective risk without prolongation of event free survival in newly diagnosed myeloma: a randomised study from the EBMT [abstract]. Blood 2000; 96:558a.

88. Gazitt Y, Reading CC, Hoffman R, et al. Purified CD 34+ Lin-thy + stem cells do not contain clonal myeloma cells. Blood 1995; 86:381–389.
89. Tricot G, Gazitt Y, Leemhuis S, et al. Collection, tumor contamination and engraftment kinetics of highly purified hematopoietic progenitor cells to support high dose therapy in multiple myeloma. Blood 1998; 91:4489–4495.
90. Barbui AM, Galli M, Dotti G, et al. Negative selection of peripheral blood stem cells to support a tandem autologous transplantation programme in multiple myeloma. Br J Haematol 2002; 116:202–210.
91. Vesole D, Barlogie B, Jagannath S, et al. High-dose therapy for refractory multiple myeloma: improved prognosis with better supportive care and double transplants. Blood 1994; 84:950–956.
92. Weaver CH, Zhen B, Schwartzberg LS, et al. Phase I-II evaluation of rapid sequence tandem high-dose melphalan with peripheral blood stem cell support in patients with multiple myeloma. Bone Marrow Transplant 1998; 22:245–251.
93. Bjorkstrand B, Ljungman P, Bird JM, et al. Double high-dose chemoradiotherapy with autologous stem cell transplantation can induce molecular remission in multiple myeloma. Bone Marrow Transplant 1995; 15:367–371.
94. Vesole D, Tricot G, Jagannath S, et al. Autotransplant in multiple myeloma: what have we learned? Blood 1996; 88:838–847.
95. Desikan R, Barlogie B, Sawyer J, et al. Results of high dose therapy for 1000 patients with multiple myeloma: durable complete remission and superior survival in the absence of chromosome 13 abnormalities. Blood 2000; 95:4008–4010.
96. Attal M, Harousseau JL, Facon T, et al. Single versus double autologous stem-cell transplantation for multiple myeloma. New Engl J Med. 2003; 349:2495–2502.
97. Cavo M, Zamagni E, Cellini C, et al. Single vs tandem autologous transplants in multiple myeloma : Italian experience [abstract]. Hematol J 2003; 4:S60.
98. Sonneveld P, Van der Holt B, Segeren CM, et al. Intensive versus double intensive therapy in untreated multiple myeloma: updated analysis of the prospective phase III study hovon 24MM [abstract]. Hematol J 2003; 4:S59.
99. Sirohi B, Powles R, Singhal S, et al. Long-term outcome of myeloma patients treated with an elective autograft with follow-up >5 years: results comparable to tandem autotransplantation [abstract]. Blood 2002; 100:179a.
100. Barlogie B, Jagannath S, Desikan KR, et al. Total therapy with tandem transplants for newly diagnosed multiple myeloma. Blood 1999; 93:66–75.
101. Facon T, Avet-Loiseau H, Guillerm G, et al. Chromosome 13 abnormalities identified by Fish analysis and serum β_2 microglobulin produce powerful myeloma staging system for patients receiving high-dose therapy. Blood 2001; 97:1566–1571.
102. Fassas A, Spencer T, Sawyer J, et al. Both hypodiploidy and deletion of chromosome 13 independently confer poor prognosis in multiple myeloma. Br J Haematol 2002; 118:1041–1047.
103. Tricot G, Spencer T, Sawyer J, et al. Predicting long-term (5 years) event-free survival in multiple myeloma patients following planned tandem autotransplants. Br J Haematol 2002; 116:211–217.
104. Bjorkstrand B. European Group for Blood and Marrow Transplantation Registry studies in multiple myeloma. Semin Hematol. 2001 38:219–225.
105. Kröger N, Schwerdtfeger R, Kiehl M, et al. Autologous stem cell transplantation followed by a dose-reduced allograft induces high complete remission rate in multiple myeloma. Blood 2002; 100:755–760.
106. Maloney DG, Molina AJ, Sahebi F, et al. Allografting with nonmyeloablative conditioning following cytoreductive autografts for the treatment of patients with multiple myeloma. Blood 2003; 102:3447–3454.

10 Allogeneic Transplantation in Multiple Myeloma

Gösta Gahrton, MD,
Kenneth C. Anderson, MD,
and William Bensinger, MD

1. INTRODUCTION

Allogeneic transplantation has proved to be the treatment of choice for many hematologic malignancies in patients younger than 50 to 55 yr. Randomized studies and studies based on the availability of a compatible donor have shown that allogeneic transplantation is superior to both autologous transplantation and conventional chemotherapy in patients with acute myeloblastic leukemia during the first remission *(1)*. Cures have apparently been obtained in approx 50 to 60% of patients with chronic myelocytic leukemia, a disease that so far has not been curable using any other treatment modalities *(2,3)*. Subgroups of patients with acute lymphoblastic leukemia *(4,5)*, chronic lymphocytic leukemia *(6,7)*, myelodysplastic syndrome *(8,9)*, and myelofibrosis *(10)* are also candidates for allogeneic transplantation.

From: *Current Clinical Oncology: Biology and Management of Multiple Myeloma*
Edited by: J. R. Berenson © Humana Press Inc., Totowa, NJ

Multiple myeloma (MM) accounts for somewhat more than 1% of new cancers *(11)*. The incidence is approx 4 out of 100,000 in the US population. The median age of patients with MM is approx 70 yr, and the fraction of patients under the age of 55 is approx 11% *(12)*. Thus, fewer than 1000 patients would be eligible for an allogeneic transplant in the United States every year. On a worldwide basis, however, this amount rises to several thousands of people.

The target malignant cell in MM is highly sensitive to both irradiation and alkylating agents, i.e., to the combination of treatment modalities typically used for conditioning before allogeneic transplantation in patients with other hematologic disorders. Furthermore, evidence has been provided in randomized studies that high-dose treatment followed by autologous transplantation is superior to conventional intermittent combination treatment, i.e., vincristine + melphalan + cyclophosphamide + prednisone (VMCP) alternating with carmustine + vincristine + doxorubicin + prednisone (BVAP) *(13)* or doxorubicin + carmustine + cyclophosphamide + melphalan *(14)*. Thus, high-dose treatment per se can improve the results. The advantage of using allogeneic stem cells over autologous stem cells is that the allogeneic graft could induce a graft-vs-myeloma effect *(15–17)* and may be free of contaminating myeloma cells that could be retransfused in the autologous setting. An early study showed that allogeneic B cells could be engrafted in a patient with myeloma *(18)*. Additionally, two small series of myeloma transplants, published independently by the Bologna *(19)* and Huddinge *(20)* groups, appeared promising. One of the Huddinge patients was a 47-yr-old woman who had been treated for 6 yr with conventional melphalan and prednisolone therapy. She was considered resistant to other types of treatment and received an allogeneic transplant in 1983. Four years after the transplant procedure, she was still in complete remission, with no signs of myeloma, and was thought to be cured. However, shortly thereafter she had a relapse, but survived with a slowly progressing disease and died 12 yr after the transplant. One of the patients in the Bologna study was still in complete remission 13 yr after the transplant. Following these promising reports, the European Group for Blood and Marrow Transplantation (EBMT) established a registry for patients who underwent allogeneic transplantation for multiple myeloma. Presently, more than 2000 patients have been reported to the registry. The International Bone Marrow Transplant Registry (IBMTR) has reports on 2216 patients (M. Horowitz, personal communication), but it includes a relatively large number of patients previously reported to the EBMT registry. The Seattle group has performed 180 transplants that have not been reported to either the EBMT or IBMTR. Thus, the total number of allogeneic transplants can only roughly be estimated at 4000 to 5000, including those that were not reported to either registry.

2. CONDITIONING

The regimens used to condition patients for allogeneic transplantation do not differ significantly from procedures used for other hematologic malignancies. The most common conditioning regimen reported to the EBMT registry is cyclophosphamide with total body irradiation (TBI), according to the usual Seattle protocol *(21)*: cyclophosphamide (60 mg/kg ^{2}) plus TBI 10–12 Gy unfractionated or fractionated and with or without lung shielding to approx 9 Gy. However, there are numerous variants of these regimens, e.g., somewhat lower doses of cyclophosphamide or TBI and variants in the fractionation. Also, regimens combining TBI and melphalan (usually 140 mg/m^2) have been used. In a small series of patients, 110 to 120 mg/m^2 of melphalan in combination with TBI 12 Gy divided in 6 fractions was used *(22)*, with promising results. The addition of other cytotoxic drugs—e.g., bleomycin + camustine (BCNU) and N-(2-chloroethyl)-N'-cyclohexyl-N-nitrosurea (CCNU), as well as etoposide—has also been attempted. No particular regimen appears to be superior in terms of response rates or outcome *(23,24)*.

The Seattle group has used busulfan and cyclophosphamide in most of their patients *(25,26)*. However, their results appear to be comparable to those reported to the EBMT registry. In a study by Cavo and colleagues *(27)*, 19 patients were conditioned with busulfan (16 mg/kg) and cyclophosphamide (200 mg/kg). Of these, 42% entered complete remission, and the overall survival and event-free survival rates at 4 yr were 26 and 21%, respectively. Four patients were in complete remission 54, 66, 80, and 94 mo after the transplant. These results are similar to those reported to the EBMT registry, as well as those presented by the Seattle group.

Low-dose conditioning (i.e., with the use of reduced intensity or nonmyeloablative regimens) has been used with increasing frequency during the last few years *(28,29)*. Interest in reduced-intensity regimens is a result of the historically high transplant-related morbidity and mortality associated with high-intensity preparative regimens. In addition, because of relatively high complications rates, allogeneic transplants have historically been offered only to patients aged 50 to 55 yr or less and who have human lymphocyte antigen (HLA)-matched family members. In practice, this limits the utility of allografting to fewer than 5% of patients with MM. A significant reduction in transplant-related complications could result in the increased applicability of this potentially curative technique.

Reduced-intensity regimens are designed to provide a greater degree of immunosuppression than cytoreduction to allow engraftment of donor hematopoetic stem cells. This technique relies on the well-known graft-vs-myeloma effect to eliminate residual disease. In studies of transplantation in dogs, Storb and coworkers found that conditioning with 200 cGy TBI was enough to promote engraftment *(30)*, although in clinical trials, graft rejection occurred in several

Table 1
Nonmyeloablative Allografting for Multiple Myeloma.

Reference	N	Auto	Donors	Regimen	TM, n	CR n	2yOS, %	EFS, %
35	54	Plan	FM	F,TBI	9	31	70	54
36	22	1-2 fail	FM/URD	F,Cy,TBI,A	5	6	26	22
37	20	None	FM/URD	F,M,Cm	3	2	71	30
38	22	9 fail	FM/URD	F,M	9	7	30	19
39	45	12plan	FM/URD	M	17	29	36[a]	13*
40	17	Plan	FM/URD/MM	F,M,A	2	12	74	56
41	21	9-Plan	URD	F,M,A	5	8	74	53

[a]3-yr follow-up

TM, transplant mortality; CR, complete response; 2yOS, overall survival at 2 yr; EFS, event-free survival at 2 yr; FM, family member; F, fludarabine; TBI, total body irradiation (2 Gy); URD, unrelated donor, Cy, cyclophosphamide; A, antithymocyte globulin; Cm, campath; M, melphalan; MM, mismatched donor.

patients with myeloma *(31)*. It was later shown that of TBI using 200 cGy combined with fludarabine 30 mg/m^2 for 3 to 5 d promoted engraftment and only occasional rejections were seen. Other so-called nonmyeloablative regimens have included melphalan + fludarabine, cyclophosphamide + fludarabine + TBI, busulfan + ATG, melphalan + CAMPATH, and busulfan + cyclophosphamide. Donors have included both matched family members and matched unrelated volunteers. Reduced-intensity allogeneic transplants have been utilized as therapy following initial treatment with conventional therapy after relapse from conventional therapy. The transplant-related mortality after reduced-intensity regimens, while lower than that seen with full-dose regimens, is still in the range of 10 to 30%. Response rates of 10 to 55% have been reported. Recently, a tandem strategy has been developed that relies on the cytoreductive effect of an autograft while separating the acute toxicities caused by high-dose chemotherapy from complications associated with an allogeneic transplant. Recently, results of a multicenter study have been reported *(31a)*. Complete remission was observed in more than half of patients, but rates of treatment-related mortality and chronic graft-vs-host disease remained high. Longer studies to evaluate this approach further are now being conducted.

These and other phase II studies show that engraftment as well as remissions can be obtained with low-dose nonmyeloablative conditioning in both previously untreated and refractory patients *(31,32–41)* (Table 1). Preliminary results suggest that remissions and survival are of longer duration in patients with responsive disease who achieve at least a partial response to conventional chemotherapy or who have had a planned autologous transplant. In contrast, relatively

Table 2
Complete Remission (CR) Following Allogeneic Transplantation

Author (reference)	Method to claim abscence of monoclonal Immunoglobulin	Bone marrow plasma cells	Required duration of response to claim CR	CR overall
Gahrton et al. (23,24)	Conventional electrophoresis or immunofixation	No apparent myeloma cells <5% plasma cells	None	54%
Alyea et al. (42,43)	Immunofixation	<5% plasma cells	3 mo	33%
Bensinger et al. (25,26)	Immunofixation	<5% plasma cells	None	35%

few patients who receive reduced-intensity allografts following a failed autologous transplant achieve a durable remission. Further follow-up will be required to confirm these observations.

3. DEFINITION OF RESPONSE

Response rates to allogeneic transplantation vary with the criteria used to define "response." In EBMT studies, the definition of a complete remission has been the disappearance of monoclonal immunoglobulin in serum or light chains in urine, based on the results of conventional electrophoresis or immunofixation, as well as the absence of myeloma cells in the marrow (23,24). This definition was originally practical, because none of the centers within the EBMT performed immunofixation to determine remission. Thus, some of the patients might have had a complete remission by conventional electrophoresis but would not have fulfilled the criteria if immunofixation had been done. Although immunofixation has been used with increased frequency in EBMT centers, however, there has been no apparent difference in complete remission rates in patients who received a transplant before 1990 vs those who receiving one thereafter. Partial remission has been defined as a reduction in monoclonal immunoglobulins or light chains by 25% or more; a decrease of less than 25% has been reported as "no response" or "no change." An increase in immunoglobulin level by 25% or more has been used to define "progressive disease."

The Seattle group has required a negative immunofixation to claim a complete remission, which might be the reason for their seemingly lower rate of complete remission than that seen in EBMT studies (25,26) (Table 2). This also applies to studies conducted at the Dana Farber Cancer Institute, where a complete remission is defined by a negative immunofixation (42,43) (Table 2).

None of the groups performing allogeneic transplants have defined complete remission on the basis of polymerase chain reaction (PCR) findings. Limited studies using this technique to detect monoclonal myeloma cells in bone marrow indicate that not all patients who have receive an allogeneic transplant and enter complete remission (defined by immunofixation) are PCR-negative Thus, the complete remission rate would be even lower if it were based on the finding of a PCR-negative marrow. Also, the sensitivity of this technique varies. The "fingerprinting" technique using VH family primers detects one monoclonal cell in 10^3 to 10^4 normal cells, and the use of patient-specific primers detects one monoclonal cell in 10^5 to 10^6 normal ones *(44)*.

It is obvious that the criteria used to define response used previously for patients treated with conventional therapy are not useful for defining complete remission or a complete response following allogeneic or autologous transplantation. For this reason, representatives of the three main registries for transplantation—the EBMT, IBMTR, and ABMTR—have united to propose criteria to be used to define response, relapse, and progression in patients with MM who are treated with high-dose therapy and stem cell transplantation *(45)*. Briefly, immunofixation is required for the definition. The original monoclonal paraprotein should be absent for a minimum of 6 wk, and less than 5% of the cells in a marrow aspirate or a trephine biopsy should be plasma cells. No increase in the size or number of lytic bone lesions is allowed. The criteria for partial remission are a reduction in monoclonal paraprotein of more than 50% that is maintained for a minimum of 6 wk. In Bence-Jones MM, the light-chain excretion in 24-h urine should either be reduced by more than 90% or to less than 200 mg maintained for a minimum of 6 wk.

Progressive disease is defined by an increase of 25% or more in the serum monoclonal paraprotein level, which must represent an absolute increase by at least 5 g/L and confirmed by at least one repeated investigation. The urinary 24-h excretion of light chains must increase by more than 25% and represent an absolute increase of at least 200 mg/24 h, which is confirmed by at least one repeated test. Plasma cells must have increased by 25%, and by a value of at least 10% of total nucleated cells in the marrow.

The definition also includes detailed proposals to define minimal response, relapse, plateau, and how to assess nonsecretory myeloma as well as plasmacytoma.

Current results may not be based on all of these criteria, although most EBMT centers in recent years seem to have followed them relatively well. Future studies will be based entirely on these proposed changes. Pretransplant response status is defined by the common response criteria for conventional chemotherapy.

Based on current response criteria, complete responses were obtained in approx 50% of the patients in previous EBMT registry studies. In the most recent study, a complete hematologic response was seen in more than 50% of the patients at 6 mo and approx 60% of the patients at 2 yr following transplantation (Table 3) *(46)*.

Table 3
Complete Remission Following Allogeneic Bone Marrow Transplantation

Response status before transplantation	No. of patients	No. and % in CR after transplantation	
CR	50	49	98%
PR	202	106	52%
NC	41	10	24%
PD	20	5	25%

CR, complete remission; PR, partial emission; NC, no change; PD, progressive disease. (From ref. *46*.)

Complete responses were lower in both the Dana Farber Cancer Institution experience *(43,44)* and the Seattle studies *(25,26)*, i.e., 33 and 35%, respectively; as mentioned above. However the difference may be associated with a stricter definition of complete response at those institutions. The complete remission rate following transplantation was dependent on the pretransplant response status and the number of treatment regimens that were given before transplantation. There was also a tendency for a better response in women and in patients who had been diagnosed at stage I, irrespective of the stage at the time of transplantation. Differences owing to gender, and stage of disease were not significant.

4. OVERALL SURVIVAL: PROGNOSTIC FACTORS

Overall survival has improved dramatically in EBMT studies conducted from 1994 compared with the results observed between 1983 and 1993*(46)*. The overall 4-yr survival was only 32% before 1994, but rose to 50% from 1994 to 1998 (Fig. 1). Several factors explain this improvement. During the later time period, patients were given a transplant earlier in the course of the disease. They also received fewer treatment regimens before the transplant, and more effective antibacterial and antiviral drugs were used both for the treatment and prevention of transplant-related complications. This has decreased transplant-related mortality (Fig. 2) and improved the overall survival rate.

As in previous studies, an important prognostic factor is the gender of the patient, i.e., women have a better outcome than men *(23,24,46)*. Another important pretransplant prognostic factor is the number of treatment regimens before transplant: patients who receive only one treatment regimen have a better outcome than those who receive two or more prior treatments. Patients with a low β_2-microglobulin level have a better outcome than patients with a high β_2-microglobulin, and patients who have progressive disease at the time of transplantation have a worse outcome than other response groups; in contrast, patients who had a complete response at the time of transplantation have the best outcome.

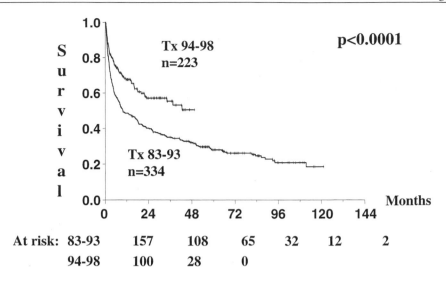

Fig. 1. Actuarial survival after bone marrow transplantation according to time periods. The Kaplan–Meier curves show a significantly better survival for patients who received the transplant during the period 1994 to 1998 as compared with the period 1983 to 1993. (Reproduced with permission from ref. 46.)

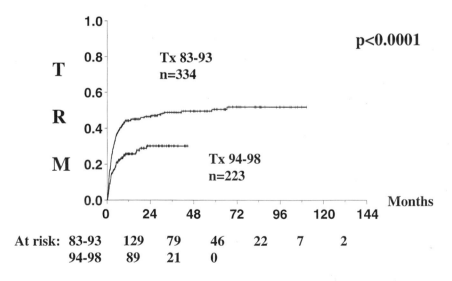

Fig. 2. Transplant related mortality according to the time period of transplantation. The Kaplan–Meier curves show a significantly lower transplant-related mortality in patients who received the transplant during the period of 1994 to 1998 compared with the period of 1983 to 1993. (Reproduced with permission from ref. 46.)

The stage at diagnosis, irrespective of the stage at the time of transplantation, tends to be a favorable prognostic factor, but the difference between stages is not statistically significant. A previous multivariate analysis of factors in patients with full reports (MED-Bs, which are later, more complete reports, in contrast to MED-As, which are early reports with relatively few variables) show that age is the most important prognostic factor, followed by gender and types of treatment before transplant. If all the information available on patients that was reported on MED-As was utilized, the number of treatment regimens before transplant could not be analyzed, because this parameter is not included in the MED-A report form. Only gender, donor–recipient relationship, response to treatment before transplant, age at transplant, and the time from diagnosis to transplant were included. Again, being a woman was the most important prognostic factor, followed by the donor–recipient relationship (with female-to-male having the worst outcome and female-to-female the best), then response status just before transplant (with patients who were in complete remission prior to the transplant having the best outcome while those with progressive disease having the worst). Age at transplant was the fourth most important factor, with younger patients (age <37 yr) having a better outcome. Time from diagnosis to transplant was not an independent prognostic factor.

In the EBMT studies, it has not been possible to detect procedural factors of prognostic importance. Attempts have been made to find conditioning regimens that would be superior to TBI + cyclophosphamide. However, the overall survival did not differ because of different treatment regimens, i.e., TBI + cyclophosphamide, TBI + melphalan, busulfan + cyclophosphamide (BuCy), or melphalan alone. However, the reports do not contain data that makes it possible to evaluate dosages or TBI fractionation data in such comparisons. Graft-vs-host disease (GVHD) is an important prognostic factor, i.e., patients with GVHD grade III or IV had worse outcomes than patients with a lower GVHD grade, and there was no significant difference between patients who did not have GVHD and those with grade I GVHD. Although T-cell depletion resulted in significantly fewer patients with severe GVHD (grade III or IV), it was not possible to detect a difference in the overall survival of patients who had received T-cell depletion for GVHD prevention compared with those who had received other treatment methods, including cyclosporine alone, cyclosporine + methotrexate, or cyclosporine + prednisolone. These observations held, regardless of whether T-cell depletion was used without further GVHD prevention or whether it was combined with cyclosporine or other GVHD prevention methods. This may be the result of higher rates of relapse with a T-cell depleted graft.

A comparison of patients who achieved complete remission and those who did not obtain complete remission but underwent engraftment indicated a significantly superior survival rate for those who entered a complete remission (Fig. 3).

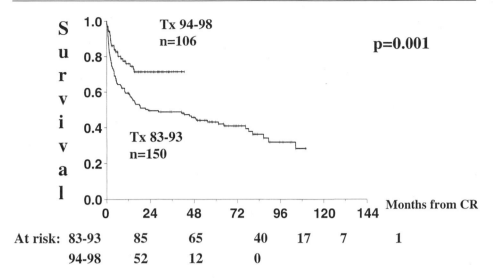

Fig. 3. Actuarial survival after bone marrow transplantation according to the response to transplantation. The Kaplan–Meier curves show significantly better survival among patients who entered complete remission after engraftment than among those who did not. (Reproduced with permission from ref. *46*.)

Patients who underwent transplantation during the time period of 1994 to 1998 and entered complete remission had a 3-yr overall survival rate of 70%; the 10-yr overall survival rate is now more than 20%.

In earlier studies, the transplant-related mortality (TRM) was high overall and significantly higher in men than in women *(23,24)*. For men, the TRM was 51% at 2 yr, whereas in women it was 34%. Since 1994, the reduction in treatment-related mortality has been significant, with an overall rate of 21% at 6 mo and 30% at 2 yr. Although the TRM is still high, it is now similar to that seen in patients with many other types of hematologic disorders.

The overall relapse rate for patients in complete remission was 36% at 3 yr and 50% at 6 yr. Later relapses did occur; there was no clear plateau in the relapse curve, and no clear improvement has been seen since 1994.

The Seattle group has performed allogeneic transplants in 80 patients *(26)*, but only 21% of them had chemotherapy-sensitive disease. All of them received busulfan and cyclophosphamide, with or without TBI with lung and liver shielding. The complete remission rate was 35%, the probability of survival at 5 yr was 20%, and the progression-free survival rate was 16%. For patients who entered a complete remission, the relapse-free survival at 5 yr was 33%. As in the EBMT study, the total TRM was high (56%). Late TRM was 15% due to chronic GVHD and infection.

The Dana Farber Cancer Institute has taken a somewhat different approach to that of the EBMT and Seattle groups *(43,44)*. Sixty-six patients received T-cell–

depleted (CD6) marrow from histocompatible sibling donors *(44)*. The median age of these patients was 45 yr, and they included 9 with stage IA disease, 17 with stage IIA, 23 with stage IIIA, 12 with stage IIIB, and 5 patients with plasmacytomas. Twenty-eight percent of the patients entered a complete remission. The overall and progression-free survival rates were 51 and 28% at 2 yr and 39 and 18% at 4 yr, respectively. At 4 yr, the cumulative incidence of nonrelapse-related mortality was 24% and the relapse incidence was 46%. The causes of nonrelapse, treatment-related mortality was mainly infectious complications and GVHD, which accounted for 24 and 7% of treatment failures, respectively. These results corroborate relatively well with EBMT and Seattle results. Therefore, it is not clear whether T-cell depletion will result in better survival than other GVHD prevention methods.

The results of the Bologna group *(27)* also corroborate those reported previously by the EBMT group *(24)*, the Seattle group *(25,26)*, and the Dana Farber group *(43)*. TRM is high in all these studies (approx 24–40%), but their patients include long-term survivors who have been without signs of disease for more than 10 yr.

The Hammersmith group has studied the results of PCR analyses to identify minimal residual disease *(47)*. Among 11 patients who entered complete remission by EBMT criteria, 8 were PCR-positive shortly after transplantation, but 7 were in molecular remission within 12 mo and another 3 achieved complete remission without further therapy. Only 1 patient died without having achieved molecular remission. Two additional patients died in complete remission, one of them with pneumonitis and the other with cancer of the esophagus.

In one study, Corradini and colleagues *(48)*, used patient-specific primers to carry out molecular analyses in two groups: one consisting of patients who had received an allogeneic transplant and the other consisting of patients who had received an autologous transplant. The frequency of molecular remission tended to be higher in the allogeneic group than in the autologous group. Recently, Corradini studied 70 patients who had received an allogeneic transplant. Clone-specific molecular markers were successfully generated in 48 of them. PCR analysis results were negative in 35 patients in this group (73%), and this negative result persisted throughout the follow-up period in 16 (33%). The PCR analysis results were positive in 13 patients (27%); the positive results persisted throughout follow-up. The cumulative incidence of relapse at 5 yr was 0% in patients with a persistently negative PCR test and 100% in patients with a persistently positive PCR test; it was 33% in those with a mixed pattern *(49)*.

The results of allogeneic transplantation using reduced conditioning are still inconclusive (Table 1). Crawly recently made a survey of patients who had received such transplants in EBMT centers *(33)*. Data were obtained on 256 patients from 38 centers; 194 of whom had received a matched sibling donor transplant and 40 of whom had received transplant from a matched but unrelated donor. A large fraction of the patients were heavily pretreated—the median time from diagnosis to transplant was 20 mo—and 29% of the patients had progressive disease. Conditioning regimens varied, but were claimed by the reporting centers to be non myeloablative or low dose. Peripheral blood stem cells were used with 205 of the transplants. Despite this relatively poor prognosis, the 1-yr treatment related mortality was only 23.5% and the 2-yr, only 26%. At 2 yr, the overall and progression-free survival rates were 50 and 39%, respectively. The prognostic parameters seemed mainly the same as for those given full-dose conditioning. The 2-yr survival in patients in complete or partial remission prior to transplant was encouraging (74%).

Other studies using nonmyeloablative conditioning seem to corroborate these findings, i.e., that transplant-related mortality is lower when reduced conditioning is used. Longer follow-up and comparative studies are warranted to determine whether nonmyeloablative regimens will result in better overall and long-term survival rates than are seen with conventional myeloablative regimens or autologous transplantation—single or double.

5. GVHD

GVHD is an important cause of death in patients with MM. In the early EBMT registry study (24), 63% of the patients developed GVHD; of these, 32% had grade I, 21% had grade II, 5% had grade III, and 5% had grade IV disease. Patients with GVHD grade III or IV had an extremely poor survival. T-cell depletion diminished the number of patients with severe GVHD; unfortunately, however T-cell depletion did not improve survival rates compared with those seen in patients treated with other GVHD prevention modalities.

Alyea and colleagues (42,43) used T-cell depletion in 66 patients who were sensitive to conventional chemotherapy before the transplant. The T cells were depleted from the allogeneic bone marrow using CD6 monoclonal antibodies and complement lysis. They did not use any other form of GVHD prevention treatment in these patients. Only 4% of the patients had grade III and 17% had grade II GVHD. These figures are favorable compared with the frequency of GVHD following other treatment modalities and similar to those that have been obtained in T-cell depleted patients in the EBMT registry. Thus, GVHD may be diminished by T-cell depletion or perhaps by positive selection of CD34-positive cells. Thus far, however, improved survival rates have not been shown using such methods.

6. GRAFT-VS-MYELOMA EFFECT: DONOR LYMPHOCYTE TRANSFUSIONS

In the EBMT data, attempts have been made to detect a graft-vs-myeloma effect by relating outcome to the degree of GVHD (23,24). Patients with grade I GVHD did not appear to perform better than those with grade 0. The difficulty in finding such an effect may in part be due to the heterogeneity of the patients. However, it has been shown that donor lymphocyte infusion (DLI) may result in a new remission or decrease in monoclonal immunoglobulin *(15–17,42,43,50,51)*.

Alyea and colleagues *(42)* used prophylactic CD4-positive DLI 6 to 9 mo after transplantation in 14 out of 24 patients who received CD6 T-cell-depleted marrow as the sole GVHD preventive method. Three patients were in complete response and 11 had persistent disease before infusion. Significant graft vs myeloma responses were noted after DLI in 10 patients with persistent disease and resulted in six complete responses and four partial responses. After DLI, 50% of the patients developed acute GVHD of grade II or greater or extensive chronic GVHD. The 2-yr estimated overall survival and progression-free survival rates for all 24 patients were 55 and 42%, respectively. The 14 patients who received DLI appeared to have an improved 2-yr survival rate compared with historical controls. Although only 58% of patients were able to receive DLI, despite T-cell depletion, the investigators concluded that DLI may be a valuable treatment method to use after transplantation, but should probably be combined with less toxic conditioning regimens.

Orsini and colleagues studied the mechanisms of the DLI effect *(51–53)*. By repeated analysis of the T-cell repertoire, using PCR amplification of 24 V_β gene families over at least 1 yr, the appearance of clonal T-cell populations was demonstrated in four patients. Some clones were noted within the first 3 mo after DLI and coincided with decreasing levels of monoclonal paraprotein, indicating an ongoing graft-vs-myeloma effect. Other clones appeared later and coincided with GVHD *(52)*. Recently, these investigators showed that the graft-vs-myeloma effect of DLI is probably mediated by donor-derived CD8 T-cell clones with anti-myeloma specificity that are present in the patient before DLI is administered. In contrast, T-cell clones associated with GVHD are expanded de novo after DLI *(53)*. These study findings indicate that it might be possible to develop an anti-myeloma cell therapy that does not result in GVHD.

7. ALTERNATIVE DONORS

Only a few patients with MM have received marrow from matched unrelated donors following myeloablative conditioning. In the EBMT registry, only six such alternative-donor transplants have been analyzed—three from HLA-mismatched related donors and three from HLA-matched unrelated donors. Five of the six patients died fewer than 75 d after the transplant. Only one patient survived more than 200 d after the transplant *(54)*.

The Seattle group has performed 26 transplants with alternative donors *(55)*. Of these, 12 were related donors, either with 1 antigen mismatch (*n* = 8) or 2 antigen mismatches (*n* = 4). Death from GVHD (*n* = 1), regimen-related toxicity ($n = 3$), and hemorrhage ($n = 1$) occurred in five of eight recipients mismatched for one HLA antigen. One patient died from progressive disease, but two out of eight patients survived disease-free for 7 and 8.5 yr after transplantation. Among the four recipients who received related marrow mismatched for two HLA antigens, two died of transplant-related complications and one of progressive disease; one is surviving disease-free 3 yr after the transplant.

Fourteen patients have received marrow from matched unrelated donors: 12 fully HLA-matched and 2 with a minor mismatch. Ten of the 12 HLA-matched recipients died because of GVHD ($n = 3$), regimen-related toxicity ($n = 3$), infection ($n = 3$), or progressive disease at 3 yr ($n = 1$). Two of the 12 HLA-matched recipients survived 1.5 and 7 yr after transplantation. One of 2 recipients of marrow from HLA-mismatched donors survived disease-free for 2 yr.

The Vancouver group has reported seven patients who received HLA-mismatched marrow from relatives ($n = 3$) or matched unrelated donors ($n = 5$) *(56)*. GVHD of grades II, III, or IV developed in all seven recipients and was the cause of death in two of them. Two patients died of chronic GVHD, and one patient died from disease progression. Only two of the seven patients survived; one was in partial remission at 4 mo and the other was in complete remission at 30 mo.

Most of the patients who received myeloablative conditioning allografts from matched unrelated donors or nonmatched related donors had been in an advanced stage of disease. Only few patients have received such allogeneic transplants so far; therefore, it is difficult to evaluate the results. An increasing number of patients have received allografts from unrelated donors after reduced-intensity conditioning. At least six studies have reported the results of using reduced-intensity regimens prior to transplants from matched unrelated donors (Table 1). Preliminary reports indicate 2-yr survival rates in the range of 26 to 74%. Longer follow-up is required for reliable conclusions. Matched unrelated transplants should therefore be done only in centers that have study protocols for allogeneic transplantation in MM.

8. PERIPHERAL BLOOD STEM CELL TRANSPLANTATION

Peripheral blood stem cell transplantation (PBSCT) is being used with increasing frequency for allogeneic transplantation *(57)*. As in autologous transplantation procedures, the time to engraftment is shorter if patients receive peripheral blood stem cells instead of marrow cells *(46,57–59)* Chronic GVHD appears to occur frequently and perhaps more severely following PBSCT *(60,61)*, but acute GVHD seems to occur at a similar rate *(46,60,61)*. The Bologna group reported a small series of patients with very low TRM *(62)*. In the EBMT registry, however, several hundred patients have received an allogeneic transplant with peripheral blood stem cells. Transplant-related mortality was not reduced and survival rates were not improved with bone marrow in the recently published study *(39)*, but later follow-up seems to indicate a marginally better survival with bone marrow. In a recent study, 30 patients with multiple myeloma received a high-dose busulfan and melphalan regimen followed by allogeneic peripheral blood cells from matched family members *(63)*. These were not all low-risk patients, given that 50% were considered treatment-resistant and 10 had a prior failed autologous transplant. Transplant-related mortality in this study was 30%, but 71% achieved complete remission. The overall survival and event-free survival rates at 6 yr were 60 and 67%, respectively. These encouraging results are at least as good as those achieved in much earlier studies using reduced-intensity regimens. Further studies are underway to clarify this point.

9. ALLOGENEIC TRANSPLANTATION VS AUTOLOGOUS TRANSPLANTATION

A comparison of allogeneic vs autologous transplantation has been made utilizing patients reported to the EBMT registry *(64)*. These patients had been matched primarily for the most important prognostic factors for allogeneic transplantation—sex and the number of treatment regimens before transplantation. A total of 189 allogeneic transplant recipients were compared with the same number of matched autotransplant recipients. Except for the median age—which was somewhat lower in the allotransplant group (43 yr) than in the autotransplant group (49 yr)—a cross-match showed well-matched prognostic factors. However, the follow-up period was shorter for the autotransplant group than for the allotransplant group, because autotransplantation did not start until 1986, whereas allotransplantation was started in 1983.

The complete remission rate and time from transplant to complete remission were similar for the two groups. The most striking difference was a higher TRM in the allogeneic transplant group compared with the autologous transplant group (41 vs 13%, respectively), which resulted in a significantly better median overall survival rate for the autologous transplant group than for the allogeneic transplant group (34 vs 18 mo, respectively). However at 4 yr and 6 yr from transplant, the fraction of surviving patients was similar. Further studies showed that the main reason for this difference was a higher TRM in allotransplanted men, and a lower difference in TRM among women between the two groups. Thus, the overall survival rate did not differ significantly after allotransplantation compared with autotransplantation in women.

The relapse rate for patients who achieved complete remission was significantly lower following allogeneic transplantation than following autologous transplantation. However, this did not result in a significant survival advantage for these patients, although there was a slight tendency for a better long-term survival in the allotransplanted patient group (50% vs 39%).

The higher TRM after allogeneic transplant was associated not only with GVHD, but also with a higher frequency of other complications, e.g., bacterial infections and veno-occlusive disease (VOD). However, there is no clear explanation for the higher TRM among men compared with women in the allotransplant group.

The difference in relapse rates may occur, as in other disorders (e.g., acute myelocytic leukemia or acute lymphoblastic leukemia), as a result of the reinfusion of malignant cells through the autologous infusate as well as the lack of a graft-vs-tumor effect in the autologous setting.

Earlier, Corradini and colleagues *(48)* presented a small series of patients who had received allotransplants or autotransplants. The same higher TRM was found in the recipients of allogeneic transplants, but a molecular analysis of minimal residual disease showed a higher proportion of PCR-negative complete responders.

The results of studies conducted by Alyea and colleagues corroborate those of EBMT-based studies *(43)*. Sixty-six patients who had received allogeneic transplants were compared with 166 patients who had received autologous transplants. The patients were relatively well matched for prognostic parameters. The patients who received autologous transplants had significantly better overall and progression-free survival rates at 2 yr (74 and 48%, respectively) compared with the recipients of allogeneic transplants (51 and 28%, respectively). However, by year 4, the outcomes were similar. As seen in the EBMT study, the nonrelapse mortality was higher in the allogeneic group (24 vs 13% at 4 yr), but the relapse rate was lower (46 vs 56%).

The improvement in outcome for allogeneic transplants from 1994 *(46)* may change the results of a comparison between autologous and allotransplantation to the advantage of allogeneic transplantation. The overall results of single autologous transplantation in the EBMT registry do not seem to have improved significantly from 1994. However, these results do not take into account the effect of double autologous transplantation. Combining autologous transplantation with nonmyeloablative allogeneic transplantation may further improve results *(31a)*.

10. SYNGENEIC TRANSPLANTS

The results of syngeneic transplants in patients with MM were first reported by the Seattle group *(65,66)*. Two of 11 recipients of syngeneic marrow tissue survived 9 and 16 yr after transplant, one with no evidence of disease and the other with a small persistent monoclonal spike without disease progression for more than 15 yr *(67)*. Two patients died early from TRM and 7 following disease progression or relapse at a median of 32 mo (range: 3.5–57 mo) after the transplant.

The EBMT has presented results on 25 twin transplants, 17 of whom were still alive at the time of the report and 13 of whom were still in complete remission at 5 to 111 mo (median: 29 mo) after the transplant *(68)*. The complete remission rate was 68% and the median overall length of survival was 72 mo.

A case-matched analysis showed a tendency toward a better overall survival for twin vs autologous transplants and a significantly better overall survival than for allogeneic transplants. The TRM was low: only two twins died as a result of TRM, one from a viral infection and the other from VOD. The relapse rate appeared to be similar to that in allogeneic transplants, but significantly lower than in autologous transplants. The difference between the syngeneic transplants and the autologous transplants could be explained by the reinfusion of malignant cells in the autologous setting. However, it is also possible that the GVHD reported in five syngeneic transplants (four cases of grade I GVHD and one with grade II) may have been associated with a graft-vs-myeloma effect. It is interesting to note that all four patients with grade I GVHD were still in complete remission 10 to 109 mo after the transplant. Thus, transplantation appears to be the treatment of choice for patients who have a syngeneic donor.

11. FUTURE CONSIDERATIONS

Allogeneic transplantation appears to be hampered by a high TRM. It seems possible, however, to reduce mortality using T-cell depletion (as was done by the Dana Farber group). An increased relapse rate that might result from this method may perhaps be countermanded by administering DLI. It is also possible that TRM can be reduced by using a less intensive conditioning regimen. Again, the increased risk for relapse could be countermanded by donor-lymphocyte transfusions at the reappearance of monoclonal immunoglobulin. Based on this new information, the EBMT has started a new prospective protocol based on genetic randomization, with the aim of reducing intensity in the conditioning regimen to counteract the possibility of a higher risk for relapse with DLIs. In that protocol, all patients receive an autologous transplant, and those with an HLA-identical sibling later receive an allogeneic transplant with reduced-intensity conditioning. DLIs will be used when monoclonal immunoglobulins reappear. GVHD may also be modulated by ex vivo transduction of T cells within donor lymphocytes, using a suicide gene, before the infusion. In case of severe GVHD following a DLI, such T cells could be killed by the administering gangcyclovir. These and other approaches may indicate that the results of allogeneic transplantation can be improved and perhaps the number of patients cured of MM can be increased.

REFERENCES

1. Zittoun RA, Mandelli F, Willemze R, et al, for the European Organization for Research and Treatment of Cancer (EORTC) and the Gruppo Italiano Malattie Ematoloigche Maligne Dell'Adulto (GIMEMA) Leukemia Cooperative Groups. Autologous or allogeneic bone marrow transplantation compared with intensive chemotherapy in acute myelogenous leukemia. N Engl J Med 1995; 332:217–223.
2. van Rhee F, Szydlo RM, Hermans J, et al. Long-term results after allogeneic bone marrow transplantation for chronic myelogenous leukemia in chronic phase: a report from the Chronic

Leukemia Working Party of the European Group for Blood and Marrow Transplantation. Bone Marrow Transplant 1997; 20:553–560.

3. Appelbaum FR, Clift RA, Radich J, Anasetti C, Buckner CD. Bone marrow transplantation for chronic myelogenous leukemia. Semin Oncol 1995; 22:405–411.

4. Herve P, Labopin M, Plouvier E, Palut P, Tiberghien P, Gorin NC. Autologous bone marrow transplantation for childhood acute lymphoblastic leukemia: a European survey. EBMT Working Party on ABMT. Bone Marrow Transplant. 1991; 8 (Suppl 1):72–75.

5. Doney K, Fisher LD, Appelbaum FR, et al. Treatment of adult acute lymphoblastic leukemia with allogeneic bone marrow transplantation: multivariate analysis of factors affecting acute graft-vs-host disease, relapse, and relapse-free survival. Bone Marrow Transplant 1991; 7:453–459.

6. Michallet M, Archimbaud E, Bandini G, et al. HLA-identical sibling bone marrow transplantation in younger patients with chronic lymphocytic leukemia. European Group for Blood and Marrow Transplantation and the International Bone Marrow Transplant Registry. Ann Int Med 1996; 124:311–315.

7. Flinn IW, Vogelsang G. Bone marrow transplantation for chronic lymphocytic leukemia. Semin Oncol 1998; 25:60–64.

8. De Witte T. Allogeneic and autologous stem cell transplantation in myelodysplastic syndromes. Pathologie Biologie 1997; 45:643–649.

9. Runde V, de Witte T, Arnold R, et al. Bone marrow transplantation from HLA-identical siblings as first-line treatment in patients with myelodysplastic syndromes: early transplantation is associated with improved outcome. Chronic Leukemia Working Party of the European Group for Blood and Marrow Transplantation. Bone Marrow Transplant. 1998; 21:255–261.

10. Anderson JE, Sale G, Appelbaum FR, Chauncey TR, Storb R. Allogeneic marrow transplantation for primary myelofibrosis and myelofibrosis secondary to polycythaemia vera or essential thrombocytosis. Br J Haematol 1997; 98:1010–1016.

11. Landis SH, Murray T, Bolden S, Wingo PA. Cancer statistics: 1998. Ca: A Cancer Journal for Clinicians 1998; 48:6–29.

12. National Board of Health and Welfare. The Cancer Registry. Cancer incidence in Sweden 2000. Statistics Health and Disease 2002; 5.

13. Attal M, Harousseau JL, Stoppa AM, et al. A prospective, randomized trial of autologous bone marrow transplantation and chemotherapy in multiple myeloma. Intergroupe Francais du Myelome. N Engl J Med 1996; 335:91–97.

14. Child JA, Morgan GJ, Davies FE, et al, for the Medical Research Council Adult Leukaemia Working Party. High-dose chemotherapy with hematopoietic stem-cell rescue for multiple myeloma. N Engl J Med 2003; 348:1875–1883.

15. Tricot, G, Vesole DH, Jagannath S, Hilton J, Munshi N, Barlogie B. Graft-versus-myeloma effect: proof of principle. Blood 1996; 87:1196–1198.

16. Verdonck LF, Lokhorst HM, Dekker AW, Nieuwenhuis HK, Petersen, EJ. Graft-versus-myeloma effect in two cases. Lancet 1996; 348:346.

17. Aschan J, Lönnqvist B, Ringdén O, Kumlien G, Gahrton, G. Graft-versus-myeloma effect. Lancet 1996; 348:346.

18. Sadamori N, Ozer H, Higby DJ, Sandberg AA. Chromosomal evidence of donor B-lymphocyte engraftment after bone-marrow transplantation in a patient with multiple myeloma. N Engl J Med 1983; 308:1423–1424.

19. Tura S, Cavo M, Baccarani M, Ricci P, Gobbi M. Bone marrow transplantation in multiple myeloma. Scand. J Haematol. 1986; 36:176–179.

20. Gahrton G, Ringdén O, Lönnqvist B, Lindquist R, Ljungman P. Bone marrow transplantation in three patients with multiple myeloma. Acta Med Scand. 1986; 219:523–527.

21. Thomas ED, Storb R, Clift RA, et al. Bone-marrow transplantation. N Engl J Med 1975; 292:823–843.

22. Russell N, Miflin G, Stainer C, et al. Allogeneic bone marrow transplant for multiple myeloma. Blood 1997; 89:2610–2617.
23. Gahrton G, Tura S, Ljungman P, et al, for the European Group for Bone Marrow Transplantation. Allogeneic bone marrow transplantation in multiple myeloma. N Engl J Med 1991; 325:1267–1273.
24. Gahrton G, Tura S, Ljungman P, et al. Prognostic factors in allogeneic bone marrow transplantation for multiple myeloma. J Clin Oncol 1995; 13:1312–1322.
25. Bensinger WI, Buckner CD, Clift RA, et al. A phase I study of busulfan and cyclophosphamide in preparation for allogeneic marrow transplant for patients with multiple myeloma. J Clin Oncol 1992; 10:1492–1497.
26. Bensinger WI, Buckner CD, Anasetti C, et al. Allogeneic marrow transplantation for multiple myeloma: an analysis of risk factors on outcome. Blood 1996; 88:2787–2793.
27. Cavo, M, Bandini, G, Benni, M, et al. High-dose busulfan and cyclophosphamide are an effective conditioning regimen for allogeneic bone marrow transplantation in chemosensitive multiple myeloma. Bone Marrow Transplant. 1998; 22:27–32.
28. Slavin S, Nagler A, Naparstek E, et al. Nonmyeloablative stem cell transplantation and cell therapy as an alternative to conventional bone marrow transplantation with lethal cytoreduction for the treatment of malignant and nonmalignant hematologic diseases. Blood. 1998; 91:756–763.
29. Sandmaier BM, McSweeney P, Yu C, Storb R. Nonmyeloablative transplants: preclinical and clinical results. Semin Oncol. 2000; 27(2 Suppl 5):78–81.
30. Zaucha JM, Yu C, Zellmer E, et al. Effects of extending the duration of postgrafting immunosuppression and substituting granulocyte-colony-stimulating factor-mobilized peripheral blood mononuclear cells for marrow in allogeneic engraftment in a nonmyeloablative canine transplantation model. Biol Blood Marrow Transplant 2001; 7:513–516.
31. Corradini P, Montefusco V, Rizzo E, et al. Myeloablative versus reduced-intensity conditioning followed by allogeneic stem cell transplantation in multiple myeloma patients [abstract]. Hematol J 2003; 4 (Suppl 1):S222. Abstract 301.
31a. Maloney DG, Molina AJ, Sahebi F, et al. Allografting with nonmyeloablative conditioning following cytoreductive autografts for the treatment of patients with multiple myeloma. Blood 2003; 102:9:3447–3454.
32. Crawley C, Szydlo R, Lalancette M, et al. Results of Reduced intensity conditioning allogeneic transplantation in Myeloma: a report from EBMT [abstract]. Hematol J 2003; 4(Suppl 1): S224. Abstract 305.
33. Carrasco A, Aleman A, de Lima M, et al. Outcomes in patients with refractory relapse multiple myeloma after reduced intensity conditioning regimen allograft or myeloablative autologous stem cell transplantation [abstract]. Hematol J 2003; 4(Suppl 1):S225. Abstract 306.
34. Einsele H, Schaefer HJ, Bader P, et al. Followup of patients with progressive MM undergoing allografts after reduced intensity conditioning [abstract]. Hematol J 2003; 4(Suppl 1):S225. Abstract 307.
35. Maloney DG, Molina AJ, Sahebi F, et al. Allografting with non-myeloablative conditioning following cytoreductive autografts for the treatment of patients with multiple myeloma. Blood. 2003; 102:3447–3454.
36. Einsele H, Schafer HJ, Hebart H, et al. Follow-up of patients with progressive multiple myeloma undergoing allografts after reduced-intensity conditioning. Br J Haematol 2003; 121:411–418.
37. Peggs KS, Mackinnon S, Williams CD, et al. Reduced-intensity transplantation with in vivo T-cell depletion and adjuvant dose-escalating donor lymphocyte infusions for chemotherapy-sensitive myeloma: limited efficacy of graft-versus-tumor activity. Biol Blood Marrow Transplant 2003; 9:257–265.
38. Giralt S, Aleman A, Anagnostopoulos A, et al. Fludarabine/melphalan conditioning for allogeneic transplantation in patients with multiple myeloma. Bone Marrow Transplant. 2002; 30:367–373.

39. Lee CK, Badros A, Barlogie B, et al. Prognostic factors in allogeneic transplantation for patients with high-risk multiple myeloma after reduced intensity conditioning. Exp Hematol. 2003; 31:73–80.

40. Kroger N, Schwerdtfeger R, Kiehl M, et al. Autologous stem cell transplantation followed by a dose-reduced allograft induces high complete remission rate in multiple myeloma. Blood. 2002; 100:755–760.

41. Kroger N, Sayer HG, Schwerdtfeger R, et al. Unrelated stem cell transplantation in multiple myeloma after a reduced-intensity conditioning with pretransplantation antithymocyte globulin is highly effective with low transplantation-related mortality. Blood. 2002; 100:3919–3924.

42. Alyea E, Weller E, Schlossman R, et al. T cell depleted allogeneic bone marrow transplantation followed by donor lymphocyte infusion in patients with multiple myeloma: induction of graft versus myeloma effect. Blood. 2001; 98:934–939.

43. Alyea E, Weller E, Schlossman R, et al. Outcome after autologous and allogeneic stem cell transplantation for patients with multiple myeloma: impact of graft versus myeloma effect. Biol Blood Bone Marrow Transpl 2003. In press.

44. Corradini PCM, Lokhorst H, Martinelli G, et al. Molecular remissions are frequently achieved in myeloma patients undergoing allografting with peripheral blood stem cells. Bone Marrow Transplantation. 2001; 27(Suppl 1):S39.

45. Bladé J, Samson D, Reece D, et al. Criteria for evaluating disease response and progression in patients with multiple myeloma treated by high-dose therapy and haematopoietic stem cell transplantation (annotation). Br J Haematol 1998; 102:1115–1123.

46. Gahrton G, Svensson H, Cavo M, et al. Progress in allogeneic bone marrow and peripheral blood stem cell transplantation for multiple myeloma: a comparison between transplants performed 1983–93 and 1994–98 at European Group for Blood and Marrow Transplantation centres. Br J Haematol. 2001; 113:209–216.

47. Owen RG, Bybee A, Cooke F, et al. Minimal residual disease after allogeneic and autologous stem cell transplant in myeloma. Br J Haematol 1996; 93(Suppl 2): no. 620.

48. Corradini P, Voena C, Tarella C, et al. Molecular and clinical remissions in multiple myeloma: role of autologous and allogeneic transplantation of hematopoietic cells. J Clin Oncol 1999; 17:208–215.

49. Corradini P, Cavo M, Lokhorst, H, et al. Molecular remission after myeloablative allogeneic stem cell transplantation predicts a better relapse-free survival in multiple myeloma. Blood 2003; 102:1927–1929.

50. Lokhorst HM, Schattenberg A, Cornelissen JJ, Thomas LL, Verdonck LF. Donor leukocyte infusions are effective in relapsed multiple myeloma after allogeneic bone marrow transplantation. Blood 1997; 90:4206–4211.

51. Orsini E, Alyea EP, Chillemi A, et al. Conversion to full donor chimerism following donor lymphocyte infusion is associated with disease response in patients with multiple myeloma. Biol Blood Marrow Transpl. 2000; 6:375–386.

52. Orsini E. Alyea E, Schlossman R, et al. Changes in T cell receptor repertoire associated with graft-versus tumor effect and graft-versus-host disease in patients with relapsed multiple myeloma receiving donor lymphocyte infusion. Bone Marrow Transpl. 2000; 25:623–632.

53. Orsini E, Bellucci R, Alyea EP, et al. Expansion of tumor specific CD8+ T cell clones in patients with relapsed myeloma after donor lymphocyte infusion. Cancer Res. 2003; 63:2561–2568.

54. Gahrton G, Tura S, Ljungman P, et al, for the European Group for Blood and Marrow Transplantation. An update of prognostic factors for allogeneic bone marrow transplantation in multiple myeloma using matched sibling donors. Stem Cells 1995; 13(Suppl 2):122–125.

55. Bensinger WI, Buckner CD, Gahrton G. Allogeneic stem cell transplantation for multiple myeloma. Hematol Oncol Clin N Am 1997; 11:147–157.

56. Reece DE, Shepherd JD, Klingemann HG, et al. Treatment of myeloma using intensive therapy and allogeneic bone marrow transplantation. Bone Marrow Transplant 1995; 15:117–123.

57. Dreger P, Suttorp M, Haferlach T, Loffler H, Schmitz N, Schroyens W. Allogeneic granulo-cyte colony-stimulating factor-mobilized peripheral blood progenitor cells for treatment of engraftment failure after bone marrow transplantation. Blood 1993; 81:1404–1407.

58. Schmitz, N, Bacigalupo, A, Hasenclever D, et al. Allogeneic bone marrow transplantation vs filgrastim-mobilized peripheral blood progenitor cell transplantation in patients with early leukaemia: first results of a randomised multicentre trial of the European Group for Blood and Marrow Transplantation. Bone Marrow Transplant 1998; 21:995–1003.

59. Bensinger, WI, Clift, RA, Martin, P, et al. Allogeneic peripheral blood stem cell transplanta-tion in patients with advanced hematologic malignancies: a retrospective comparison with marrow transplantation. Blood 1996; 88:2794–2800.

60. Urbano-Ispizua A, Garcia-Conde J, Brunet S, et al. High incidence of chronic graft versus host disease after allogeneic peripheral blood progenitor cell transplantation. The Spanish Group of Allo-PBPCT. Haematologica 1997; 82:683–669.

61. Storek J, Gooley T, Siadak M, et al. Allogeneic peripheral blood stem cell transplantation may be associated with a high risk of chronic graft-versus-host disease. Blood 1997; 90:4705–4709.

62. Cavo M, Bandini G, Lemoli RM, et al. Allogeneic transplantation with bone marrow or periph-eral blood stem cells for multiple myeloma: a multivariate analysis of risk factors on outcome. Molecular and clinical remissions in multiple myeloma: the role of auto/allografting of hemato-poietic cells. Abstract presented at: 24th Annual Meeting European Group for Blood and Mar-row Transplantation; Courmayeur, Italy; March 22–26, 1998. Abstract No. 746, p. S213.

63. Majolino I, Corradini P, Scime R, et al. High rate of remission and low rate of disease recur-rence in patients with multiple myeloma allografted with PBSC from their HLA-identical sibling donors. Bone Marrow Transplant 2003; 31:767–773.

64. Björkstrand B, Ljungman P, Svensson H, et al. Allogeneic bone marrow transplantation versus autologous stem cell transplantation in multiple myeloma: a retrospective case-matched study from the European Group for Blood and Marrow Transplantation. Blood 1996; 88:4711–4718.

65. Fefer A, Cheever MA, Greenberg PD. Identical-twin (syngeneic) marrow transplantation for hematologic cancer. J Natl Cancer Inst 1986; 76:1269–1273.

66. Osserman ED, DiRe LB, Sherman WH, Hersman JA, Storb R. Identical twin marrow trans-plantation in multiple myeloma. Acta Haematologica 1982; 68,215–223.

67. Bensinger WI, Demierer T, Buckner CD, et al. Syngeneic marrow transplantation in patients with multiple myeloma. Bone Marrow Transplant 1996; 18:527–531.

68. Gahrton G, Svensson H, Björkstrand B, et al. Syngeneic transplantation in multiple myeloma: a case-matched comparison with autologous and allogeneic transplantation. Bone Marrow Transplant 1999; 24:741–745.

11 Immunological Approaches to Multiple Myeloma

Hakan Mellstedt, MD, PhD,
Maurizio Bendandi, MD,
Anders Österborg MD, PhD,
and Larry W. Kwak, MD, PhD

1. INTRODUCTION

Tumor cells express tumor-associated protein antigens on the cell surface, as well as peptides of the protein presented in the groove of the major histocompatibility complex (MHC). Although most tumor antigens are shared self-antigens, they can be regarded as tumor-specific antigens and used as targets for immunotherapy.

The tumor clone in multiple myeloma (MM) consists of plasma cells and clonogenic B lymphocytoid precursors. Plasma cells express usually only MHC class I molecules on the surface, whereas B lymphocytes exhibit both MHC class I and class II antigens. In myeloma, clone-specific idiotypic immunoglobulin structures are expressed on the surface of the malignant

From: *Current Clinical Oncology: Biology and Management of Multiple Myeloma*
Edited by: J. R. Berenson © Humana Press Inc., Totowa, NJ

cells; these structures might be an ideal target for immunotherapy *(1)*. Idiotypic immunoglobulins are unique antigens, in that they are normally involved in immune regulation. Other surface-bound antigens in MM may also be considered immunotherapy targets, including MAGE-1, the interleukin (IL)-6 receptor, B-cell-associated CD antigens, sperm-17, etc.

2. PRINCIPLES OF IMMUNOTHERAPY

There are two major forms of immunotherapy: specific and unspecific. Unspecific immunotherapy involves immune effector functions that do not recognize the specific tumor cells; natural killer cells, monocytes, neutrophils, and various soluble factors released from activated cells of the immune system they are activated to kill the tumor cells. Specific immunotherapy involves immune effectors that recognize and bind to specific antigens on the tumor cells and are activated to kill the malignant cells.

There are two major approaches in specific immunotherapy: active immunotherapy (tumor vaccination) and passive immunotherapy (e.g., monoclonal antibodies [MAbs]). Unconjugated MAbs induce tumor cell death by activating various immune functions, e.g., antibody-dependent cellular cytotoxicity (ADCC), complement dependent cytotoxicity (CDC), and the induction of an idiotypic response network that results in tumor-specific humoral and cellular immunity. Antibodies can also induce apoptosis and bystander killing through a local inflammatory response that involves the release of proinflammatory cytokines from activated cells. Antibodies can also be used as carriers of cytotoxic substances.

When a tumor-derived antigen is used to vaccinate patients, the antigen is taken up by the cell, processed within the cell, and presented on the MHC molecules of antigen-presenting cells (APCs), i.e., dendritic cells, monocytes and macrophages, and B lymphocytes. APCs have to be activated to present the antigen and to induce an immune response. Exogenous antigens most frequently use the class II antigen presentation pathway. After degradation in the endosomes, the peptides are bound to MHC class II molecular complexes and then transported to the cell surface. Exogenous antigens may also enter proteosomes using the ubiquitin system. Processed peptides are then transported to the endoplasmic reticulum, where they bind with MHC class I complexes, which are then transported to the surface of APC. This process seems to be facilitated by granulocyte-macrophage colony-stimulating factor (GM-CSF) *(2)*. Thus, both MHC class II-restricted (CD4) helper T (T_H) cells and MHC class I-restricted (CD8) T lymphocytes can be induced when tumor antigens are used for vaccination. Both T-cell populations are mandatory for the induction of a fully competent and effective anti-tumor response. Consequently, the immunogen should contain T_H epitopes as well as cytotoxic T lymphocyte (CTL) epitopes. T_{H1} cells are instrumental for inducing a CD8–CTL response, as well as for inducing humoral immunity by switching to a T_{H2} response. T_H cells are essential for a memory response, while T_{H1} and $_{H2}$ cells might also mediate tumor-cell killing. T_{H1} cells have been shown to directly lyse tumor cells and produce γ-interferon (IFN), which activates monocytes to release nitrogen oxide and hydrogen superoxide, both of which are toxic to tumor cells. T_{H2} cells secrete IL-4 upon antigen specific activation; this cytokine stimulates eosinophils to produce molecules that are toxic to tumor cells *(3)*.

Adjuvants have to be added to induce an effective immune response. Several adjuvants for human use are available, including chemical compounds, products derived from various microorganisms, and cytokines. GM-CSF seems to be a key cytokine for the induction of an immune response *(4)*, as it activates APC, up-regulates MHC complexes and costimulatory molecules, and promotes migration to the local lymph nodes, where the immune response is initiated. Other cytokines (e.g., IL-2 and IL-12) might also be important for the amplification of a T-cell response.

3. IDIOTYPE IMMUNIZATION IN ANIMAL MODELS

Eisen and colleagues were the first to prove that syngeneic BALB/c mice that have been immunized with purified myeloma immunoglobulin proteins obtained from mineral-oil-induced plasmacytomas (MOPCs) and coupled with complete Freund's adjuvant developed a sustained humoral response specific for the individual idiotype used for the immunization *(5–7)*. Moreover, these animals were capable of rejecting a specific tumor challenge involving the parental neoplasm, but were not resistant to other MOPC tumors. This suggests idiotypic specificity for this anti-tumor immunity. A few years later, Jorgensen and colleagues showed that immunization with MOPC-315 plasmacytoma-derived light chains alone was sufficient to confer protection against a subsequent tumor challenge *(8)*. In this system, tumor resistance correlated with splenocyte proliferation in vitro, with no apparent antibody production.

Subsequently, idiotype-specific, protective anti-tumor immunity was reproduced in several animal models of myeloma, leukemia, and lymphoma *(9–12)*, but studies of the cellular mechanisms involved in tumor resistance have yielded mixed results. For example, in studies of BCL-1 or 38C13 lymphoma, tumor protection could be transferred from immune mice to naive mice by mixing serum taken from the immune mice with tumor cells before challenging naive mice; this phenomenon suggests an essential role for antibodies *(10,12)*, although protection against a subsequent tumor challenge could also be reversed by treating immunized mice with MAbs against T cells *(12)*.

Additional insight into the role of T cells in the response to tumor idiotype has been gained through experiments using cloned, idiotype-specific T cells. Immunization of mice with light chains derived from MOPC-315 elicited MHC class II-restricted CD4$^+$ T-cell clones of both T_H1 and T_H2 *(13)*. When either of these clones was administered subcutaneously, together with a challenge of syngeneic cells transfected with the cognate idiotype, it protected the mouse in an idiotypic-specific and dose-dependent manner. To mimic more closely the in vivo situation—wherein naive lymphocytes are able to interact with target tumor cells immediately following activation and in the complete absence of preformed antibodies—mice transgenic for the T-cell receptor (TCR) isolated from these T-cell clones were generated. Such transgenic mice were found to be resistant to challenge with immunoglobulin-secreting tumor *(14)*. Furthermore, because the tumor was MHC class II-negative, an indirect mechanism of tumor cell neutralization was postulated *(15)*. Finally, the transfer of lymphocytes obtained from these transgenic mice into mice with severe combined immunodeficiency (SCID) that were devoid of B cells resulted in resistance to MOPC-315, which demonstrated that such idiotype-specific T cells were sufficient for tumor resistance.

Perhaps the best evidence of a role for CD8-positive idiotype-specific T cells was provided by the unexpected finding of cross-reactivity between murine influenza virus hemagglutinin-specific T-cell clones and a 9 amino-acid epitope contained in the CDR-2 region of an immunoglobulin heavy-chain variable region in myeloma *(16)*.

Kwak and colleagues screened a series of selected recombinant cytokines for their ability to enhance the protective effect of tumor-derived idiotypic immunoglobulin conjugated with keyhole limpet hemocyanin (KLH) in a murine model *(17)*. It had previously been demonstrated that conjugation with an immunogenic carrier protein (e.g., KLH) was required to elicit protection against a subsequent tumor challenge in this model *(11)*. For such studies, a single dose of Id-KLH was injected subcutaneously, then free recombinant murine GM-CSF was administered intraperitoneally as close as possible to the initial immunization site as possible. GM-CSF was administered for 4 d, starting on the vaccination day. Fourteen days later, immunized mice were challenged with 10,000 tumor cells (i.e., 100 times the minimum lethal dose) and followed to determine survival. All of the mice that received GM-CSF had a significantly prolonged survival and an increased number of long-term survivors compared with the mice that had been immunized with the Id-KLH conjugate alone. Moreover, GM-CSF administered locally (i.e., subcutaneously) was more effective than that administered systemically (i.e., intraperitoneally), and a reproducible trend approaching statistical significance with lower doses was observed.

The overall results of other studies using other cytokines have been generally disappointing. The administration of human IL-2, murine IFN-γ, human IL-1α or IL-1β, or murine IL-12 by various routes, doses, and schedules failed to augmented protection following tumor challenge significantly compared with a single subcutaneous dose of Id-KLH alone. Combinations of murine GM-CSF with IL-2, IL-12, IFN-γ, or human tumor necrosis factor (TNF)-α also failed to demonstrate an additional protective effect compared with GM-CSF alone plus a single dose of Id-KLH. On further investigation, the mechanism involved in the additive tumor protection provided using GM-CSF was found to be critically dependent on effector CD4-positive and CD8-positive T cells, was demonstrated in vivo by the abrogation of protection in immunized mice after either T-cell subset was depleted using with monoclonal antibodies. The clear-out requirement for T cells was not associated with any apparent increase in antibody response directed against idiotype, which suggests that the mechanism of augmented protective anti-tumor immunity provided by GM-CSF was dependent on selective activation of the T-cell arm of the immune response.

3.1. Natural Idiotype Immunity in Monoclonal Gammopathies in MAN

3.1. T Cells in Multiple Myeloma and Monoclonal Gammopathies of Undetermined Significance

Although a relatively low number of T cells has been observed in the blood of patients with MM and monoclonal gammopathies of undetermined significance MGUS (18), the total number of T lymphocytes was within the normal range in most studies (19,20). A consistent finding in these studies was a low CD4–CD8 ratio, which was most pronounced in patients with advanced disease (19,20). An increase in the CD4-positive/CD45RO-positive (suppressor/inducer T cell) subset in MGUS (21) and a low number of cells in MM (22) have also been described. The presence of T lymphocytes that are cytotoxic for autologous plasma cells (23) and an increased number of CD8-positive T cells with Fc receptors for the myeloma immunoglobulin isotype (24) have also been reported.

The presence of activated human lymphocyte antigen ([HLA])-DR-positive) T cells in patients with myeloma has also been reported (25). These T cells produced large amounts of IL-2 and IFN-γ, and were able to recognize myeloma plasma cells in vitro after stimulation with CD3. Clonal expansion of CD4-positive as well as CD8-positive T cells has also been noted (26,27). CD8-positive clonal T-cell populations were seen more frequently in patients with a low tumor burden compared with those with advanced disease (28). The relevance of such clonal T cells to the recognition of malignant B cells is not known. In one patient, two large expansions within CD8-positive subsets displayed no reactivity against the idiotype. Idiotype recognition was confined to a small, unexpanded T-cell population, but with the use of a monoclonal-restricted TCR (TCRBV22) (28).

The susceptibility of T cells to apoptosis in patients with MM has been analyzed by determining the cell-surface expression of the fas antigen and the intracellular exhibition of the bcl-2 protein (29). The number of FAS-positive cells were significantly higher in patients than in controls. Spontaneous and triggered apoptosis was higher in patients with MM than in controls and mainly restricted to HLA-DR-positive T cells *(29)*. An increase in CD8-positive/CD57-positive cells with a suppressive effect on T-cell activity was also found in patients with myeloma *(30)*. Thus, an increase in suppressor T-cell activity and T-cell susceptibility to apoptosis may prevail in patients with myeloma *(30)*. Furthermore, co-stimulatory molecules and intracellular signaling proteins down-regulated in the T cells of patients with myeloma became increasingly abnormal as the stage of the disease advanced *(31)*. These abnormalities may contribute an impaired T-cell activity in patients with monoclonal gammopathies.

Recent studies of the V_b repertoire in the T cells from patients with MM show marked skewing *(31a)*. These results suggest a limited ability of these cells to respond to antigens including those expressed on tumor cells.

3.1.1. IDIOTYPE-SPECIFIC IMMUNITY

The presence of idiotype-specific T cells in the blood of patients with MM or MGUS has been studied by activating T cells with an autologous myeloma-derived idiotypic immunoglobulin. Activation of these T cells has been analyzed by DNA synthesis (^{3}H-thymidine incorporation), cytokine secretion (IFN-γ, IL-2, IL-4), or both *(32)*. The number of specific cytokine-secreting cells can also be determined using an enzyme-linked immunospot (ELISPOT) assay *(33)*. Naturally occurring idiotype-specific T cells were frequently detected in patients with indolent myeloma or MGUS *(32)*. An idiotype-specific type I T-cell response (characterized by the secretion of IFN-γ and IL-2) predominated in patients with MGUS or early-stage myeloma, whereas a type II response (characterized by the production of IL-4) was seen more often in patients with a high tumor load *(32)*. Idiotype reactivity was confined to both CD4-positive and CD8-positive T-cell subsets as well as MHC class I- and II-restricted T cells *(34)*. The median total blood levels of idiotype-specific T cells approx 20^5 and 10^5 peripheral blood mononuclear cell (PBMC), which corresponds roughly to 1:5000 mononuclear cells *(33)*. The fine specificity of idiotype-reactive T cells was mapped using peptides corresponding to the complete CDR1-3 regions of the heavy and light chains as well as to MHC-restricted sequences of the CDR2 and CDR3 heavy-chain regions. T cells reacting specifically with peptides that corresponded with each of the three CDRs of the heavy-chain variable part of the idiotype were found *(35,36)*. Peptides corresponding to the CDRs of the variable part of the light chain of the monoclonal immunoglobulin or other unrelated immunoglobulin fragments were also found, but were not efficient in eliciting an idiotype-specific immune response *(35,37,38)*. Taken together, these findings support the existence of MHC-restricted idiotype-specific T cells that may target immunogenic CDR peptides in monoclonal gammopathies. Such T cells might be an important part of a naturally occurring, anti-tumor-specific immune response. Humoral immunity, conveyed by anti-idiotypic antibodies, has also been detected by using ELISPOT assay, especially in patients with MGUS or stage I MM *(39)*. Such antibodies are most likely to form complexes in vivo with the tremendous number of excess of circulating free monoclonal immunoglobulins, but may not be of importance for an immune defense against the tumor.

4. IDIOTYPE IMMUNIZATION IN PATIENTS WITH MULTIPLE MYELOMA

As indicated above, tumor-derived idiotypic immunoglobulins may elicit both humoral and cellular anti-idiotypic responses, the latter having been shown to confer resistance to tumor cell challenges in animal models. A rewarding therapeutic approach might thus be to immunize patients with myeloma with the autologous idiotype.

One of the first studies of immunoglobulin immunization in patients with MM suggested a novel strategy for the successful transfer of tumor antigen-specific T-cell immunity from a healthy immunized donor to a recipient with MM who was undergoing bone marrow transplant (BMT) *(40)*. The patient was a 43- yr-old woman with progressive myeloma refractory to chemotherapy using vinblastine and dexamethasone (VAD chemotherapy) who presented with considerable tumor burden, characterized by a serum M-protein level of 3.9 g/dL and 50% bone marrow plasmacytosis. Myeloma immunoglobulin protein was isolated from the plasma of the recipient, chemically conjugated with KLH to enhance its immunogenicity, and mixed with a water-in-oil adjuvant formulation. Her 47-yr-old HLA-matched male sibling BMT donor received two subcutaneous immunizations of myeloma immunoglobulin KLH at 1-wk intervals before marrow harvest. Longer intervals between immunizations had been planned, but were not feasible because of the recipient's deteriorating health. Nevertheless, successful immunization of the donor against the myeloma idiotype and the KLH carrier was achieved and demonstrated by significant in vitro lymphoproliferative responses.

In the recipient, the lack of preexisting anti-idiotypic immunity was demonstrated prior to the BMT. On the contrary, 30 and 60 days after conditioning with busulfan and cyclophosphamide and the transfer of unmanipulated donor marrow, significant lymphoproliferative responses against idiotype as well as KLH were detected in the recipient. Additional evidence of the transfer of T-cell immunity was provided by the successful isolation of a CD4-positive T-cell line generated from PBMC obtained in bulk from the recipient. The unique specificity of this T-cell line for the myeloma idiotype was demonstrated by the lack of response to a panel of isotype-matched human myeloma immunoglobulin proteins. Blocking experiments demonstrated that idiotype recognition occurred in an MHC class II-restricted manner. Finally, this T-cell line was shown by fluorescent *in situ* hybridization with a Y-chromosome specific probe to be unequivocally of donor origin. The patient experienced only grade II skin graft-vs-host disease, which was resolved by means of corticosteroid therapy. Examination of the bone marrow on day 90 revealed no residual myeloma, and by day 220 serum M-protein levels had been reduced by more than 90%; this reduction persisted for 3.5 yr. These encouraging results led to a clinical trial to confirm the potential for marrow donor immunization in MM. This trial is still in progress.

The autologous idiotypic immunoglobulin isolated from serum can also be used to vaccinate patients. In our first series, consisting of five patients with stage I MM, immunization with autologous serum M-protein precipitated in alum only resulted in a modest, short-lived idiotype-specific T-cell immunity in two patients *(41)*. In our second series, five patients with indolent MM were immunized with the autologous idiotypic immunoglobulin (precipitated in alum) at day 1 together with GM-CSF (a potent inducer of a specific antitumor immunity *(4, 17,42)*) 75 µg/d subcutaneously on days 1 through 4. GM-CSF was administered at the same site as the idiotypic immunoglobulin. The immunization procedure was repeated at weeks 2, 4, 6, 8, and 14. An idiotype specific T-cell immunity was induced in all five patients. In four of these patients, CD8-positive MHC class I-restricted idiotype-specific T cells were predominant, although CD4-positive MHC II-restricted T cells were also induced. Epitope mapping revealed reactivity against peptides corresponding to the CDR 1, 2, and 3 regions of the heavy chains but not to CDR peptides from idiotypic proteins obtained from other patients with myeloma. The magnitude of the T-cell response was higher and the duration of specificity of T-cell immunity was longer compared with that of the first series of patients, because they did not GM-CSF. In one of the patients in the second series, the M-component concentration was reduced by 65%. No other treatment was given *(43)*.

We have begun a more extensive prospective clinical trial to explore the effectiveness of idiotype immunization in eliminating minimal residual disease (MRD) after high-dose therapy in patients with MM *(44)*. Fifteen patients who were selected on the basis of minimal prior treatment (>1 yr) and chemosensitive disease prior to autologous peripheral stem cell transplantation (PSCT) have been enrolled in this study; to date, five are evaluable for immunological responses. Two to 15 mo (median: 5 mo) after the PSCT, patients received a series of three monthly vaccinations with M protein 0.5 mg made immunogenic by conjugation to KLH and administered locally by SC injection with free GM-CSF (250 µg/m^2 for 4 d) as an immunological adjuvant. To determine whether immunity could be induced against the unique myeloma idiotype, fresh PBMCs were isolated by Ficoll-Hypaque centrifugation before and at the time of each vaccination and observed in a culture medium alone or in a medium to which KLH or unconjugated autologous myeloma immunoglobulin proteins were added. After 6 d, supernatants were assayed for TNF-α and GM-CSF level or cells pulsed with ^{3}H-thymidine. Despite prior exposure to immunosuppressive transplant conditioning regimens, vigorous postvaccination responses against the KLH carrier were observed in all patients (TNF-α median: 818 pg/mL; range: 322–998 pg/mL) compared with medium alone (78 pg/mL; range: 31–138 pg/mL). Furthermore, cell-mediated responses against autologous myeloma immunoglobulin were elicited in four of the five patients (median TNF-α: 745 pg/mL; range: 207–1000 pg/mL). These responses were specific for the idiotype, as demonstrated by the lack of response to control isotype-matched myeloma immunoglobulin proteins. By ELISA, serum anti-KLH antibodies were also uniformly observed, but an idiotype-specific antibody response was observed in only one patient (endpoint titer >1:500). No responses to KLH or myeloma immunoglobulin were recorded prior to vaccination. As with preclinical experiments (45), these results suggest that host immune recovery, occurring as soon as 2 mo following a PSCT, may be sufficient for active immunotherapy in the MRD setting.

Another vaccine strategy involves the use of dendritic cells—antigen-presenting cells capable of presenting idiotype antigen in the context of MHC class I and class II molecules as well as inducing co-stimulatory molecules that mediate signals for T-cell activation. Although present in low numbers in the blood, dendritic cells can be generated ex vivo from their precursors by culturing them in the presence of GM-CSF and IL-4 (46). When pulsed with the tumor antigen in vitro, dendritic cells have shown promise as an adjuvant for vaccination. Dendritic cells generated from the blood of patients with myeloma have been shown to have a normal functional capacity (47) and have induced a stronger in vitro predominantly type-I T-cell idiotype-specific response than monocytes (38).

In the first report, autologous dendritic cells were cultured ex vivo with GM-CSF and IL-4 obtained from a patient with myeloma, incubated with the idiotypic immunoglobulin, then infused intravenously in the patient. An idiotype-specific MHC class I- and II-restricted T-cell response was induced and classical tumor-recognizing cytotoxic T lymphocytes could be expanded from the blood. A 20% reduction in the serum M component was noted (48). Several ongoing studies using idiotype-loaded dendritic cells in patients in remission after high-dose chemotherapy and in refractory patients are ongoing as of this writing (Table 1). All studies have shown the induction of idiotype-specific T cells; in some cases, classical cytotoxic T cells were generated. It is, however, too early to evaluate the clinical impact.

Taken together, these results indicate that an idiotype-specific T-cell response can be induced in patients at an early stage of the disease and after intensive chemotherapy. Several issues remain to be addressed in future clinical studies in MM. The potential effect of large amounts of circulating antigens or the induction of tolerance to idiotype should be considered in the design of vaccination trials (59). Such obstacles may favor the use of vaccination in the MRD setting or very early in the course of the disease. The problem of circulating antigen

Table 1
Summary of Recent Idiotype-Vaccine Clinical trials in Multiple Myeloma

Treatment	Clinical setting	Anti-tumor effect (proportion of patients)
Id-KLH+GM-CSF or IL-2 (29)	First remission after HDCT and PBSCT	(0/12)
ID-KLH+GM-CSF (49)	Remission after HDCT and PBSCT	NE (n = 8)
ID-KLH+GM-CSF (44,50)	First remission after HDCT and PBSCT	CR (2/11)
ID+GM-CSF (43)	IgG MM (stage 1)	PR (1/5)
ID-pulsed DC (Id-KLH) (51)	First remission after HDCT and PBSCT	→ M protein (1/12)
ID-pulsed DC (Id-KLH + GM-CSF) (52)	Remission after HDCT and PBSCT	→ M-protein (3/10)
ID-pulsed DC (53)	Remission after HDCT and PBSCT	CR (3/17) PR (2/17)
ID-pulsed DC (54)	Remission after HDCT and PBSCT	→ M-protein (1/5)
ID- or Id-KLH-pulsed DC → Id-KLH (48)	Remission after HDCT and PBSCT	CR (2/21) → M protein (8/21)
ID-KLH-pulsed DC (55)	IgG MM	→ M-protein (1/6)
ID-pulsed DC → ID+GM-CSF (56)	Advanced stage	→ Bone marrow plasma-cell infiltration (1/10)
ID-pulsed DC (57)	Advanced stage	→ M-protein (6/42)
ID-pulsed DC (47)	Advanced stage	→ M-protein
ID-KLH-pulsed DC + GM-CSF (58)	Advanced stage	No effect (n = 2)

KLH, keyhole limpet hemozyanine; GM-CSF, granulocyte-macrophage colony-stimulating factor; HDCT, high-dose chemotherapy; PBSCT, peripheral blood stem cell transplantation; CR, complete remission; PR, partial remission; NE, not evaluable; DC, dendritic cells.

214

underscores the importance of focusing on the induction of a T-cell response rather than antibodies, which may be easily blocked by the M protein. It also remains to be formally demonstrated that myeloma tumor cells express idiotype within an MHC–peptide complex on the cell surface, such that they can serve as targets for a T-cell response. Another important question is whether idiotype-specific T cells may provide T- to B-cell help and thus drive the B-cell clone *(60)*. This has not been observed so far in idiotype-immunized patients. However, in an animal model, T cells were described that specifically facilitated terminal tumor B-cell differentiation, with a shift from a B-cell lymphoma to a plasmocytoma *(61)*. Idiotype-specific T cells may also be clonally deleted, resulting in the tumor escaping T-cell immunosurveillance *(62)*.

5. MAb-BASED THERAPY

Reports on MAb therapy in patients with MM are few.

IL-6 is an essential growth factor for myeloma cells. A mouse MAb against human IL-6 was used to treat 10 patients with myeloma. In several patients, an antiproliferative effect was characterized by a reduction in the plasma cell-labeling index within the bone marrow. One patient achieved a 30% reduction in tumor mass, but no other patients had a significant clinical response *(63)*.

Many myeloma cell-specific antigens have been identified as targets for antibody therapy, including CD19, CD20, CD38, MUC-1, HM1.24. During one phase II trial, a mouse monoclonal antibody against CD19 was coupled with blocked ricin to inhibit nonspecific binding. CD19 is not expressed on the malignant myeloma plasma cells, but on the clonogenic myeloma tumor cells that appear early in the B-cell ontogeny. Many side effects were noted, including elevated hepatic transaminase levels, myalgia, thrombocytopenia, nausea, vomiting, capillary syndromes, and neurotoxicity. No clinical effects were seen *(64)*.

CD20 is expressed in approx 20% of patients with MM, often in a heterogenous fashion; its expression can also be induced in vitro with IFN-γ. Following the demonstration of a transient partial response to rituximab in a patients with relapsed CD20-positive light-chain myeloma, rituximab was evaluated in several clinical studies in myeloma. Rituximab was combined with melphalan–prednisolone (MP) in a study of patients with newly diagnosed myeloma, the rationale being that it induced chemosensitization and B-cell depletion in vivo *(65)*. Five of 22 patients demonstrated a response to initial rituximab therapy prior to the initiation of MP; 4 of these patients had CD20-positive plasma cells. The inference of a role for rituximab in the achievement of complete remission following MP and progression-free survival cannot be evaluated, however. In another report of 18 evaluable patients previously treated for myeloma received rituximab monotherapy *(66)*, only 1 patient achieved partial remission. However, 5 patients had stable disease, with a median time to treatment failure of 5 mo. Five of these six patients had CD20-positive bone marrow plasma cells.

Because circulating CD20-positive B cells represent the proliferative compartment of myeloma plasma-cell overproduction, rituximab has also been used in vivo to "purge" the blood of B cells before collecting autologous stem cells. This approach is feasible and is associated with prolonged B-cell depletion. Unfortunately, no data are available that support the use of this technique outside clinical trials (67,68). Rituximab appears to limited activity in myeloma. IFN-γ may increase the expression of CD20, although the feasibility of doing so in vivo has not yet been demonstrated.

A humanized HM1.24 MAb is in a phase I trial. Clinical information is not yet available.

Angiogenesis is of fundamental importance for the growth of tumor cells, including myeloma plasma cells, in bone marrow. Treatment approaches directed against neoangiogenesis is attracting great interest. A key factor in angiogenesis is vascular endothelial growth factor (VEGF) and its receptors. A MAb against VEGF—bevacizumab—has been produced and is currently being tested for its efficacy, with or without thalidomide, in patients treated for myeloma who have experienced a relapse.

6. DONOR LEUKOCYTE INFUSIONS

Donor leukocyte infusions (DLIs) have been shown to induce sustained remissions in patients with acute and chronic myeloid leukemia who relapse after an allogeneic BMT (allo-BMT). The existence of graft-vs-myeloma reactions has been suggested by remissions occurring after DLIs in patients with myeloma who experience a relapse following allo-BMT (69,70). In a recent study, 13 patients with relapsed myeloma after allo-BMT were treated with DLIs. The T-cell doses ranged from 1×10^6/kg to 33×10^7/kg. Repetitive courses were given in some cases. A complete remission was achieved in four patients and a partial remission in four. The only prognostic factors for response were a T-cell dose greater than 1×10^8/kg and the occurrence of graft-vs-host disease (71). The exact mechanism for the cell-mediated immune response is not known, but probably involves T-cells recognition of minor histocompatibility complexes.

7. AUTOLOGOUS T LYMPHOCYTE INFUSIONS

Because patients with myeloma show impaired T-cell responses (31a,72,73), techniques have been developed to generally activate and expand autologous T cells for use in these patients (31a). The first study involved 38 patients undergoing high-dose therapy. The T lymphocytes were obtained from a steady-state leukapheresis collection. The T cells were expanded using magnetic beads harboring antibodies that activate and expand T cells (anti-CD3 and anti-CD28

Table 2
Principles of Ongoing Immunotherapeutic Studies in Multiple Myeloma

Type of immunotherapy	Immunotherapeutic technique	Phase of disease
Passive specific	• Anti-IL-6 MAb • Anti-CD19 MAb • Anti-CD20 MAb • Anti-IL-6R MAb • Anti-VEGF MAb • Anti-HM.1.24 MAb	Advanced disease
Active specific	• Free idiotypic Ig protein or • Loaded onto DCs (vaccination cells) GM-CSF and/or IL-2 and/or IL-12	• Advanced disease, in complete remission • After chemotherapy or • During early phase of disease
Donor leukocyte infusions (adoptive cell transfer)	• Donor T lymphocytes	• Relapse after allo-BMT • Genetic bone marrow transplantation
Autologous T-cell infusion	• Ex vivo activated autologous T lymphocytes	• After high-dose therapy • Relapse from other therapy

MAb, monoclonal antibody; Ig, immunoglobulin; DC, dendritic cell; GM-CSF, granulocyte-macrophage colony-stimulating factor; IL, interleukin; allo-BMT, allogenic bone marrow transplant.

antibodies). The cell were reinfused 3 d after autologous stem cell infusion as part of a high-dose therapy procedure. The early results were promising with a rapid increase in high levels of peripheral T cells and correction of V_β repertoire abnormalities. Although response rates assessed early appeared promising, further follow-up is required to better assess the efficacy of this modality. Moreover, the assessment of the anti-MM effects of the T-cell infusion are confounded by the high-dose chemotherapy. Thus, a trial evaluating these expanded T cells in the setting of relapsing myeloma has begun.

8. CONCLUSION

Immunotherapy for malignant diseases is an expanding therapeutic field. MM might be an ideal tumor for immunotherapy, because it expresses a unique idiotypic antigen and other shared self tumor antigens; additionally the normal counterparts of the myeloma tumor cells are regulated by immune effector functions. A summary of current immunotherapeutic principles appears in Table 2.

Very promising clinical results have already been demonstrated with DLIs. Idiotypic vaccination can induce a relevant cellular immunity; however, the clinical results have so far been scanty. Immunization in B-cell non-Hodgkin's lymphoma using the autologous idiotype has shown very encouraging clinical results, which might give hope for myeloma. Therapeutic vaccination will, without a doubt, be most effective in the MRD setting or early in the course of the disease. Given time, immunotherapy might become part of the therapeutic arsenal in MM during this decade. Great efforts are being made at several institutions to develop these concepts.

ACKNOWLEDGMENTS

These studies were supported by grants from the Swedish Cancer Society, the Cancer Society in Stockholm, the Cancer and Allergy Foundation, the Multiple Myeloma Research Foundation, the National Cancer Institute.

REFERENCES

1. Stevenson GT, Stevenson FK. Antibody to a molecularly-defined antigen confined to a tumor cell surface. Nature 1975;254:714–716.
2. Paglia P, Chiodoni C, Rodolfo M, Colombo MP. Murine dendritic cells loaded in vitro with soluble protein prime cytotoxic T lymphocytes against tumor antigen in vivo. J Exp Med 1996;183:317–322.
3. Pardoll DM, Topalian SL. The role of CD4+ T cell responses in antitumor immunity. Curr Opin Immunol 1998;10:588–594.
4. Samanci A, Yi Q, Fagerberg J, Strigard K, Smith G, Ruden U, et al. Pharmacological administration of granulocyte/macrophage-colony-stimulating factor is of significant importance for the induction of a strong humoral and cellular response in patients immunized with recombinant carcinoembryonic antigen. Cancer Immunol Immunother 1998;47:131–142.
5. Sirisinha S, Eisen HN. Autoimmune-like antibodies to the ligand-binding sites of myeloma proteins. Proc Natl Acad Sci U S A 1971;68:3130–135.
6. Lynch RG, Graff RJ, Sirisinha S, Simms ES, Eisen HN. Myeloma proteins as tumor-specific transplantation antigens. Proc Natl Acad Sci U S A 1972;69:1540–1544.
7. Hannestad K, Kao MS, Eisen HN. Cell-bound myeloma proteins on the surface of myeloma cells: potential targets for the immune system. Proc Natl Acad Sci U S A 1972;69:2295–2299.
8. Jorgensen T, Gaudernack G, Hannestad K. Immunization with the light chain and the VL domain of the isologous myeloma protein 315 inhibits growth of mouse plasmacytoma MOPC315. Scand J Immunol 1980;11:29–35.
9. Sugai S, Palmer DW, Talal N, Witz IP. Protective and cellular immune responses to idiotypic determinants on cells from a spontaneous lymphoma of NZB-NZW F1 mice. J Exp Med 1974;140:1547–1558.
10. George AJ, Tutt AL, Stevenson FK. Anti-idiotypic mechanisms involved in suppression of a mouse B cell lymphoma, BCL1. J Immunol 1987;138:628–634.
11. Kaminski MS, Kitamura K, Maloney DG, Levy R. Idiotype vaccination against murine B cell lymphoma. Inhibition of tumor immunity by free idiotype protein. J Immunol 1987;138:1289–1296.
12. Campbell MJ, Esserman L, Byars NE, Allison AC, Levy R. Idiotype vaccination against murine B cell lymphoma. Humoral and cellular requirements for the full expression of antitumor immunity. J Immunol 1990;145:1029–1036.

13. Lauritzsen GF, Weiss S, Bogen B. Anti-tumour activity of idiotype-specific, MHC-restricted Th1 and Th2 clones in vitro and in vivo. Scand J Immunol 1993;37:77–85.
14. Lauritzsen GF, Weiss S, Dembic Z, Bogen B. Naive idiotype-specific CD4+ T cells and immunosurveillance of B-cell tumors. Proc Natl Acad Sci U S A 1994;91:5700–5704.
15. Lauritzsen GF, Bogen B. The role of idiotype-specific, CD4+ T cells in tumor resistance against major histocompatibility complex class II molecule negative plasmacytoma cells. Cell Immunol 1993;148:177–188.
16. Cao W, Myers-Powell BA, Braciale TJ. Recognition of an immunoglobulin VH epitope by influenza virus-specific class I major histocompatibility complex-restricted cytolytic T lymphocytes. J Exp Med 1994;179:195–202.
17. Kwak LW, Young HA, Pennington RW, Weeks SD. Vaccination with syngeneic, lymphoma-derived immunoglobulin idiotype combined with granulocyte/macrophage colony-stimulating factor primes mice for a protective T-cell response. Proc Natl Acad Sci U S A 1996;93: 10972–10977.
18. Bergmann L, Mitrou PS, Kelker W, Weber KC. T-cell subsets in malignant lymphomas and monoclonal gammopathies. Scand J Haematol 1985;34:170–176.
19. Mellstedt H, Holm G, Pettersson D, Bjorkholm M, Johansson B, Lindemalm C, et al. T cells in monoclonal gammopathies. Scand J Haematol 1982;29:57–64.
20. San Miguel JF, Caballero MD, Gonzalez M. T-cell subpopulations in patients with mono-clonal gammopathies: essential monoclonal gammopathy, multiple myeloma, and Waldenstrom macroglobulinemia. Am J Hematol 1985;20:267–273.
21. Shapira R, Froom P, Kinarty A, Aghai E, Lahat N. Increase in the suppressor-inducer T cell subset in multiple myeloma and monoclonal gammopathy of undetermined significance. Br J Haematol 1989;71:223–225.
22. Serra HM, Mant MJ, Ruether BA, Ledbetter JA, Pilarski LM. Selective loss of CD4+ CD45R+ T cells in peripheral blood of multiple myeloma patients. J Clin Immunol 1988;8:259–265.
23. Paglieroni T, MacKenzie MR. In vitro cytotoxic response to human myeloma plasma cells by peripheral blood leukocytes from patients with multiple myeloma and benign monoclonal gammopathy. Blood 1979;54:226–237.
24. Hoover RG, Hickman S, Gebel HM, Rebbe N, Lynch RG. Expansion of Fc receptor-bearing T lymphocytes in patients with immunoglobulin G and immunoglobulin A myeloma. J Clin Invest 1981;67:308–311.
25. Massaia M, Attisano C, Peola S, P, et al. Rapid generation of antiplasma cell activity in the bone marrow of myeloma patients by CD3-activated T cells. Blood 1993;82:1787–1797.
26. Janson CH, Grunewald J, Osterborg A, et al. Predominant T cell receptor V gene usage in patients with abnormal clones of B cells. Blood 1991;77:1776-1780.
27. Moss P, Gillespie G, Frodsham P, Bell J, Reyburn H. Clonal populations of CD4+ and CD8+ T cells in patients with multiple myeloma and paraproteinemia. Blood 1996;87:3297–3306.
28. Halapi E, Werner A, Wahlstrom J, et al. T cell repertoire in patients with multiple myeloma and monoclonal gammopathy of undetermined significance: clonal CD8+ T cell expansions are found preferentially in patients with a low tumor burden. Eur J Immunol 1997;27:2245–2252.
29. Massaia M, Borrione P, Attisano C, et al. Dysregulated Fas and Bcl-2 expression leading to enhanced apoptosis in T cells of multiple myeloma patients. Blood 1995;85:3679–3687.
30. Frassanito MA, Silvestris F, Cafforio P, Dammacco F. CD8+/CD57 cells and apoptosis suppress T-cell functions in multiple myeloma. Br J Haematol 1998;100:469–477.
31. Mozaffari F, Hansson L, Kiaii S, et al. Signalling molecules and cytokine production in T cells of multiple myeloma: increased abnormalities by advancing stage. Br J Haematol 2004; 124:315–326.
31a. Vij R, Borrello IM, Martin T, et al. A phase I/II study of Xcellerated T cells™ after autologous peripheral blood stem cell transplantation in patients with multiple myeloma. Blood 2003; 102:Abstract 139.

32. Osterborg A, Yi Q, Bergenbrant S, Holm G, Lefvert AK, Mellstedt H. Idiotype-specific T cells in multiple myeloma stage I: an evaluation by four different functional tests. Br J Haematol 1995;89:110–116.

33. Yi Q, Bergenbrant S, Osterborg A, et al. T-cell stimulation induced by idiotypes on monoclonal immunoglobulins in patients with monoclonal gammopathies. Scand J Immunol 1993;38:529–534.

34. Yi Q, Eriksson I, He W, Holm G, Mellstedt H, Osterborg A. Idiotype-specific T lymphocytes in monoclonal gammopathies: evidence for the presence of CD4+ and CD8+ subsets. Br J Haematol 1997;96:338–345.

35. Fagerberg J, Yi Q, Gigliotti D, et al. T-cell-epitope mapping of the idiotypic monoclonal IgG heavy and light chains in multiple myeloma. Int J Cancer 1999;80:671–680.

36. Hansson L, Rabbani H, Fagerberg J, Osterborg A, Mellstedt H. T-cell epitopes within the complementarity-determining and framework regions of the tumor-derived immunoglobulin heavy chain in multiple myeloma. Blood 2003;101:4930–4936.

37. Wen YJ, Ling M, Lim SH. Immunogenicity and cross-reactivity with idiotypic IgA of VH CDR3 peptide in multiple myeloma. Br J Haematol 1998;100:464–468.

38. Dabadghao S, Bergenbrant S, Anton D, He W, Holm G, Yi Q. Anti-idiotypic T-cell activation in multiple myeloma induced by M-component fragments presented by dendritic cells. Br J Haematol 1998;100:647–654.

39. Bergenbrant S, Osterborg A, Holm G, Mellstedt H, Lefvert AK. Anti-idiotypic antibodies in patients with monoclonal gammopathies: relation to the tumour load. Br J Haematol 1991;78:66–70.

40. Kwak LW, Taub DD, Duffey PL, et al. Transfer of myeloma idiotype-specific immunity from an actively immunised marrow donor. Lancet 1995;345:1016–1020.

41. Bergenbrant S, Yi Q, Osterborg A, et al. Modulation of anti-idiotypic immune response by immunization with the autologous M-component protein in multiple myeloma patients. Br J Haematol 1996;92:840–846.

42. Dranoff G, Jaffee E, Lazenby A, et al. Vaccination with irradiated tumor cells engineered to secrete murine granulocyte-macrophage colony-stimulating factor stimulates potent, specific, and long-lasting anti-tumor immunity. Proc Natl Acad Sci U S A 1993;90:3539–3543.

43. Osterborg A, Yi Q, Henriksson L, M, et al. Idiotype immunization combined with granulocyte-macrophage colony-stimulating factor in myeloma patients induced type I, major histocompatibility complex-restricted, CD8- and CD4-specific T-cell responses. Blood 1998;91:2459–2466.

44. Kwak LW, Sternas L, Jagannath S, Siegel D, Munchi N, Barlogie B. T-cell responses elicited by immunization of multiple myeloma patients with idiotypic M-protein plus GM-CSF in remission after autologous transplantation. Blood 1997;90(Suppl. 1):579a.

45. Kwak LW. Tumor vaccination strategies combined with autologous peripheral stem cell transplantation. Ann Oncol 1998;9(Suppl 1):S41–S46.

46. Caux C, Liu YJ, Banchereau J. Recent advances in the study of dendritic cells and follicular dendritic cells. Immunol Today 1995;16:2–4.

47. Wen YJ, Ling M, Bailey-Wood R, Lim SH. Idiotypic protein-pulsed adherent peripheral blood mononuclear cell-derived dendritic cells prime immune system in multiple myeloma. Clin Cancer Res 1998;4:957–962.

48. Liso A, Stockerl-Goldstein K, Reichardt V, et al. Idiotype vaccination using dendritic cells after autologous peripheral blood progenitor cell transplantation for multiple myeloma. Blood 1998;92(suppl. 1):105 a.

49. Schuetze S, Smith B, Bensinger W, Appelbaum F, Maloney DG. Myeloma idiotype vaccination post allogenic or autologous transplant can amplify idiotype-specific cellular immunity [abstract]. Blood 1999;94(suppl. 1):122.

50. Munchi N, Desikan R, Siegal D. Preliminary report of clinical efficacy of patient (pt) specific vaccination using purified idiotype protein in myeloma [abstract]. Blood 1999;94(suppl. 1):704.

51. Reichardt VL, Okada CY, Liso A, et al. Idiotype vaccination using dendritic cells after autologous peripheral blood stem cell transplantation for multiple myeloma: a feasibility study. Blood 1999;93:2411–2419.

52. Reichardt VL, Milazzo C, Brugger W, Einsele H, Kanz L, Brossart P. Specific immunotherapy of multiple myeloma patients using idiotype pulsed serum-free generated dendritic cells [abstract]. Blood 2001;98(suppl. 1):374).

53. Lacy M, Wettstein P, Gertz M. Dendritic cell-based idiotypic vaccination in post transplant multiple myeloma [abstract]. Blood 2000;96(suppl. 1):374.

54. Yi Q, Desikan R, Barlogie B, Munchi N. Optimizing dendritic cell-based immunotherapy in multiple myeloma [abstract]. Blood 2001;98(suppl. 1):374.

55. Lim SH, Bailey-Wood R. Idiotypic protein-pulsed dendritic cell vaccination in multiple myeloma. Int J Cancer 1999;83:215–222.

56. Titzer S, Christensen O, Manzke O, et al. Vaccination of multiple myeloma patients with idiotype-pulsed dendritic cells: immunological and clinical aspects. Br J Haematol 2000;108:805–816.

57. MacKenzie MR, Peshwa M, Wun T. Immunotherapy of advanced refractory multiple myeloma with idiotype-pulsed dendritic cells (mylovenge) [abstract]. Blood 2000;96(Suppl. 1):166.

58. Cull G, Durrant L, Stainer C, Haynes A, Russell N. Generation of anti-idiotype immune responses following vaccination with idiotype-protein pulsed dendritic cells in myeloma. Br J Haematol 1999;107:648–655.

59. Bogen B. Peripheral T cell tolerance as a tumor escape mechanism: deletion of CD4+ T cells specific for a monoclonal immunoglobulin idiotype secreted by a plasmacytoma. Eur J Immunol 1996;26:2671–1679.

60. Clark EA, Ledbetter JA. How B and T cells talk to each other. Nature 1994;367:425–428.

61. Hilbert DM, Shen MY, Rapp UR, Rudikoff S. T cells induce terminal differentiation of transformed B cells to mature plasma cell tumors. Proc Natl Acad Sci U S A 1995;92:649–653.

62. Lauritzsen GF, Hofgaard PO, Schenck K, Bogen B. Clonal deletion of thymocytes as a tumor escape mechanism. Int J Cancer 1998;78:216–222.

63. Bataille R, Barlogie B, Lu ZY, et al. Biologic effects of anti-interleukin-6 murine monoclonal antibody in advanced multiple myeloma. Blood 1995;86:685–691.

64. Grossbard ML, Fidias P, Kinsella J, et al. Anti-B4-blocked ricin: a phase II trial of 7 day continuous infusion in patients with multiple myeloma. Br J Haematol 1998;102:509–515.

65. Hussein M, Carma M, Maclain D, et al. Biological and clinical evaluation of rituxan in the management of newly diagnosed multiple myeloma patients. Blood 1999;94(Suppl 1):331a.

66. Treon SP, Raje N, Anderson KC. Immunotherapeutic strategies for the treatment of plasma cell malignancies. Semin Oncol 2000;27:598–613.

67. Waples I, Guaeltieri R, Hoon J, et al. High dose chemotherapy in stem cell transplantation in patients with multiple myeloma treated with monoclonal antibody against CD20 prior to stem cell collection. Blood 2000;96(Suppl. 1):326 b.

68. Cremer F, Gemmel C, Witzens M, et al. Treatment with the anti-CD20 antibody rituximab as consideration therapy for patients with multiple myeloma after proliferative stem cell transplantation. Blood 2000;96(Suppl. 1):298b.

69. Tricot G, Vesole DH, Jagannath S, Hilton J, Munshi N, Barlogie B. Graft-versus-myeloma effect: proof of principle. Blood 1996;87:1196–1198.

70. Verdonck LF, Lokhorst HM, Dekker AW, Nieuwenhuis HK, Petersen EJ. Graft-versus-myeloma effect in two cases. Lancet 1996;347:800–801.

71. Lokhorst HM, Schattenberg A, Cornelissen JJ, Thomas LL, Verdonck LF. Donor leukocyte infusions are effective in relapsed multiple myeloma after allogeneic bone marrow transplantation. Blood 1997;90:4206–4211.

72. Raitakari M, Brown RD, Gibson J, Joshua DE. Review Article: T cells in myeloma. Hematol Oncol 2003; 21:33–42.

73. Maecker B, Anderson KS, von Bergwelt-Baildon MS, et al. Viral antigen-specific CD8+ T-cell responses are impaired in multiple myeloma. Br J Haematol 2002; 121:842–848.

12 Remission Maintenance in Multiple Myeloma

Heinz Ludwig, MD and Niklas Zojer, MD

CONTENTS

1. INTRODUCTION

The maintenance phase is defined as the time period between best response to induction chemotherapy and relapse. It is characterized by a stable—"plateau"—phase of variable length, a cytokinetically quiescent state *(1)* in which myeloma cell proliferation is balanced by myeloma cell death. Complete or partial remission is not an absolute prerequisite for a plateau phase, which can be observed in patients whose best response to induction treatment is achievement of stable disease. Not surprisingly, a long plateau phase is a strong indicator of long survival in multiple myeloma (MM) *(2–4)*. Short plateau phases are associated with short doubling times of the patients' M-component and frequent resistance to salvage chemotherapy after relapse *(3)*.

Average remission duration after induction chemotherapy is approx 12 mo, but there are wide individual variations in length, with some patients relapsing shortly after onset of remission and others enjoying tumor control for 1 to 2 yr, or even longer. The frequency of remissions, particularly complete remissions,

From: *Current Clinical Oncology: Biology and Management of Multiple Myeloma*
Edited by: J. R. Berenson © Humana Press Inc., Totowa, NJ

is significantly higher and remission duration is longer after high-dose chemotherapy and autologous stem cell transplantation *(5)*, and still longer after allogeneic transplantation *(6)*. Sooner or later, however, relapse occurs in all patients, with the potential exception of a few patients who are cured after allogeneic transplantation or at least remain in long-lasting (>5–10 yr) remission.

Despite considerable improvements in induction treatment in recent years, with higher rates of complete remissions achievable, the length of the plateau phase and, thus, survival seems to be still determined mostly by characteristics intrinsic to the tumor cell. Specific chromosome aberrations are among the most important biologic variables determining aggressiveness of disease (*see* Chapters 4 and 7 for details). It is conceivable that chromosomal aberrations also confer susceptibility or resistance to different kinds of maintenance treatment, although such data are lacking to date. It certainly would be desirable to have guidelines at hand to include biological features in the process of decision making on the "if" and "how" of maintenance treatment.

Patients in remission usually enjoy a lack of symptoms of their disease, but may be anxious about the threat of relapse and the burden, toxicity, and uncertain outcome of second-line chemotherapy. This explains why during the 1970s and 1980s, an induction chemotherapy regimen was often applied continuously from onset of treatment until relapse. Significant bone marrow toxicity and other adverse effects, restriction of the patient's autonomy and reduction of quality of life, as well as an increased financial burden were the negative consequences of this strategy. Therefore, several attempts have been made to evaluate the optimal design and duration of induction chemotherapy and to develop alternative strategies to prolong remission.

2. MAINTENANCE CHEMOTHERAPY

The optimal length of induction chemotherapy is still unknown. Some treatment centers apply chemotherapy for roughly 1 yr, some treat longer, and others follow a more individualized approach, with adaptation of treatment duration to response to treatment.

The first prospective, randomized trial on the effect of terminating chemotherapy in responsive patients after 1 yr was published in 1975 by the Southwest Oncology Group *(7)*. Ninety-six patients who had responded to melphalan–prednisolone (MP), MP–procarbazine, or MP–vincristine after 1 yr of induction therapy were randomized to 1,3-bis-(2-chloroethyl)-1-nitrosurea (BCNU)–prednisolone, continued MP, or no chemotherapy. No differences were found among these three maintenance groups with regard to frequency of relapse, remission duration, and survival time. However, the frequencies of pneumonia and herpes zoster infections were significantly higher in patients receiving continuous chemotherapy. These observations prompted further studies that confirmed similar survival times in chemotherapy-treated and nonmaintained myeloma patients *(8,9)*. These studies reported high frequencies of second remissions in patients who had experienced a relapse from a nonmaintained first remission.

In the British Medical Research Council's IVth trial on myelomatosis *(10)*, 226 patients who had achieved stable disease for at least 4 mo taking MP or MP–vincristine induction chemotherapy were randomly assigned to another yr of the same chemotherapy or to a nonmaintained control group. In contrast to the expected outcome, a slight but nonsignificant survival advantage was observed in the control group, in which patients had not received chemotherapy during the plateau phase of their disease. No data on remission duration were reported.

Cohen and colleagues *(11)* randomized 286 patients who had achieved remissions while taking BCNU–cyclophosphamide–prednisone (BCP) induction therapy to MP or prednisone–adriamycin–azathioprine–vincristine (PAIV) or to no maintenance treatment. The majority of patients had received BCP treatment for 3 to 8 mo prior to randomization, but 10% had only one or two cycles and 13% received 10 to 20 courses of induction chemotherapy. Remission duration was slightly longer in patients on MP or PAIV maintenance therapy compared with nonmaintained controls, but these differences failed to reach statistical significance. Overall survival was comparable in patients with and without maintenance treatment. The authors concluded that both the toxicity and the financial burden argue against chemotherapeutic treatment during maintenance.

Similar findings were reported by Canadian investigators *(12)* who enrolled 497 patients for MP induction treatment. Of these, 210 achieved responses that were stable for at least 4 mo and 185 were randomized to continued chemotherapy until relapse or controls. Median time to progression was significantly longer in the chemotherapy arm (31 vs 23 mo; $p = 0.0011$), but 57% of the nonmaintained patients achieved a second response after reinstitution of chemotherapy and seven patients achieved a third response to another resumption of MP. The overall result was a slightly increased time to eventual melphalan failure in nonmaintained patients (39 vs 31 mo), although this difference failed to reach statistical significance. Overall survival was similar in both groups (51 vs 46 mo for nonmaintained and MP-maintained patients, respectively; $p = 0.59$) (Fig. 1). Two additional randomized trials with different experimental designs *(13,14)* also failed to show a survival advantage for prolonged induction treatment in patients who were responsive to first-line treatment.

In summary, the results of six randomized trials showed no benefit for maintenance chemotherapy in terms of improving overall survival (Table 1), although continuation of cytotoxic therapy might prolong the duration of remission. Of

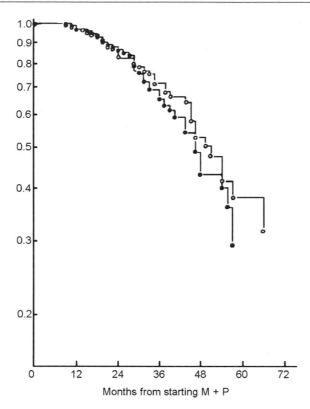

Fig. 1. Similar median survival in patients maintained with melphalan–prednisone (MP) (closed circles) and controls (51 and 46 mo in unmaintened and MP maintained patients respectively) *(12)*.

note, the concept of "consolidation" chemotherapy has gained increased interest recently. Barlogie's group *(15)* is currently evaluating the impact of intensive posttransplant consolidation chemotherapy on disease-free patients and on the overall survival of patients with myeloma. The rationale is analogous to that for the treatment of acute leukemias, i.e., eradication of the malignant clone—at least as completely as possible.

Currently, however, there is no indication that complete eradication of disease can be achieved by intensive treatment protocols (with the possible exception of allogeneic transplantation), and there is no clear evidence supporting the extension of therapy beyond what is necessary to achieve complete remission outside clinical trials. Up to -two-thirds of nonmaintained patients achieved second responses upon reinstitution of therapy at relapse, which results in equal or possibly even longer time periods to chemotherapy failure compared with patients on continuous chemotherapy.

Table 1
Major Randomized Trials on Chemotherapy as Maintenance Treatment

| First author | | Outcome | |
(Reference)	Treatment	RFS	Survival
SWOG (7)	BCNU+P	n.s.	n.s.
	cont. MP		
	controls		
MacLennan (10)	MP(V) 1 yr	n.d.	n.s.
	n.s.controls		
Cohen (11)	PAIV × 8	16.2 mo	41 mo
	MP × 6	14.9 mo	38 mo
	controls	11.5 mo	35 mo
Belch (12)	MP until relapse	16.2 mo	51 mo
	controls	11.2 mo	45 mo

RFS, relapse-free survival; SWOG, Southwest Oncology Group; BCNU, 1,3-bis-(2-chloroethyl)-1-nitrosurea; P, prednisone; MP, melphalan–prednisone; PAIV, prednisone + adriamycin + azathioprine + vincristine; n.s., not significant; n.d., no data.

3. INTERFERON-α MAINTENANCE THERAPY

3.1. Biological Effects of Interferon-α

Interferon (IFN)-α is a pleiotropic cytokine with various effects on myeloma cells, as well as on cells of the immune system. When directly applied to freshly isolated myeloma cells grown either in clonogenic assays or in tissue culture, IFN-α usually exerts a significant inhibitory effect on cell growth (16), particularly when higher concentrations are used, but it may also stimulate cell proliferation under certain conditions (17). IFN-α down-regulates the expression of interleukin (IL)-6 receptors on myeloma cells (18) and, thus, may reduce their sensitivity to their most important growth and differentiation factor. IFN-α has also been shown to enhance autocrine IL-6 production in myeloma cells (19).

Controversial findings have also been reported regarding IFN-induced effects on fas-mediated apoptosis. In one study, IFN-α inhibited cell death stimulated by anti-fas monoclonal antibody (MAb) (20); in another investigation, IFN-α increased the sensitivity of myeloma cells to fas-induced apoptosis (21). The authors of the latter study showed that IFN-α activates Stat1 and attenuates IL-6-induced activation of Stat3. These effects were followed by up-regulation of the fas protein and would explain why IFN-α can sensitize myeloma cells to fas-induced apoptosis (22).

IFN-α was also shown to protect myeloma cells from dexamethasone-induced apoptosis (23) and to induce apoptosis in myeloma cell lines in a dose-dependent manner (24). Other biological effects of IFN-α, which may be clinically relevant, relate to its ability to increase the expression of MHC antigens on tumor cells *(25)*, to activate NK cells in vitro *(26)* and in vivo *(27)*, to activate macrophages *(28)*, and to stimulate the terminal differentiation of dendritic cells *(28)*. Furthermore, IFN-α has been shown to stimulate the production of IL-1, IL-2, IL-6, IFN-γ, and tumor necrosis factor (TNF) in different cell types *(29)*. It is also a potent inhibitor of angiogenesis *(30)*, which—in the light of the recently observed association between angiogenesis and progression of myeloma—could be therapeutically relevant.

3.2. First Applications of IFN-α in Myeloma

The first observation that IFN-α has anti-myeloma activity was published by Mellstedt and colleagues in 1979 *(31)*. Two out of four chemotherapy-resistant myeloma patients who had been treated with daily injections of natural leukocyte IFN-α achieved a complete response; the other two patients achieved a partial response. Large-scale studies were limited at that time owing to the shortage of IFN-α, which had to be extracted from leukocytes. Despite these limitations, a small number of studies of natural IFN could be carried out. Clinical research was greatly facilitated by the introduction of genetically engineered IFN-α2a and IFN-α2b. In phase II studies, response rates of 20 to 50% were reported with IFN monotherapy. Subsequently, IFN monotherapy was compared with MP or VMCP chemotherapy in two prospective, randomized phase III trials. In the trial conducted by Ahre and colleagues, *(32)* IFN-α yielded a response rate of 14% compared with 44% for MP-treated patients. In our own study, *(33)* a response rate of 14% and of 58% was obtained with IFN-α and with VMCP, respectively. Despite the significantly lower response rate obtained with interferon alone, no difference in survival was seen because IFN-failing patients could be effectively treated with second-line chemotherapy.

3.3. IFN-α Maintenance Therapy

The results of the trials described above and data obtained from studies on the combined use of IFN-α and chemotherapy indicated that IFN might be most active in patients with a low tumor mass and relatively benign disease. Both features are more prominent in patients who have responded to initial chemotherapy and entered a "plateau phase." Furthermore, the plateau phase resembles the G_0 phase of the cell cycle, which can be prolonged by IFN-α in vitro *(34)*. Thus, it was only a question of time for IFN-α to be tested as maintenance treatment for myeloma. Mandelli and colleagues *(35)* were the first to report a prolongation of remission-duration by use of IFN-α. Patients who had responded to initial chemotherapy by tumor reduction or at least stabilization of disease were randomized to receive either 5 Mega U/m^2 IFN-α2 or no treatment. IFN-treated patients showed significant prolongations of remission duration as compared with patients in the control arm (26 vs 14 mo; $p < 0.0002$). In their first publication the authors also reported a tendency toward increased overall survival in the IFN group ($p = 0.053$), which reached statistical significance in the subgroup of patients with complete or partial response to induction chemotherapy. In a follow-up report, however, this difference failed to retain its statistical significance *(36)*.

Subsequently, several other randomized studies were published in which IFN-α maintenance treatment was compared with no treatment (Table 2). Four of these studies *(37-40)* reported significant benefits for the IFN arm in terms of prolonged remission duration. There was also a tendency toward a prolonged overall survival, but statistical significance was only achieved in one study *(38)*. Another study *(41)* reported a trend toward prolonged remission duration but no difference in survival, another study a trend toward prolonged overall survival with no data given on remission duration *(42)*, and two studies *(43,44)* found no benefits for IFN-α maintenance treatment. A negative impact of IFN maintenance treatment on disease outcome was not observed in any of these studies, however, inconsistent benefit observed in randomized trials led to a considerable debate in the medical community, with some physicians being strongly in favor of IFN maintenance therapy, others opposing it strictly.

Recently, a large randomized US trial evaluated IFN-α maintenance treatment for patients treated with upfront conventional therapy or high-dose therapy *(44a)*. Pateints who received maintenance of IFN-α owed no benfit, and no difference was observed in either patients treated upfront with conventional or high-dose therapy.

3.4. Meta-Analysis of Randomized Trials

The reason for the divergent results reported from randomized trials on IFN-α maintenance treatment is the limited statistical power of studies that involve relatively small numbers of patients (284 patients in the largest trial). In order to detect a significant 5% increase of an anticipated median remission duration of 12 mo in untreated controls or of an anticipated median overall survival of 36 mo in conventionally treated patients, more than 900 patients would have to be enrolled. We, therefore, conducted a meta-analysis that overcomes the limitations of single trials, and developed a new statistical approach which allows analysis of published data on median remission duration and overall survival times, and, thus, yields reliable results much faster than meta-analysis based on individual patient data. Our first meta-analysis was published in 1995 *(38)*. It has recently been updated, and is now based on the results derived from 1615 patients enrolled in 13 trials in which IFN maintenance treatment was compared with nonmaintained controls *(45)*. The updated results confirm the earlier findings: IFN-α maintenance treatment significantly prolongs remission duration and overall survival. The respective median gains were 4.4 mo in remission duration and 7 mo in overall survival. Similar findings were obtained by the Oxford group of investigators *(46)* who conducted a meta-analysis based on individual patient

Table 2
Large Randomized Trials on IFN Maintenance Treatment in Myeloma

| First author (reference) | Number of patients | | Induction regimen | Response to induction treatment | IFN dose (MU/ m^2/wk) | RFS | IFN arm superior Survival |
	IFN	Controls					
Drayson (41)	143	141	ABCM	Plateau phase	5.6	Trend	n.s.
Salmon (43)	97	96	VMCP/VBAP or VAD	CR	5.6	n.s.	n.s.
Browman (39)	85	91	MP	CR, PR	6.0	$p < 0.05$	$p < 0.05$
Grosbois (42)	80	66	MP	Plateau	9.0	n.d.	Trend
Westin (37)	61	64	MP	CR, PR	9.4	$p < 0.0001$	n.s.
Peest (44)	52	65	MP or VBAMDex	CR, PR, stable disease	9.4	n.s.	n.s.
Mandelli (35)	50	51	MP or VMCP/VBAP	CR, PR, stable disease	14.0	$p < 0.0002$	$p < 0.05$
Ludwig (38)	46	54	VMCP or IFN+VMCP	CR, PR, stable disease	3.8	$p < 0.01$	$p < 0.05$
Blade (40)	50	42	VMCB/VBAP	CR, PR	9.0	$p < <0.05$	Trend

IFN, interferon; RFS, relapse-free survival; ABCM, adriamycin, BCNU, cyclophosphamide, melphalan; VMPC, vincristine, melphalan, cyclophosphamide, prednisone; VBAP, vincristine, BCNU, adriamycin, prednisone; VAD, vincristine, adriamycin, dexamethasone; VBAMD, vincristine, BCNU, adriamycin, melphalan, dexamethasone; MP, melphalan–prednisone; CR, complete remission; PR, partial remission; n.s., not significant; n.d., no data.

data. They reported an estimated gain of 7 mo for both relapse-free survival and for overall survival in patients treated with IFN maintenance therapy. The absolute improvement in overall survival was 4.3% and the relative reduction for the risk of death 12% in interferon maintained patients (Fig. 2). However, the results of these meta-analyses are limited by the heterogenerity of patients enrolled and different regimens between different trials.

3.5. Candidates for IFN-α Treatment

Clinical experience from other IFN-sensitive cancers, such as melanoma or renal cell cancer, indicates that patients with good prognostic factors are the most likely candidates to benefit from IFN-α treatment. If this situation also applies to myeloma, patients with good performance status, less-aggressive disease, and relatively young age would be preferential candidates for IFN-α treatment. However, no solid scientific basis exists for this recommendation. Subgroup analysis by the Oxford investigators (46) failed to identify a group of patients more likely to benefit from interferon treatment-α.

3.6. Dose and Schedule of IFN-α

It is not known yet what particular dose and treatment schedule is required for IFN-α to exert its optimal therapeutic efficacy. In melanoma, higher doses seem to translate into better clinical results (47), into significant stimulation of natural killer cell activity, and into increases in CD3 and CD4 cells, as well as increases in the CD4–CD8 ratio (48). In myeloma, such a dose–response relation has only been suggested by a single randomized trial enrolling 52 patients (49). Data from the latter trial indicate that patients who tolerate at least 30×10^6 U/mo have a significantly superior outcome compared with those who are on lower doses. In their seminal study Mandelli and co-workers used a starting dosage of 5×10^6 U/m^2 thrice weekly, (35) but this dose induced considerable adverse effects and could not be maintained for long. Consequently, it was reduced to 3×10^6 U/m^2 for the rest of the trial. Based on these experiences and the failure to demonstrate a clear-cut dose–response effect in myeloma, a treatment regimen of 3×10^6 U thrice weekly, flat dose, is now commonly used. As expected, combination of interferon maintenance treatment with chemotherapy, e.g., alternating application of IFN-α (3×10^6 U, thrice weekly) and cycles of vinblastine, adriamycin, and dexamethasone (VAD), MP, and CP resulted in no advantages over maintenance treatment with IFN-α alone (50).

3.7. Combined IFN-α-Prednisone Maintenance Treatment

Glucocorticoids, particularly dexamethasone and prednisone, have considerable activity in myeloma and lead to complete or partial remissions in approx 20 to 40% of newly diagnosed patients. Steroids have additional beneficial effects in myeloma patients: they reduce bone pain, improve the sense of well-being,

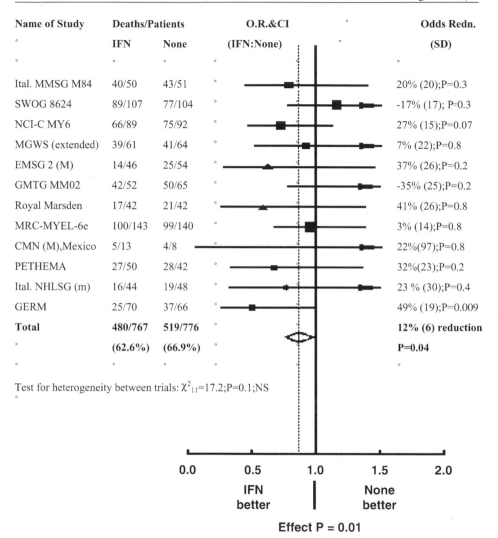

Name of Study	Deaths/Patients		O.R.&CI	Odds Redn.
	IFN	None	(IFN:None)	(SD)
Ital. MMSG M84	40/50	43/51		20% (20);P=0.3
SWOG 8624	89/107	77/104		-17% (17); P=0.3
NCI-C MY6	66/89	75/92		27% (15);P=0.07
MGWS (extended)	39/61	41/64		7% (22);P=0.8
EMSG 2 (M)	14/46	25/54		37% (26);P=0.2
GMTG MM02	42/52	50/65		-35% (25);P=0.2
Royal Marsden	17/42	21/42		41% (26);P=0.8
MRC-MYEL-6e	100/143	99/140		3% (14);P=0.8
CMN (M),Mexico	5/13	4/8		22%(97);P=0.8
PETHEMA	27/50	28/42		32%(23);P=0.2
Ital. NHLSG (m)	16/44	19/48		23 % (30);P=0.4
GERM	25/70	37/66		49% (19);P=0.009
Total	**480/767**	**519/776**		**12% (6) reduction**
	(62.6%)	**(66.9%)**		**P=0.04**

Test for heterogeneity between trials: χ^2_{11}=17.2;P=0.1;NS

```
0.0        0.5        1.0        1.5        2.0
          IFN                   None
         better                 better
```

Effect P = 0.01

Fig. 2. Mortality in trials on interferon (IFN) maintenance therapy. Large squares indicate trials that provide more information and hence have narrower 99% confidence intervals (CI). If the square is to the left of the solid line then mortality is lower in the group allocated to IFN (vs no maintenance), but if the CI crosses this line then this result is not statistically significant ($p < 0.01$). An arrow at the right-hand end of the CI indicates that the CI extends further than the plotting area. The total for maintenance trials is represented as diamond centered on the odds ratio (OR) estimate, with 95% CI shown by the width of the diamond. The vertical dotted line shows the overall odds ratio estimate, i.e., the center of the diamond. (Modified from The Myeloma Trialists' Collaborative Group [46].)

increase appetite, and may ameliorate adverse effects induced by IFN therapy. These facts and in vitro findings of additive inhibitory effects of steroids and interferon on myeloma colony formation *(51)* make both drugs almost ideal choices for combined use in an attempt to prolong remission duration. Indeed, the combination of IFN-α and steroids was found to yield increases in plateau-phase duration *(52)*. These findings were confirmed in a prospective, randomized trial, in which IFN-α–prednisone was compared with IFN-α alone *(53)*. Remission duration was significantly longer in the combined treatment than in the monotherapy arm (19 vs 9 mo; $p < 0.008$). Median survival from the start of maintenance was unusually long in both arms but only marginally longer with IFN-α–prednisone as compared with IFN alone (57 vs 46 mo; $p = 0.36$).

3.8. IFN-α After High-Dose Therapy and Autologous Transplantation

In theory, patients subjected to high-dose chemotherapy and transplantation are ideal candidates for IFN-α maintenance therapy. Tumor burden is substantially reduced, and myeloma-cell proliferation is slowed to a minimum. In fact, the data available to date seem to support this notion, although not uniformly. The only prospective, randomized trial on the impact of interferon maintenance treatment following high-dose treatment and transplantation involved 85 patients. Early results revealed significant prolongations of remission duration (46 vs 27 mo; $p < 0.025$) and overall survival, with 14 deaths in the control arm compared with 5 deaths in the treatment arm ($p < 0.006$) at a median follow-up of 52 mo *(54)*, although in a recent follow-up, the differences between the arms had ceased to be statistically significant because most patients ultimately succumbed to their disease *(55)*. Of three retrospective comparisons, two yielded positive results and one brought negative results. Bjorkstrand and colleagues *(56)* conducted a matched-pair analysis using data from the European Group for Blood and Bone Marrow Transplantation database, and found a significantly superior outcome in terms of remission duration and overall survival in the patients treated with interferon. Multivariate analysis of data from the Spanish Registry for Transplant in Multiple Myeloma identified posttransplant IFN-α treatment as being significantly associated with longer progression-free and overall survival *(57)*. No such benefits were observed by the analysis of data from the French Registry on Autologous Bone Marrow Transplantation in Multiple Myeloma *(58)*. The recent large randomized US trial showed no benefit of maintenance IFN in either patients randomized to upfront high-dose therapy or conventional therapy (*see* Subheading 3.3.) *(44a)*.

3.9. Adverse Effects of IFN-α Treatment

Side effects of IFN-α therapy vary greatly among individual patients. Younger patients with excellent performance status experience few adverse effects and may continue receiving treatment for several years. A prominent side effect is the occurrence of fever 4 to 8 h after administration of the drug. This complication

Table 3
Adverse Effects of Interferon
Reported by Myeloma Patients

Fever (2–3 wk)	34%
Flu-like symptoms	50%
Fatigue	36%
Muscle pain	21%
Nausea	17%
Neurologic/psychological	12%
Leukopenia	7%
Loss of appetite	5%
Thrombocytopenia	2%
Other	each <1%

From ref. 66.

is seen in approximately two-thirds of patients and usually subsided after 2 to 3 wk of treatment. It is frequently associated with flu-like symptoms, such as chills, myalgias, headache, and malaise, which also cease in many patients despite continuation of treatment. In approx 30% of patients, however, these symptoms persist and may require temporary dose reduction or even discontinuation of therapy. Hematologic toxicity includes leukopenia and thrombocytopenia, which are dose dependent and have also been described as a reason for discontinuation of treatment. However, we think that there is no reason to taper the dose or even stop treatment because of hematotoxicity unless the leukocyte count falls below 1500/μL and/or the thrombocyte count falls below 50,000/μL. Other adverse effects are fatigue, weakness, anorexia, weight loss, depression, and, rarely, alopecia (Table 3). Autoimmune diseases, particularly autoimmune thyroiditis and hypothyroidism, may be induced or enhanced by IFN-α in individual patients. Preliminary data suggest that pegylated IFN-α (PEG-IFN), which has a longer half-life compared with conventional IFN-α and thus is applied once weekly only, has a more favorable toxicity profile (59). However, data on efficacy of PEG-IFN as maintenance treatment for myeloma are lacking to date.

There are few systematic studies on how to best ameliorate IFN-related adverse effects (60–62). Acute IFN-α toxicity, such as fever, may respond to treatment with paracetamol or other nonsteroidal anti-inflammatory drugs. Long-term sequelae of IFN-α treatment, such as anorexia and fatigue, can sometimes be improved by low doses of steroids, and patients with depressions may respond to serotonin-reuptake inhibitors, psychostimulants, or steroids. (61). Even with such interventions at hand, some patients discontinue IFN-α owing to toxicity rather early after the onset of therapy. In the Medical Research Council trial, 90% of patients were still taking IFN 6 mo after allocation to this treatment (41); in

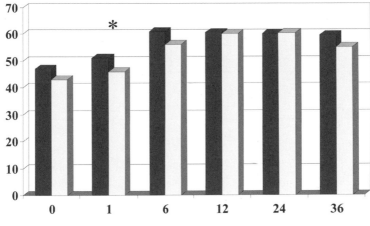

Time after start of treatment (months)

Fig. 3. Quality of life in patients randomized to either melphalan–prednisone (MP) (solid bars) or interferon plus MP (white bars). Interferon maintenance treatment is associated with significantly reduced quality of life shortly after initiation of treatment ($p = 0.01$). After 1 yr there is no difference in global quality of life between the two study arms. Patients who suffer from interferon toxicity tend to discontinue treatment early. The asterisk (*) indicates a statistically significant difference. (Modified from Wisloff et al. [63].)

our trial, the figure at 12 mo was 80% (38); 60% of patients were still taking IFN after 2 yr in the Nordic study (63).

3.10. Quality of Life

Quality of life (QOL) under treatment with IFN-α has been systematically studied in two trials. In the Nordic trial (64), 90% of the 583 patients randomized to MP or MP–IFN-α (5×10^6 U, three times/wk) participated in the quality of life study, and 83% completed all questionnaires (63). QOL was moderately reduced during the first treatment year on IFN, mainly because of higher frequencies of chills, fever, fatigue, anorexia, nausea, vomiting, and dry skin (Fig. 3). After the first yr, however, there was practically no difference in QOL in both groups. Probably a large proportion of patients tolerated interferon quite well from the onset of treatment or developed excellent tolerance during the course of treatment, whereas those who suffered from considerable toxicity discontinued interferon therapy within the first year. In the Canadian trial, (65) three different health states were assessed and compared among IFN-treated and untreated patients. Time without symptoms of disease, relapse, and toxicity (TWiST) was used as an overall indicator of QOL and was related to time with toxicity and the period following disease relapse. A significantly longer TWiST, indicating a superior QOL, was observed in the IFN arm. IFN-α treatment was associated

Table 4
Myeloma Patient Choice of Interferon As Maintenance Treatment

Proposed Benefit (Median Gain)	Yes	Responses Possibly	No
+7 mo remission duration	57.5%	18.9%	23.4%
+3 mo survival	32.1%	13.0%	54.9%

with more toxicity that, on the average, lasted for 4.1 mo. This burdensome time was clearly compensated by a significant prolongation of median relapse-free survival amounting to 9.8 mo.

3.11. Patients' Perceptions of IFN-α

An improvement of remission duration and survival in the magnitude of 4 to 7 mo at the expense of more toxicity and inconvenience, with possible additional financial costs, may be quite differently viewed by individual patients. Some may eagerly accept, whereas others may decide to refrain from such treatment. To better understand the viewpoints of myeloma patients, we undertook an interview study on conditions that have to be offered as a trade-off for patients to be willing to accept IFN treatment (66). The findings matched our anticipations: the longer the presumable gain in survival, the higher the proportion of patients willing to undergo therapy. When the presumable gain in remission duration or survival was said to be 3 mo, only 37% of the interviewed patients would have opted for the treatment. However, when the prospective gain was increased to 7 mo, 57% of the patients would have agreed to be treated (Table 4). It also became clear that patients who accepted the proposed hypothetical treatment differed in their personality profiles from those who declined it. Patients who would have accepted treatment—the risk takers—were younger, had more advanced myeloma, and came from a higher socioeconomic background (Table 5).

Interestingly, 37% of the 356 patients interviewed had already been treated with IFN, mainly for prolongation of their maintenance phase. The frequency of IFN use in patients who previously had been transplanted was 51% (66).

Overall, IFN-α may have minimal benefit for patients with MM as maintenance therapy. However, the high cost of the drug, significant side effects, and recent negative results of large clinical trials should be taken into consideration before committing patients to long-term treatment with this agent.

4. PREDNISONE MAINTENANCE THERAPY

As mentioned above, a prolonged remission duration with combined IFN–prednisone maintenance treatment compared with IFN alone was reported by Salmon and colleagues (53). Because there was no arm evaluating the effect of

Table 5
Description of Interferon (IFN)-Treated and Nontreated Myeloma Patients

Patients With MM Who Opt for IFN Treatment	Patients With MM Who Reject IFN Treatment
• are younger than 60 yr	• are older than 60 yr
• have experience with IFN	• lack experience with IFN
• suffer from advanced myeloma	• suffer from early-stage myeloma
• have poor feelings of well-being	• have good feelings of well-being
• are educated above high school level	• are educated below college level

prednisone monotherapy, the exact contribution of each of the two agents to the superior outcome of combined treatment remained to be defined. This issue was clarified in 2002, when Berenson and colleagues *(67)* published the results of a randomized study establishing the value of glucocorticoid therapy as maintenance treatment for myeloma. Patients responding to a VAD-like regimen with or without oral quinine induction therapy were randomized to oral prednisone at two different dose levels: a pharmacologic dose of 50 mg on alternate days ($n = 51$) or a physiologic dose of 10 mg ($n = 61$) taken on alternate days until disease progression began. Both progression-free survival (14 vs 5 mo; $p = 0.003$) and overall survival (37 vs 26 mo; $p = 0.5$) were significantly improved in patients receiving 50 mg compared with 10 mg of prednisone taken on alternate days (Fig. 4). Toxicities and the side-effect profile were similar between the arms. In general, the treatment was well tolerated.

These results show that 50 mg of alternate-day prednisone offers an effective, safe, and inexpensive alternative to IFN maintenance therapy. Indeed, results seen with prednisone treatment in this single study compared favorably with results obtainable by IFN maintenance treatment, as suggested by meta-analysis (9 vs 4.4–6 mo increase in remission duration; 11 vs 7 mo improvement of overall survival). So far, no randomized comparison of glucocorticoid maintenance therapy alone vs combined glucocorticoid–IFN treatment has been published. We randomized more than 150 patients in such a trial and hope to soon be able to report the outcome of this study.

5. THALIDOMIDE ALONE OR THALIDOMIDE COMBINATIONS AS MAINTENANCE TREATMENT

Thalidomide was introduced as effective treatment of patients with myeloma who have had a relapse and patients with refractory myeloma in 1999 *(68)*. Since then, several trials have confirmed its activity as a single agent and in combination with dexamethasone or with cytotoxic drugs.

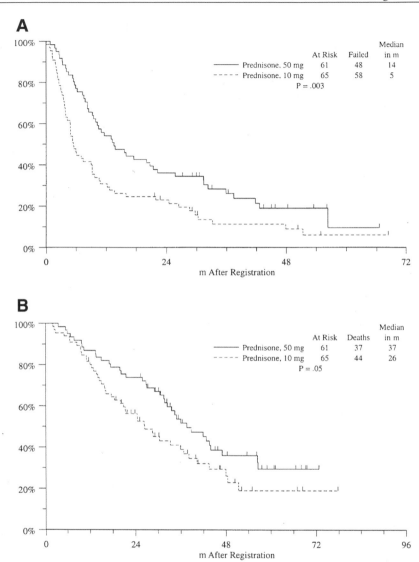

Fig. 4. Progression-free ([A] 14 vs 5 mo; $p = 0.003$) and overall survival ([B] 37 vs 26 mo; $p = 0.5$) was significantly superior with 50 mg alternate day prednisone as compared to 10 mg alternate day. (From ref. 67.)

Several studies that are ongoing as of this writing are evaluating the tolerability and efficacy of thalidomide alone as maintenance treatment following conventional or high-dose therapy. A United Kingdom Myeloma Forum Phase 2 Study (69) is using thalidomide maintenance treatment after high-dose melphalan-based autografting at five dose levels: 50 mg, 100 mg, 200 mg, 250 mg, and 300 mg. Treatment commences 3 mo after an autograft. Twenty patients have been recruited to each cohort, for a target total recruitment of 100. Eighty-four patients were recruited as of August 2003 and interim results have been reported in an abstract *(70)*. At a median follow-up of 6 mo, 18 out of 84 patients (21%) had stopped taking thalidomide, 7 following disease progression, and 11 because of toxicity, including neuropathy *(4)*, rash *(3)*, nonspecific side effects *(3)* and thrombosis *(1)*. A significant number of patients (approx 50%) reported side effects—including constipation, rash, and lethargy—but continued the treatment. Only 58% continued the allotted dose above 200 mg compared with 82% taking 200 mg or less.

Similar dose levels were achieved by Sahebi and colleagues *(71)*. Patients started maintenance thalidomide at 50 mg/d 6 to 8 wk after a single cycle of autografting, and the dose was gradually increased to a target dose of 400 mg/d. The median tolerated dose was 200 mg/d, and only 14% of patients were able to achieve the target dose of 400 mg/d.

Thalidomide–dexamethasone combinations are even more effective than thalidomide alone and induce responses in up to 40% of pretreated and up to 70% of newly diagnosed patients. It has to be noted that patients on thalidomide–dexamethasone or thalidomide–chemotherapy combinations are at increased risk of thromboembolic complications and might benefit from prophylactic anticoagulation with low-molecular-weight heparin.

Alexanian and colleagues *(72)* provided first evidence of the efficacy of thalidomide–dexamethasone as consolidation therapy for patients in continuous partial remission after autologous transplantation. Thalidomide was initiated at a daily dose of 100 mg, which was escalated to a maximum of 300 mg. Dexamethasone 20 mg/m^2 days 1 through 4 was applied on a pulse schedule. A further marked reduction (90%) of paraprotein was seen in 12 out of 21 of patients (57%), with 4 out of 21 (19%) achieving complete remission. Although this is a small study and thalidomide–dexamethasone was administered as consolidation rather than maintenance treatment, these results appear promising.

Currently, a Canadian multicenter trial *(73)* is evaluating prednisone 50 mg on alternate days + thalidomide 200 mg as maintenance treatment for myeloma after autologous transplantation, and our study group (CEMSG) is comparing thalidomide (maximum dose: 200 mg/d) + IFN with single-agent IFN maintenance in nontransplant patients initially randomized to thalidomide–dexamethasone or MP for induction treatment. Results will be presented in 2005.

6. NOVEL APPROACHES TO IMPROVEMENT OF REMISSION DURATION

Newer treatment strategies for myeloma aim to increase the rate of complete remission, thereby achieving longer periods of good QOL for more patients. For the same reason, remissions need to be maintained as long as possible, with the number of residual myeloma cells curbed to a minimum. If it became possible to eradicate residual disease during the plateau phase, multiple myeloma might even become a curable disease. Several strategies are presently being pursued to achieve these goals (Table 6).

6.1. Cytokines

IL-2 activates natural killer cells, (74,75) fosters lymphokine-activated killer (LAK) activity, (75,76) and promotes the release of cytokines, including IFN-γ and TNF (77). These effects might help control residual disease in patients who have achieved remission following induction treatment.

Therapeutic activity of IL-2 in chemoresistant myeloma has been shown in a number of small studies (unpublished data) (75,78). In a study evaluating the effects of IL-2 maintenance treatment following autologous stem cell transplantation, two out of six myeloma patients remained in partial remission, tolerating IL-2 well (79). In another study, patients after bone marrow transplantation for hematologic malignancies were treated with either IL-2 "maintenance" doses $(0.3 \times 10^6 \text{ U/m}^2/\text{d}$, days 12–21) or, in addition, escalating IL-2 "induction" doses $(0.3–4.5 \times 10^6 \text{ U/m}^2/\text{d}$, days 1–5). Pronounced immunomodulatory effects were observed in patients treated with higher IL-2 doses, but patients in this group also experienced mild to moderate adverse effects, such as fever, nausea, diarrhea, and local skin rashes. Dose-limiting toxicities were hypotension and thrombocytopenia (80). The activity of IL-2 maintenance treatment is further evaluated in a prospective, randomized trial (81).

6.2. Small Molecules and Immunomodulatory Drugs

Bortezomib (Velcade™), the first representative of a new class of anti-cancer drugs that inhibit the proteasome, has recently been shown to exert a 35% response rate in heavily pretreated myeloma patients (82). Similarly, Revlimid™ and Activimid™ have shown excellent activity in advanced disease. These later drugs belong to the group of immunomodulatory drugs, which are derivatives of thalidomide but show different biologic activities and offer the advantage of oral administration. All the above-mentioned new drugs are likely to be tested for their potential as maintenance treatment soon.

6.3. Vaccination Strategies

Vaccines have been used to induce an active immune response directed against epitopes on the surface of tumor cells or their precursors, which reduces or eliminates residual cells of the tumor clone. The most specific epitope on myeloma cells is the immunoglobulin idiotype, which should, therefore, be the ideal antigenic target. Because the myeloma immunoglobulin idiotype is patient-specific, a drawback of this therapeutic modality is the necessity to prepare vaccines individually. Although in principle this approach is interesting, prepa-

Table 6
New Approaches to Myeloma Treatment
That Might be Applied During Maintenance

New drugs
    Thalidomide
    Proteasome inhibitors
    ImiDs

Monoclonal antibodies against
    myeloma markers
    CD38
    cytokines (IL-6)
    VEGF

Vaccinations with
    individual immunoglobulin idiotypes
    antigen-pulsed dendritic cells
    plasmid-DNA encoding idiotypes
    myeloma cells + transfected fibroblasts
    enhanced by the addition of
        adjuvants
        stimulatory cytokines (GM-CSF,IL-12)

Inhibition of angiogenesis
    Thalidomide
    VEGF inhibitors

Immune effector cells
    Allogeneic T cells
    Primed autologous T cells
    Xcellerated T cells™

ImiDs, immunomodulatory drugs; IL, interleukin; VEGF, vascular endothelial growth factor; GM-CSF, granulocyte-macrophage colony-stimulating factor.

ration of idiotype-based protein vaccines is cumbersome and expensive, considering presently available technologies. Thus, data on idiotype protein vaccines for myeloma are limited *(83)*; in addition, they have not been proven similarly successful as in patients with B-cell lymphomas *(84)*.

Presentation of the idiotype to the immune system may be enhanced by means of antigen-pulsed dendritic cells. The clinical efficacy of this concept has been investigated by several study groups *(85,86)*. An even newer and fascinating vaccination technique is the use of plasmid DNA encoding the idiotype *(87)*, which has proven successful in animal models and is being evaluated in clinical trials as of this writing. Vaccination with a combination of myeloma cells and transfected fibroblasts, which produce high levels of granulocyte-macrophage colony-stimulating factor, is also presently being investigated. This approach also has already effected pronounced tumor reductions in an animal model *(85)*.

6.4. MAbs

Another potential target is the CD38 surface molecule, which has the advantage of being expressed on virtually all myeloma cells in all patients. Treatment with MAbs against CD38 was already tested clinically, but the outcome remained unsatisfactory *(88)*. CD20, a B-cell antigen, has been described as expressed on mature tumor cells in approx 20% of myeloma patients *(89)*; however, this figure is controversial. The CD20 antigen is strongly expressed on bone marrow cells in rare patients with lymphoplasmacytic myeloma, however, and may exist on a substantial fraction of circulating myeloma precursor cells. Unfortunately, treatment of advanced myeloma patients with anti-CD20 antibody has shown very limited success *(90)*. Also, the application of anti-CD20 antibody after autologous transplantation was reported to be associated with a shortened plateau phase *(91)*. It seems that the adverse effect of anti-CD20 treatment is due to temporary eradication of normal functional B cells and, thus, attenuation of humoral and cellular anti-tumor immunity.

Suppression of stimulatory cytokines by monoclonal antibodies or by receptor-blocking molecules is another promising novel approach. Antibodies against IL-6 were the first to enter clinical trials. Phase I results showed a transient inhibition of tumor growth in some patients with advanced disease, but eventually all patients experienced disease progression on this therapy *(92)*. The clinical relevance of anti-IL-6 maintenance therapy being studied by the Intergroupe Francophone du Myelome (IFM99) as of this writing. Patients who underwent autologous transplantation are randomized into a cohort receiving an intermittent treatment regimen with anti-IL-6 antibodies + dexamethasone or dexamethasone only (Harrosseau JL, personal communication).

6.5. Mini-Allografts and Autologous T Cells

Mini-allografts require less aggressive conditioning regimens—e.g., fludarabine *(93)* and/or low-dose irradiation—and thus may considerably decrease early transplant-related mortality rates compared with conventional allogeneic transplantation. This procedure often includes the use of donor lymphocyte infusions to obtain and maintain a graft-vs-myeloma effect *(94)*.

Infusion of activated and in vitro expanded autologous T cells (Xcellerated™ T cells) is another interesting approach for remission maintenance treatment. Lymphocytes from heavily pretreated patients can successfully be expanded several fold in vitro ($5-10 \times 10^{10}$ T cells/patient and culture) and re-infused with few side effects. As this treatment was shown to have anti-myeloma activity *(95)*, it seems attractive to exploit this concept for remission maintenance treatment.

6.6. Bisphosphonates

The potential of bisphosphonates (zoledronic acid) to prevent or delay the transition from monoclonal gammopathies of undetermined significance to active myeloma is being studied by Berenson and colleagues as of this writing. A similar approach is considered for patients with smoldering myeloma *(96)*. Patients are randomized to receive either zoledronic acid in combination with thalidomide or zoledronic acid only. Bisphosphonates may also have beneficial effects as remission maintenance treatment, especially in terms of reducing skeletal events and bone pain. Recently, the American Society of Clinical Oncology published guidelines on the use of bisphosphonates in myeloma (97). The panel recommended that patients with lytic bone disease should receive either intravenous zolendronate 4 mg infused over 15 min or pamidronate 90 mg delivered over 120 min every 3 to 4 wk. The panel also believes that it is reasonable to start these agents in patients with osteopenia, but without clear evidence of lytic bone disease.

The manifold anti-myeloma effects of bisphosphonates observed in vitro however do not seem to translate into a survival benefit clinically *(97)*. Possibly, new bisphosphonates or new inhibitors of osteoclast stimulators—e.g., the NF-κB ligand (RANKL), MIP-1α, or substances that neutralize the recently defined inhibitors of osteoblast activity (DKK, FrzB)—will provide better control of myeloma-induced microenvironmental changes and thereby mitigate tumor progression.

7. SUMMARY

The benefits of maintenance treatment in myeloma are comparable in magnitude to the effects of adjuvant chemotherapy in patients with moderate-risk breast or colon cancer, for which adjuvant therapy is standard. Thus, there are several arguments suggesting that maintenance treatment should be offered to myeloma patients after successful induction therapy. For patients with unsatisfactory responses to induction treatment (e.g., achievement of stable disease, only) more intensive "consolidation" chemotherapy should be considered. Currently there are no established guidelines for selecting the maintenance treatment that is best suited for the individual patient. Prednisone (50 mg orally qod) clearly shows a survival benefit as maintenance treatment in a single large randomized trial. It should be considered the first choice of treatment for patients who achieve a partial or complete remission with conventional chemotherapy that contains steroids. It should be noted that no data exist so far on the safety and efficacy of prednisone for maintenance after autologous transplantation. In contrast, results of IFN-α trials have been mixed and the recent largest US trial shows no benefit with this expensive drug. If IFN is considered as maintenance therapy, (a) in a patient with good response to conventional therapy, relatively young age (<70 yr), good performance status, and favorable tumor characteristics (slowly progressive disease); and (b) in a patient who has achieved a complete or partial response after transplantation. As of this writing, thalidomide is being investigated for maintenance therapy after autografting, but no data on efficacy are available yet. Thus, IFN-α is an attractive choice for the maintenance treatment after autografting outside clinical trials. Combinations of these three agents might yield even better disease control, and data of ongoing studies are eagerly awaited.

ACKNOWLEDGMENT

This research was supported by the Wilhelminen Cancer Research Institute of the Austrian Forum Against Cancer.

REFERENCES

1. Durie BG, Russell DH, Salmon SE. Reappraisal of plateau phase in myeloma. Lancet 1980; 2:65-68.
2. Bataille R, Souteyrand P, Sany J. Clinical evaluation of response or escape to chemotherapy and of survival of patients with multiple myeloma: a prospective study of 202 patients (1975–1982). Anticancer Res 1984; 4:339–345.
3. Oivanen TM. Prognostic value of serum M-protein doubling time at escape from plateau of multiple myeloma. The Finnish Leukaemia Group. Eur J Haematol 1996; 57:247–253.
4. Corso A, Nozza A, Lazzarino M, et al. Plateau phase in multiple myeloma: an end-point of conventional-dose chemotherapy. Haematologica 1999; 84:336–341.
5. Attal M, Harousseau JL. Standard therapy versus autologous transplantation in multiple myeloma. Hematol Oncol Clin North Am 1997; 11:133–146.
6. Kulkarni S, Powles RL, Treleaven JG, et al. Impact of previous high-dose therapy on outcome after allografting for multiple myeloma. Bone Marrow Transplant 1999; 23:675–680.
7. Southwest Oncology Group Study. Remission maintenance for multiple myeloma. Arch Intern Med 1975; 135:147–152.
8. Alexanian R, Gehan E, Haut A, Saiki J, Weick J. Unmaintained remissions in multiple myeloma. Blood 1978; 51:1005–1011.
9. Paccagnella A, Cartei G, Fosser V, et al. Treatment of multiple myeloma with M-2 protocol and without maintenance therapy. Eur J Cancer Clin Oncol 1983; 19:1345–1351.
10. MacLennan IC, Cusick J. Objective evaluation of the role of vincristine in induction and maintenance therapy for myelomatosis. Medical Research Council Working Party on Leukaemia in Adults. Br J Cancer 1985; 52:153–158.
11. Cohen HJ, Bartolucci AA, Forman WB, Silberman HR. Consolidation and maintenance therapy in multiple myeloma: randomized comparison of a new approach to therapy after initial response to treatment. J Clin Oncol 1986; 4:888–899.
12. Belch A, Shelley W, Bergsagel D, et al. A randomized trial of maintenance versus no maintenance melphalan and prednisone in responding multiple myeloma patients. Br J Cancer 1988; 57:94–99.
13. Riccardi A, Ucci G, Luoni R, et al. Treatment of multiple myeloma according to the extension of the disease: a prospective, randomised study comparing a less with a more aggressive cystostatic policy. Cooperative Group of Study and Treatment of Multiple Myeloma. Br J Cancer 1994; 70:1203–1210.
14. Peest D, Deicher H. Induktions- und Erhaltungstherapie beim multiplen Myelom: Ergebnisse einer multizentrischen Studie. Onkologie 1988; 11:39–43.

15. Barlogie BJr, Shaughnessy JD. Early results of total therapy II in multiple myeloma: implication of cytogenetics and FISH. Int J Hematol. 2003; 76(suppl 1):337–339.
16. Palumbo A, Battaglio S, Napoli P, et al. Recombinant interferon-gamma inhibits the in vitro proliferation of human myeloma cells. Br J Haematol 1994; 86:726–732.
17. Ludwig CU, Durie BG, Salmon SE, Moon TE. Tumor growth stimulation in vitro by interferons. Eur J Cancer Clin Oncol 1983; 19:1625–1632.
18. Anthes JC, Zhan Z, Gilchrest H, Egan RW, Siegel MI, Billah MM. Interferon-alpha down-regulates the interleukin-6 receptor in a human multiple myeloma cell line, U266. Biochem J 1995; 309:175–180.
19. Jourdan M, Zhang XG, Portier M, Boiron JM, Bataille R, Klein B. IFN-alpha induces autocrine production of IL-6 in myeloma cell lines. J Immunol 1991; 147:4402–4407.
20. Egle A, Villunger A, Kos M, et al. Modulation of Apo-1/Fas (CD95)-induced programmed cell death in myeloma cells by interferon-alpha 2. Eur J Immunol 1996; 26:3119–3126.
21. Spets H, Georgii-Hemming P, Siljason J, Nilsson K, Jernberg-Wiklund H. Fas/APO-1 (CD95)-mediated apoptosis is activated by interferon-gamma and interferon- in interleukin-6 (IL-6)-dependent and IL-6-independent multiple myeloma cell lines. Blood 1998; 92:2914–2923.
22. Nilson K. The regulation of Fas induced apoptosis in multiple myeloma. 9th International Myeloma Workshop, Salamanca, May 23–27, 2003 Hematology J 4 (suppl 1):S29: P3.5.
23. Liu P, Oken M, Van Ness B. Interferon-alpha protects myeloma cell lines from dexamethasone-induced apoptosis. Leukemia 1999; 13:473–480.
24. Otsuki T, Yamada O, Sakaguchi H, et al. Human myeloma cell apoptosis induced by interferon-alpha. Br J Haematol 1998; 103:518–529.
25. Hermann P, Rubio M, Nakajima T, Delespesse G, Sarfati M. IFN-alpha priming of human monocytes differentially regulates gram-positive and gram-negative bacteria-induced IL-10 release and selectively enhances IL-12p70, CD80, and MHC class I expression. J Immunol 1998; 161:2011–2018.
26. Einhorn S, Blomgren H, Strander H. Interferon and spontaneous cytotoxicity in man. I. Enhancement of the spontaneous cytotoxicity of peripheral lymphocytes by human leukocyte interferon. Int J Cancer 1978; 22:405–412.
27. Hall PD, Self SE, Hall RK. The interaction of maintenance interferon with cytolytic cells in patients with multiple myeloma who responded to cytotoxic chemotherapy. Pharmacotherapy 1997; 17:248–255.
28. Luft T, Pang KC, Thomas E, et al. Type I IFNs enhance the terminal differentiation of dendritic cells. J Immunol 1998; 161:1947–1953.
29. Taylor JL, Grossberg SE. The effects of interferon -alpha on the production and action of other cytokines. Semin Oncol 1998; 25(suppl 1):23–29.
30. Sidky YA, Borden EC. Inhibition of angiogenesis by interferons: effects on tumor- and lymphocyte-induced vascular responses. Cancer Res 1987; 47:5155–5161.
31. Mellstedt H, Aahre A, Bjorkholm M, et al. Interferon therapy in myelomatosis. Lancet 1979; 2:697.
32. Ahre A, Bjorkholm M, Mellstedt H, et al. Human leukocyte interferon and intermittent high-dose melphalan-prednisone administration in the treatment of multiple myeloma: a randomized clinical trial from the Myeloma Group of Central Sweden. Cancer Treat Rep 1984; 68:1331–1338.
33. Ludwig H, Cortelezzi A, Scheithauer W, et al. Recombinant interferon alfa-2C versus polychemotherapy (VMCP) for treatment of multiple myeloma: a prospective randomized trial. Eur J Cancer Clin Oncol 1986; 22:1111–1116.
34. Arora T, Jelinek DF. Differential myeloma cell responsiveness to interferon -alpha correlates with differential induction of p19(INK4d) and cyclin D2 expression. J Biol Chem 1998; 273:11799–11805.
35. Mandelli F, Avvisati G, Amadori S, et al. Maintenance treatment with recombinant interferon alfa-2b in patients with multiple myeloma responding to conventional induction chemotherapy. N Engl J Med 1990; 322:1430–1434.

36. Pulsoni A, Avvisati G, Teresa Petrucci M, et al. The Italian experience on interferon as maintenance treatment in multiple myeloma: ten years after [letter]. Blood 1998; 92: 2184–2186.

37. Westin J, Rodjer S, Turesson I, Cortelezzi A, Hjorth M, Zador G. Interferon alfa-2b versus no maintenance therapy during the plateau phase in multiple myeloma: a randomized study. Cooperative Study Group. Br J Haematol 1995; 89:561–568.

38. Ludwig H, Cohen AM, Polliack A, et al. Interferon-alpha for induction and maintenance in multiple myeloma: results of two multicenter randomized trials and summary of other studies. Ann Oncol 1995; 6:467–476.

39. Browman GP, Bergsagel D, Sicheri D, et al. Randomized trial of interferon maintenance in multiple myeloma: a study of the National Cancer Institute of Canada Clinical Trials Group. J Clin Oncol 1995; 13:2354–2360.

40. Blade J, San Miguel JF, Escudero ML, et al. Maintenance treatment with interferon alfa-2b in multiple myeloma: a prospective randomized study from PETHEMA (Program for the Study and Treatment of Hematological Malignancies, Spanish Society of Hematology). Leukemia 1998; 12:1144–1148.

41. Drayson MT, Chapman CE, Dunn JA, Olujohungbe AB, Maclennan IC. MRC trial of alpha2b-interferon maintenance therapy in first plateau phase of multiple myeloma. MRC Working Party on Leukaemia in Adults. Br J Haematol 1998; 101:195–202.

42. Grosbois B, Mary JY, Michaux JL, et al. Interferon maintenance therapy in multiple myeloma patients achieving plateau phase after induction therapy: a multicenter randomized trial. VI International Workshop on Multiple Myeloma, Boston, MA, June 14–18, 1997.

43. Salmon SE, Crowley JJ, Grogan TM, Finley P, Pugh RP, Barlogie B. Combination chemotherapy, glucocorticoids, and interferon alfa in the treatment of multiple myeloma: a Southwest Oncology Group study. J Clin Oncol 1994; 12:2405–2414.

44. Peest D, Deicher H, Coldewey R, et al. A comparison of polychemotherapy and melphalan/prednisone for primary remission induction, and interferon -alpha for maintenance treatment, in multiple myeloma: a prospective trial of the German Myeloma Treatment Group. Eur J Cancer 1995; 31A:146–151.

44a. Barlogie B, Kyle R, Anderson K, et al. Comparable survival in multiple myeloma (MM) with high dose therapy (HDT) employing MEL 140 mg/m^2 + TBI 12 Gy autotransplants versus standard dose therapy with VBMCP and no benefit from interferon (IFN) maintenance: Results of Intergroup Trial S9321. Blood 2003; 102:Abstract 135.

45. Fritz E, Ludwig H. Interferon-α treatment in multiple myeloma: meta-analysis of 30 randomized trials among 3,948 patients. Ann Oncol. 2000; 11:1427–1436.

46. The Myeloma Trialists' Collaborative Group. Interferon as therapy for multiple myeloma: an individual patient data overview of 24 randomized trials and 4012 patients. Br J Haematol. 2001; 113:1020–2034.

47. Kirkwood JM. Systemic adjuvant treatment of high-risk melanoma: the role of interferon alfa-2b and other immunotherapies. Eur J Cancer 1998; 34(suppl 3):S12–S17.

48. Zarour, H. Richards T, Whiteside J, et al., E2690: intergroup immunological evaluation of IFNα2b dose-response in patients (Pts) with high-risk melanoma. Proc Am Soc Clin Oncol 1999; 18:538a.

49. Offidani M, Olivieri A, Montillo M, et al. Two dosage interferon -alpha 2b maintenance therapy in patients affected by low-risk multiple myeloma in plateau phase: a randomized trial. Haematologica 1998; 83:40–47.

50. Zervas K, Pouli A, Perifanis V, et al. Maintenance therapy with interferon-alpha (IFN-alpha) versus IFN-alpha plus chemotherapy in multiple myeloma (MM). The Greek Myeloma Study Group. Eur J Haematol 1996; 57:142–148.

51. Welander CE, Morgan TM, Homesley HD, Trotta PP, Spiegel RJ. Combined recombinant human interferon alfa 2 and cytotoxic agents studied in a clonogenic assay. Int J Cancer 1985; 35:721–729.

52. Palumbo A, Boccadoro M, Garino LA, Gallone G, Frieri R, Pileri A. Interferon plus gluco-corticoids as intensified maintenance therapy prolongs tumor control in relapsed myeloma. Acta Haematol 1993; 90:71–76.
53. Salmon SE, Crowley JJ, Balcerzak SP, et al. Interferon versus interferon plus prednisone remission maintenance therapy for multiple myeloma: a Southwest Oncology Group Study. J Clin Oncol 1998; 16:890–896.
54. Powles R, Raje N, Cunningham D, et al. Maintenance therapy for remission in myeloma with Intron A following high-dose melphalan and either an autologous bone marrow transplantation or peripheral stem cell rescue. Stem Cells 1995; 13(suppl 2):114–117.
55. Cunningham D, Powles R, Malpas J, et al. A randomized trial of maintenance interferon following high-dose chemotherapy in multiple myeloma: long-term follow-up results. Br J Haematol 1998; 102:495–502.
56. Bjorkstrand B, Svensson H, Goldschmidt H, et al. Alpha-interferon maintenance treatment is associated with improved survival after high-dose treatment and autologous stem cell transplantation in patients with multiple myeloma: a retrospective registry study from the European Group for Blood and Marrow Transplantation (EBMT). Bone Marrow Transplant. 2001; 27:511–515.
57. Alegre A, Diaz-Mediavilla J, San-Miguel J, et al. Autologous peripheral blood stem cell transplantation for multiple myeloma: a report of 259 cases from the Spanish Registry. Spanish Registry for Transplant in MM (Grupo Espanol de Transplante Hematopoyetico-GETH) and PETHEMA. Bone Marrow Transplant 1998; 21:133–140.
58. Harousseau JL, Attal M, Divine M, et al. Autologous stem cell transplantation after first remission induction treatment in multiple myeloma. A report of the French Registry on Autologous Transplantation in Multiple Myeloma. Stem Cells 1995; 13(suppl 2): 132–139.
59. Sirohi B, Powles R, Lawrence D, et al. An open, randomized, controlled, phase II, single centre, 2-period cross over study to compare the quality of life (QoL) and toxicity experienced on PEG interferon (P-IFN) with interferon -alpha2b (IFN) in patients with multiple myeloma (MM) maintained on a steady dose of IFN. 9th International Myeloma Workshop, Salamanca, May 23–27, 2003. Hematology J, 4 (suppl 1):S195:242.
60. Valentine AD, Meyers CA, Talpaz M. Treatment of neurotoxic side effects of interferon-alpha with naltrexone. Cancer Invest 1995; 13:561–566.
61. Valentine AD, Meyers CA. Successful treatment of interferon -alpha-induced mood disorder with nortriptyline. Psychosomatics 1995 36:418–419.
62. Valentine AD, Meyers CA, Kling MA, Richelson E, Hauser P. Mood and cognitive side effects of interferon -alpha therapy. Semin Oncol 1998 1(suppl 1):39–47.
63. Wisloff F, Hjorth M, Kaasa S, Westin J. Effect of interferon on the health-related quality of life of multiple myeloma patients: results of a Nordic randomized trial comparing melphalan–prednisone to melphalan–prednisone + alpha interferon. The Nordic Myeloma Study Group. Br J Haematol 1996; 94:324–332.
64. Nordic Myeloma Study Group. Interferon-alpha 2b added to melphalan–prednisone for initial and maintenance therapy in multiple myeloma. A randomized, controlled trial. The Nordic Myeloma Study Group. Ann Intern Med 1996; 124:212–222.
65. Zee B, Cole B, Li T, et al. Quality-adjusted time without symptoms or toxicity analysis of interferon maintenance in multiple myeloma. J Clin Oncol 1998; 16:2834–2839.
66. Ludwig H, Fritz E, Neuda J, Durie BG. Patient preferences for interferon alfa in multiple myeloma. J Clin Oncol 1997; 15:1672–1679.
67. Berenson JR, Crowley JJ, Grogan TM, et al. Maintenance therapy with alternate-day prednisone improves survival in multiple myeloma patients. Blood 2002; 99:3163–3168.
68. Singhal S, Mehta J, Desikan R, et al. Antitumor activity of thalidomide in refractory multiple myeloma N Engl J Med. 1999; 341:1565–1571.

69. Feyler S, Jackson G, Rawstron A, et al. Thalidomide maintenance following high dose therapy in multiple myeloma: a UK Myeloma Forum Phase II Study. American Society of Hematology 45th Annual Meeting, San Diego, Dec. 6–9, 2003. Blood 102, 11:2558.

70. Feyler S, Jackson G, Rawstron A, EL-Sherbiny YM, Snowden JA, Roderick JJ. Thalidomide maintenance following high dose therapy in multiple myeloma: a UK Myeloma Forum Phase 2 Study. Presented at: the American Society of Hematology 45th Annual Meeting; December 6–9, 2003; San Diego, Calif.

71. Sahebi F, Somlo G, Kogut NM, et al. Feasibility and toxicity of maintenance thalidomide following single cycle autologous peripheral blood stem cell transplant in patients with multiple myeloma. Presented at: the American Society of Hematology 45th Annual Meeting; December 6–9, 2003; San Diego, Calif. Blood 102, 11:3662.

72. Alexanian R, Weber D, Giralt S, Delasalle K. Consolidation therapy of multiple myeloma with thalidomide–dexamethasone after intensive chemotherapy. Ann Oncol 2002; 13:1116–1119.

73. Stewart AK, Chen C, Howson-Jan K, et al. A multi-center randomized phase 2 trial of thalidomide and prednisone as maintenance therapy for multiple myeloma following autologous stem cell transplant. Presented at: the 9th International Myeloma Workshop; May 23–27, 2003; Salamanca. Hematol J; 4(suppl 1):S208.

74. Heslop HE, Duncombe AS, Reittie JE, et al. Interleukin 2 infusion induces haemopoietic growth factors and modifies marrow regeneration after chemotherapy or autologous marrow transplantation. Br J Haematol 1991; 77:237–244.

75. Peest D, Leo R, Deicher H. Tumor-directed cytotoxicity in multiple myeloma: the basis for an experimental treatment approach with interleukin 2. Stem Cells 1995; 13(suppl 2):72–76.

76. Gottlieb DJ, Prentice HG, Mehta AB, et al. Malignant plasma cells are sensitive to LAK cell lysis: pre-clinical and clinical studies of interleukin 2 in the treatment of multiple myeloma. Br J Haematol 1990; 75:499–505.

77. Heslop HE, Gottlieb DJ, Bianchi AC, et al. In vivo induction of gamma interferon and tumor necrosis factor by interleukin-2 infusion following intensive chemotherapy or autologous marrow transplantation. Blood 1989; 74:1374–1380.

78. Togawa A, Sawada S, Amano M, Oshimi K, Satoh H, Takaku H. Treatment of multiple myeloma with LAK cells plus interleukin 2 or interleukin 2 alone [article in Japanese]. Rinsho Ketsueki 1989; 30:650–658.

79. Robinson N, Benyunes MC, Thompson JA, et al. Interleukin-2 after autologous stem cell transplantation for hematologic malignancy: a phase I/II study. Bone Marrow Transplant 1997; 19:435–442.

80. Higuchi CM, Thompson JA, Petersen FB, Buckner CD, Fefer A. Toxicity and immunomodulatory effects of interleukin-2 after autologous bone marrow transplantation for hematologic malignancies. Blood 1991; 77:2561–2568.

81. Peest D, Hannover, Germany. Personal communication.

82. Richardson PG, Barlogie B, Berenson J, et al. A phase 2 study of bortezomib in relapsed, refractory myeloma. N Engl J Med. 2003; 348:2609–2617.

83. Mellstedt H, Osterborg A. Active idiotype vaccination in multiple myeloma: GM-CSF may be an important adjuvant cytokine. Pathol Biol (Paris) 1999; 47:211–215.

84. Kwak LW, Campbell MJ, Czerwinski DK, Hart S, Miller RA, Levy R. Induction of immune responses in patients with B-cell lymphoma against the surface-immunoglobulin idiotype expressed by their tumors. N Engl J Med 1992; 327:1209–1215.

85. Turner JG, Tan J, Crucian BE, et al. Broadened clinical utility of gene gun-mediated, granulocyte-macrophage colony-stimulating factor cDNA-based tumor cell vaccines as demonstrated with a mouse myeloma model. Hum Gene Ther 1998; 9:1121–1130.

86. Reichardt VL, Okada CY, Liso A, et al. Idiotype vaccination using dendritic cells after autologous peripheral blood stem cell transplantation for multiple myeloma: a feasibility study. Blood 1999; 93:2411–2419.

87. Stevenson FK, Zhu D, King CA, Ashworth LJ, Kumar S, Hawkins RE. Idiotypic DNA vaccines against B-cell lymphoma. Immunol Rev 1995; 145:211–128.
88. Maloney DG, Donovan K, Hamblin TJ. Antibody therapy for treatment of multiple myeloma. Semin Hematol 1999; 36(suppl 3):30–33.
89. Ruiz-Arguelles GJ, San Miguel JF. Cell surface markers in multiple myeloma. Mayo Clin Proc 1994; 69:684–690.
90. Treon SP, Pilarski LM, Belch AR, et al. CD20-directed serotherapy in patients with multiple myeloma: biologic considerations and therapeutic applications. J Immunother. 2002; 25:72–81.
91. Musto P, Carella AM Jr, Greco MM, et al. Short progression-free survival in myeloma patients receiving rituximab as maintenance therapy after autologous transplantation. Br J Haematol. 2003; 123:746–747.
92. Van Zaanen HC, Lokhorst HM, Aarden LA, Rensink HJ, Warnaar SO, Van Oers MH. Blocking interleukin-6 activity with chimeric anti-IL6 monoclonal antibodies in multiple myeloma: effects on soluble IL6 receptor and soluble gp130. Leuk Lymphoma 1998; 31:551–558.
93. Garban F, Attal M, Rossi JF, Payen C, Fegueux N, Sotto JJ: Intergroupe Francophone du Myelome. Immunotherapy by nonmyeloablative allogeneic stem cell transplantation in multiple myeloma: results of a pilot study as salvage therapy after autologous transplantation. Leukemia. 2001; 15:642–646.
94. Bethge WA, Hegenbart U, Stuart MJ, et al. Adoptive immunotherapy with donor lymphocyte infusions after allogeneic hematopoietic cell transplantation following nonmyeloablative conditioning. Blood 2003, [Epub ahead of print].
95. Vij R, Borrello IM, Martin T, et al. A phase I/II study of Xcellerated T cells(tm) after autologous peripheral blood stem cell transplantation in patients with multiple myeloma. Presented at: the American Society of Hematology 45th Annual Meeting; Dec. 6–9, 2003; San Diego, Calif. Blood 102,11:139.
96. Greipp PR, Vesole D, Rajkumar SV, Kyle RA. Use of Zoledronic acid in early stage disease, MGUS and indolent myeloma. Presented at: the 9th International Workshop on Multiple Myeloma; May 23–27, 2003; Salamanca. Hematol J; 4(suppl 1):S11.
97. Berenson JR, Hillner BE, Kyle RA, et al. American Society of Clinical Oncology clinical practice guidelines: the role of bisphosphonates in multiple myeloma. J Clin Oncol. 2002; 20:3719–3736.

13 Myeloma Bone Disease

James R. Berenson, MD

CONTENTS

1. INTRODUCTION

The major clinical manifestation of multiple myeloma (MM) is related to osteolytic bone destruction *(1)*. Even patients who respond to chemotherapy may have progression of skeletal disease *(2,3)*, and recalcification of osteolytic lesions is rare. Bone disease can lead to pathologic fractures, spinal cord compression, hypercalcemia, and pain, and is a major cause of morbidity and mortality in these patients *(4)*, who frequently require radiation therapy or surgery. These complications result from asynchronous bone turnover, wherein increased osteoclastic bone resorption is not accompanied by a comparable increase in bone formation. The increase in osteoclast activity in MM is mediated by the release of osteoclast-stimulating factors *(5,6)* produced locally in the bone marrow microenvironment by cells of tumor and nontumor origin *(5,7)*. The enhanced bone loss is a result of the interplay between among osteoclasts, tumor cells, and other nonmalignant cells in the bone marrow microenvironment.

Bisphosphonates are specific inhibitors of osteoclast activity and are effective in the treatment of hypercalcemia associated with malignancy *(8–10)*. These agents have been evaluated as monotherapy and as adjunctive to primary anticancer treatment in patients with cancer involving the bone, including MM *(11–15)*. Bisphosphonates have been evaluated in several large randomized trials in patients with myeloma who are also receiving chemotherapy. Oral

From: *Current Clinical Oncology: Biology and Management of Multiple Myeloma*
Edited by: J. R. Berenson © Humana Press Inc., Totowa, NJ

etidronate given daily showed no clinical benefit *(4)* and oral clodronate taken daily produced variable clinical results in three randomized trials *(11,16)*. Oral pamidronate was ineffective in reducing the skeletal complications of these patients *(17)*. A large, randomized, double-blind study was conducted in patients with stage III MM who received either pamidronate 90 mg or placebo as a 4-h infusion every 4 wk for 21 cycles, in addition to anti-myeloma chemotherapy *(18,19)*. This intravenously administered bisphosphonate significantly reduced the development of skeletal complications and improved the survival of patients who had failed first-line chemotherapy. Recently, large Phase II randomized studies have evaluated more potent third-generation bisphosphonates for patients with MM. Ibandronate proved unsuccessful when given monthly at a 2 mg dose *(19a)*. In contrast, 4 mg zoledronic infused over 15 min every 3–4 wk was safe and effective at preventing skeletal complications *(19b,19c)*. A number of other types of new anti-bone resorptive agents are also in early clinical development.

2. BIOLOGY OF MYELOMA BONE DISEASE

Much progress has been made over the past few years to better define the biological basis of bone loss in patients with myeloma. Using bone histomorphometry, investigators have observed increased bone resorption with both increased eroded surfaces and mean erosion depth in patients with myeloma *(20,21)*. This excessive bone resorption has been shown to occur in the proximity of tumor cells, even in patients without obvious signs of lytic bone disease *(22)*. Patients who are in remission and the uninvolved marrow of patients with solitary plasmacytomas do not show this excessive bone resorption *(6)*. This observation suggests the importance of the bone marrow microenvironment in local destruction of bone in myeloma and that this destructive process may be mediated by direct intercellular means as well as the local release of bone-resorbing factors. Even patients who present with early myeloma show this phenomenon. In patients with monoclonal gammopathy of undetermined significance (MGUS), the presence of increased bone resorption is associated with a greater likelihood of developing full-blown MM *(23)*. Although osteoclast size appears to be normal in these patients, there appears to be increased recruitment, survival and activation of these cells *(24)*.

Obviously, enhanced osteoclastic activity would not be associated with enhanced bone loss if it were not accompanied by a reduction in bone formation *(6,22)*. This uncoupling bone process (i.e., increased bone resorption in the presence of reduced bone formation) is the hallmark of MM in patients with osteolytic bone disease. Interestingly, in the one out of four patients who present without these lesions, this uncoupling process has not been observed *(25)*. These patients often have both enhanced bone resorption and bone formation. In addition, osteocalcin (a marker of bone formation activity) has been shown to be decreased in patients with lytic bone disease, whereas patients without evidence of lytic disease had higher osteocalcin levels *(26)*. In support of the important relationship between bone disease and overall outcome in these patients, serum osteocalcin levels were shown to be inversely related to survival in one study *(27)*.

2.1. Bone-Resorbing Factors

The landmark studies of Mundy and colleagues suggested the presence of osteoclast-activating factors in supernatants derived from cultures of both human myeloma cell lines and freshly obtained myeloma bone marrow *(28)*. Although early work suggested that these factors are interleukin (IL)-β and lymphotoxin (tumor necrosis factor [TNF]-β, other factors have been implicated in more recent studies, including IL-6, IL-11, transforming growth factor (TGF)-β, macrophage colony stimulating factor (M-CSF), hepatocyte growth factor (HGF), metalloproteinases (MMPs), macrophage inflammatory protein (MIP)-1α, and a receptor for activation of NF-κB (RANK; a new member of the TNF receptor family) and its ligand, RANKL. Most recently, dickkopf-1 (dkk1), an inhibitor of Wnt signaling, has been shown to be important in myeloma bone disease.

2.1.1. IL-1β

The importance of IL-1β in myeloma bone resorption is controversial, as are the cells that produce this cytokine in the myeloma microenvironment. Although IL-1β is clearly increased in supernatants from unseparated fresh myeloma bone marrow samples *(29)*, recent attempts to determine whether the malignant cells themselves were producing this factor have had conflicting results *(30–34)*. The role of IL-1β in stimulating bone resorption has been shown in some studies using bone organ cultures; this activity has been blocked by antibodies to this cytokine *(30–32)*. The inhibitors of IL-1β function, the soluble IL-1 receptor and IL-1 receptor antagonist have been shown to be able to completely inhibit the bone resorption generated by supernatants derived from unfractionated myeloma bone marrow *(35)*. However, the importance of IL-1β in stimulating bone resorption in patients with myeloma has not been confirmed by other investigators *(36)*.

2.1.2. TNFs

Early studies suggested that lymphotoxin was the important factor in enhancing bone resorption in these patients *(37)*. More recent studies have failed to confirm these initial studies, however, and have not even shown increased secretion of this cytokine from bone marrow cells obtained from these patients *(28,29)*. TNF-β has been shown to be an important bone-resorbing cytokine and has been found in increased amounts in the supernatant from unfractionated myeloma bone marrow *(28,29)*; recent studies have also suggested that it is produced by the malignant cells *(34)*.

The effects of TNF and several other cytokines (including IL-1) are mediated by their ability to stimulate the proteolytic breakdown of IκB that leads to the release of NFκB. This enhancer translocates into the nucleus, where it induces transcription of specific genes, some of which are involved in the enhancement of bone resorption as well as increasing myeloma tumor burden. The importance of NFκB in bone resorption is supported by recent studies showing that NFκB knock-out mice have osteopetrotic bones (38). A number of other proteins involved in bone resorption, including RANK (discussed later in this chapter), also utilize the NFκB signaling pathway. This enhancer protein represents a new therapeutic target for reducing both tumor burden and bone loss in patients with myeloma.

2.1.3. IL-6

IL-6 has been shown to be critical for stimulating growth and preventing apoptosis in malignant myeloma cells (39). Although early studies suggested that myeloma tumor cells produce IL-6, (40) most studies have shown that IL-6 is produced in large amounts by bone marrow stromal cells and that its production is enhanced by the adhesion of tumor cells (41). In addition, this cytokine has been shown to play a major role in bone disease (42), inhibiting bone formation (43) and stimulating the development of osteoclasts (41), but also promoting osteoblast activity. Interestingly, IL-6 is produced in large quantities by both osteoclasts and osteoblasts (42,44) The use of anti-IL-6 antibodies clinically has demonstrated the importance of this cytokine in stimulating bone loss in patients with myeloma (45). It has also been shown that both IL-1 and TNF stimulate IL-6 activity (46), and that IL-6 is capable of working synergistically with IL-1 to stimulate osteoclast activity (47). The soluble IL-6 receptor, gp80, is also important in this process. Specifically, when gp80—which is present in large amounts in myeloma bone marrow—becomes associated with IL-6, it stimulates myeloma growth (48) and osteoclast formation (49). Thus, IL-6 and gp80 together provide dual roles, both increasing tumor burden as well as bone loss in patients with myeloma.

2.1.4. TGF-β

Recently, TGF-β has been shown to be produced by both tumor cells and stromal cells in the bone marrow of patients with myeloma (50). Recently, this cytokine was also shown to play an important role in the pathogenesis of metastatic bone disease in breast cancer (51). TGF-β in the bone milieu is capable of stimulating the release of parathyroid thyroid hormone-releasing peptide (PTHRP) from breast cancer cells which, in turn, stimulates bone resorption and the release of more TGF-β from the bone microenvironment. Recently, it has been shown that this cytokine greatly increases the differentiation of osteoclast precursors from monocyte precursors by RANKL and M-CSF (discussed later in this chapter) (52). In patients with myeloma, TGF-β has been shown to stimulate IL-6 production by tumor cells and stromal cells that may similarly enhance bone resorption and stimulate tumor growth *(50)*. Interestingly, another member of the TGF-β family—bone morphogenetic protein (BMP)-2—has been shown to be capable of both enhancing bone formation *(53)* and inducing apoptosis in myeloma cells *(54)*. This protein may also enhance osteoclast activity *(55)*.

2.1.5. RANK AND RANKL

A recently identified receptor for activation of NF-κB (RANK), a member of the TNF receptor family, and its ligand, RANKL, have been shown to be key players in the development of osteoclasts *(56)*. Unlike other soluble bone-resorbing factors, the activity of these molecules requires direct cell–cell contact. It has been known for some time that osteoclastogenesis requires the direct interaction of osteoblasts or stromal cells with osteoclasts. The identification of RANK expressed on the surface of osteoclasts and RANKL on osteoblasts and stromal cells explains how this interaction leads to osteoclast development. TNF is capable of stimulating osteoblasts to increase their expression of RANKL, but may stimulate osteoclast differentiation by a mechanism independent of the RANKL–RANK interaction *(57)*. Malignant plasma cells obtained from patients with myeloma have recently been shown to express RANKL *(58,59,59a)*; thus, it is possible that the tumor cells themselves may directly stimulate osteoclast development in the bone marrow of patients with myeloma.

Importantly, a soluble decoy receptor called osteoprotegerin (OPG) binds RANKL and prevents it from binding with RANK *(55)*. In fact, animals lacking OPG show profound osteoporosis *(60)*. It is the delicate balance between soluble OPG and RANKL that determines the amount of bone loss. In two separate studies involving murine models, OPG prevented and reversed hypercalcemia of malignancy *(61)* and blocked cancer-induced bone destruction and bone pain without obvious toxicity *(62)*. Because of these promising preclinical results, OPG is now being evaluated in early clinical trials in myeloma and in patients with breast cancer that has metastasized to bone. Because myeloma tumor cells express RANKL, it is possible that blockage of the RANKL–RANK interaction may not only reduce osteoclast stimulation but also have inhibitory effects on the tumor cells themselves. Two recent studies showed that inhibition of the RANK–RANKL interaction by either RANK-Fc or TR-Fc reduces both bone loss and tumor burden in murine models of myeloma in human severe combined immunodeficiency syndrome (SCID-hu) *(63,64)*.

Recently, it has been shown that the ratio of circulating OPG:RANKL in patients with MM not only predicts the amount of bone disease but overall survival as well *(64a)*.

2.1.6. OTHER FACTORS

M-CSF is present in increased amounts in the serum of patients with myeloma and correlates with tumor load *(65,66)*. This cytokine is capable of attracting osteoclast

Table 1
Cytokines in Myeloma Bone Disease

| | | Effect on | | |
Protein	Source	Growth	Apoptosis	Bone Disease
IL-1β	stroma/?tumor			+++
TNF-α	stroma	±	–	+
IL-6	stroma/occas. tumor	++	—	+
HGF	tumor	++		++
TGF-β	stroma			+
M-CSF	stroma			+
MMPs	stroma/tumor			+
Sydecan-1	tumor	–	+	–
MIP-1α	stroma/tumor			+++
RANKL	stroma/tumor	+?	+?	+++

IL, interleukin; TNF, tumore necrosis factor; HGF, hepatocyte growth factor; TGF, transforming growth factor; M-CSF, macrophage colony-stimulating factor; MMps, metalloproteinases; MIP, macrophage inflammatory protein; RANKL, NF-κ ligand.

precursors as well as enhancing the survival of osteoclasts (67–56). Although M-CSF, along with RANKL (see below), is all that is required for osteoclastogenesis to occur in vitro, its role in myeloma bone disease remains unclear.

IL-11 stimulates osteoclastogenesis and inhibits bone formation (70). It has been shown to be produced by osteoblasts and appears in culture supernatants of bone marrow cells obtained from patients with myeloma (71). This cytokine stimulates RANKL expression by osteoblasts. In addition, recent studies have shown that HGF, which recently has been shown to be produced by malignant plasma cells, (72) may also induce IL-11 secretion by osteoblasts (70). HGF is a potent stimulator of bone resorption (73,74). Other cytokines such as IL-1 are capable of potentiating the effect of HGF on IL-11 secretion. High serum levels of HGF are associated with a poor prognosis in patients with myeloma (75).

MMPs have been shown to have an increasingly important role in stimulating bone resorption, because their inhibitors (tissue inhibitors of metalloproteinases [TIMPs]) can prevent bone resorption (76–78). Specifically, MMP-9 has been shown to be expressed by tumor cells in patients with myeloma, whereas the bone marrow stromal cells produce MMP-1 and MMP-2 (79). In addition, co-culture of stromal cells with myeloma cells upregulates MMP-1 secretion. These specific MMPs have been shown to play a critical role in the direct degradation of bone matrix and promotion of metastasis (80). The amount of MMP-2 secretion predicted the progression of myeloma in one clinical study (81).

Syndecan-1, a heparan sulfate proteoglycan, has recently been shown to be expressed on the surface of myeloma cells (82). This molecule is actively released from the cell surface of the tumor cells, and has been demonstrated to both reduce tumor burden as well as bone destruction in animal and in vitro myeloma models (83). Syndecan-1 inhibits osteoclast differentiation while stimulating osteoblast formation. SCID mice injected with the human myeloma cell line ARH-77 transfected with this gene were less likely to develop lytic bone disease.

Recently, MIP-1α was identified as an important factor involved in myeloma bone disease (84). Levels of this cytokine are also elevated in the bone marrow of patients with myeloma. This chemokine is capable of inducing osteoclast formation in vitro; antibodies to this protein block the induction of osteoclast formation by fresh bone marrow plasma obtained from patients with myeloma. The importance of MIP-α in inducing myeloma bone loss has been reinforced by a recent study showing that an antisense construct to this molecule reduces bone loss in SCID mice containing a human myeloma cell line (85). Induction of MIP-1α activity in MM cells has also been shown not only to increase bone disease, but also to accelerate tumor growth in a murine MM model (85a). In addition, this chemokine attracts and activates monocytes, and is a potent inhibitor of early hematopoiesis.

There is evidence for an increasing role of angiogenesis in the pathogenesis of multiple myeloma (80,86). It is clear that vascular endothelial growth factor (VEGF) is produced by malignant plasma cells and that the receptors that bind this factor are expressed on bone marrow stromal cells (87). Recent study results showed that VEGF increases IL-6 production by bone marrow stromal cells obtained from patients with myeloma (88). This may indirectly lead to increased bone loss in these patients. Until recently, it was not clear that VEGF had any direct role in bone resorption. However, it is now clear that VEGF can replace M-CSF in leading to early osteoclast development (89).

An intracellular protein that inhibits osteoblast formation, dkk1 has been recently found highly elevated in MM bone marrow and blood (89a). Dkk1, an inhibitor of Wnt signaling, is highly expressed in MM bone marrow and serum levels are elevated, expecially among patients with MM who have more extensive disease.

3. ASSESSMENT OF MYELOMA BONE DISEASE

3.1. Plain Radiographs and Bone Scans

Because the major clinical manifestations of myeloma are related to bone disease, the importance of assessing its status cannot be overestimated. A variety of techniques have been used to evaluate patients with myeloma-related bone disease (Table 2). Early detection of lesions at risk to result in fracture or cord compression allows prompt use of prophylactic surgery or radiotherapy. In addition, determination of changes in bone disease is an important part of assessing the patient's response to systemic treatment. The gold standard has been the use

Table 2
Assessing Myeloma Bone Disease

Plain radiograph skeletal survey

Bone scan

Magnetic resonance imaging

Bone densitometry

MIBI scan (experimental)

PET scan

Bone resorption markers: pyridinoline, deoxypyridinoline, ICTP, N-telopeptide

Bone formation markers: alkaline phosphatase, osteocalcin, PINP

MIBI, methoxyisobutylisonitrile; PET, positron emission tomography; ICTP, C-terminal telopeptide of type I collagen; PINP, amino-terminal propeptide of type I procollagen.

of plain radiographs of the skull, spine, pelvis, and long bones of the upper and lower extremities. One study has suggested that patients without either osteoporosis or lytic bone disease have the worst survival, whereas patients with minimal lytic changes have the longest survival (90). Although older studies suggest that the lytic lesions that make up myeloma bones are not well demonstrated using bone scans (91,92), recent studies suggest that this modality may be useful, especially in lesions in the ribs, vertebral bodies, and sternum (93). On the other hand, the skull, the extremities, and the pelvic bones were better evaluated with plain radiographs in this study. In most cases, bone scans are really unnecessary as part of the routine evaluation of bone disease in myeloma.

3.2. Bone Histomorphometry

Although bone histomorphometry may be effective for assessing the extent of bone loss at individual sites (7), its usefulness is limited by its invasiveness and the heterogeneous nature of bone involvement in these patients. The expertise of an experienced bone pathologist is required for an accurate interpretation of the results.

3.3. Bone Densitometry

Dual-energy X-ray absorptiometry (DXA) has now been evaluated in some centers for its effectiveness in clarifying general bone status in patients with myeloma (94,95). This technique has clearly provided important information about patients with osteoporosis with respect to the risk of fractures and response to therapeutic interventions (96). Early studies in patients with myeloma have shown marked bone loss, and suggested changes in bone density correlate with the clinical stage and risk for fractures (94,95). Although treatment with oral glucocorticoids effectively lowers tumor burden in these patients, its use has also been associated with the loss of bone mineral density (BMD) *(95)*. DXA has recently been used to assess changes in BMD in patients with myeloma treated with bisphosphonates. During an ongoing phase II trial *(97)*, and showed marked increases in BMD in patients whose anti-myeloma therapy consisted of intravenous pamidronate alone. In a recently completed randomized phase II clinical trial evaluating pamidronate and three doses of zoledronic acid for 280 patients with myeloma and breast cancer accompanied by osteolytic bone disease, marked increases in BMD were also seen in patients receiving either of these bisphosphonates *(98,99)*. Patients receiving the lowest dose of zoledronic acid (0.4 mg) showed the smallest increases in BMD and were most likely to develop skeletal bone complications. These studies have begun to suggest the usefulness of bone densitometry for evaluating BMD in patients receiving bisphosphonate therapy for bone disease in myeloma. However, whether bone densitometry will be useful for predicting the efficacy of bisphosphonate therapy or the risk of developing skeletal complications during the course of the disease in each patient remains to be determined.

3.4. Magnetic Resonance Imaging (MRI)

MRI is being used with increased frequency to assess patients with myeloma. It is much more sensitive in detecting lesions that are not identified by plain radiographs. In the small subset of patients with normal MRI scans (approx 20%), the clinical features suggest earlier stage disease and the prognosis appears to be better *(100)*. When the MRI scan is abnormal, it generally demonstrates three patterns: diffuse involvement without the appearance of a normal marrow signal, nodular or focal areas in which normal marrow tissue has been replaced, or multiple tiny areas of replaced tissue *(101)*. Studies demonstrate that patients with diffuse involvement have the worst outlook, with decreased hemoglobin and increased plasma cell loads *(99)*. Recent studies by Moulopoulos showed that MRI may be particularly useful in determining which patients with early myeloma will develop active disease *(102)*. Approximately 2% of patients with plasma cell dyscrasias present with a solitary bony lesion. Although radiotherapy may effectively eliminate this tumor, most patients eventually develop MM *(103)*. It is in these patients that MRI may be especially useful in predicting outcome. The presence of other bone lesions on an MRI scan is associated with an earlier progression to multiple myeloma than in those patients with normal MRI scans *(104)*. However, no studies have shown that additional interventions at the time of diagnosis change the clinical outcome for this subset of patients.

In patients with more advanced myeloma, MRI is particularly useful in the evaluation of spinal cord compression; however, its usefulness as a routine procedure in these patients has not been well established. In two studies, the presence of more than 10 focal lesions or diffuse involvement in the spine predicted earlier development of vertebral compression fractures *(105,106)*. However, another study showed a lack of correlation between MRI-identified lesions and risk for vertebral fracture *(107)*.

With the increasing use of MRI in evaluating patients with myeloma at diagnosis, the modality has also been used to assess response to treatment. Despite effective chemotherapy, most MRI scans remain abnormal, although there does appear to be an improvement in their appearance in responding patients *(107–109)*. However, until the cost this procedure is reduced, it is unlikely to gain widespread use in the routine follow-up of patients with myeloma.

3.5. Other Radionuclide Scans

Recently, a new radionuclide tracer was shown to predict overall disease status in patients with myeloma. Patterns of uptake of a new radionuclide tracer, technetium-99m 2-methoxyisobutylisonitrile (^{99m}Tc-MIBI), have been useful in predicting the stage of disease and the current clinical status of patients with myeloma *(110,111)*. The positron emission tomography scan is now being used to evaluate patients with myeloma-related bone disease, but its role remains unknown.

3.6. Markers of Bone Resorption and Bone Formation

A variety of markers of bone resorption and formation have been used to assess bone disease in patients with myeloma. Patients with MM show the expected increase in bone resorption markers such as C-terminal telopeptide of type I collagen, pyridinoline, and deoxypyridinoline, and decrease in bone formation markers such as osteocalcin *(25,26,112,113)*. In addition, a decrease in osteocalcin levels or increase in C-terminal telopeptide of type I collagen (ICTP) concentrations predicted a shortened survival in myeloma. In a recent placebo-controlled, randomized Finnish clinical trial involving oral clodronate *(114)*, higher baseline levels of the amino-terminal propeptide of type I procollagen (PINP; a product of growing osteoblasts), ICTP and alkaline phosphatase (AP) were associated with a worse survival. PINP and ICTP levels decreased dramatically during clodronate treatment. Similarly, treatment with oral risedronate reduced urinary pyridinoline:creatinine and deoxypyridinoline:creatinine ratios as well as AP and osteocalcin plasma levels *(115)*. Monthly administration of intravenous pamidronate is also associated with a decrease in both bone resorption and bone formation markers *(17)*. A decrease in these markers during clodronate therapy was associated with a better survival. Current clinical trials of newer bisphosphonates are being conducted to determine whether baseline values or changes in these markers can be used to predict the development of new skeletal complications or whether these agents will be clinically effective in individual cases. In a recent study in patients with myeloma undergoing high-dose therapy and autologous transplantation, bone-resorption markers were elevated, even in patients in remission before transplantation *(116)*. However, bone-resorption markers normalized in most patients several months following the transplant procedure.

4. TREATMENT OF MYELOMA BONE DISEASE

Until the early 1950s, radiotherapy and surgery were the only treatment modalities available to the myeloma patient. Although both modalities could effectively palliate the majority of patients, they had little impact on the overall course of the disease. With the development of effective chemotherapy, these modalities became of secondary importance in the overall management of myeloma. With the recent use of hemibody irradiation, total body irradiation, and bone-seeking radionuclides as part of high-dose therapy regimens, radiation treatment may become recognized as an important part of the systemic management of these patients' disease.

4.1. Radiation Therapy

Early studies showed the exquisite sensitivity of myeloma cells to irradiation *(117)*. This treatment modality may be curative in some patients with solitary plasmacytoma of bone or extramedullary sites, although in the majority of these patients the disorder will eventually progress to multiple myeloma. Most patients with MM will require radiotherapy at some time during the course of their disease. The most common indication for radiotherapy is a painful lesion *(118,119)*. The vast majority of patients achieve pain relief with local radiotherapy at a dose of approx 3000 cGy given in 10 to 15 fractions *(117)*. Some patients with more extensive bone pain may benefit from more extensive hemibody irradiation *(120,121)*. Other indications for radiotherapy may include treatment of impending or actual pathologic fractures, spinal cord compression, tumors causing local neurological problems, and large soft tissue plasma cell tumors *(121)*. Approximately 10% of patients with MM will develop spinal cord compression, and the immediate use of systemic glucocorticosteroids and radiotherapy is important to prevent a permanent neurological deficit. Radiotherapy has also been evaluated for its use in preventing new vertebral fractures in patients with myeloma with neurological complications *(122)*. In a small nonrandomized study, investigators found some evidence suggesting that fewer vertebral fractures occurred in irradiated vertebrae than in nonirradiated ones, as assessed by MRI. However, caution must be used in the application of radiotherapy, because it will result in permanent bone marrow damage in treated areas. The importance of this point cannot be overemphasized in the patient whose overall clinical status depends on chemotherapeutic agents that cause a loss of bone marrow function. In a recently published study, investigators found that radiation of the entire shaft of the long bone is probably not necessary in most cases *(123)*. However, even in the few cases showing recurrence outside the previously irradiated field, palliation with radiotherapy was effective.

A novel radiotherapeutic approach to myeloma that is based on the bone-seeking nature of phosphonates was recently initiated within the context of high-dose therapy and autologous peripheral blood stem cell transplantation (PBSCT) *(124)*. The radionuclide holmium-166 was attached to a tetraphosphonate and given to patients with myeloma prior to high-dose melphalan ± total body irradiation followed by PBSCT. Preliminary results evaluating its anti-myeloma effect are encouraging, with high rates of complete remission rates. Its specific role in bone disease management was not evaluated, however.

4.2. Surgery

Surgical intervention may be required in patients with an impending or actual fracture or a destabilized spine. Several recent reports suggested that this modality is underutilized in patients with myeloma who have fractures in the long bones or vertebrae. In some patients, the presence of myeloma that is not evident radiographically in areas adjacent to the surgical site may impede the success of the procedure. Most patients also require radiotherapy in conjunction with the surgical procedure. Importantly, consideration must be given to the patient's overall clinical status when decisions are made regarding the timing of surgery.

Recently, it has become increasingly recognized that vertebral compression fractures (VCFs) are a significant cause of morbidity among patients with MM. The use of vertebroblasty *(124a)* and the newer minimally invasive surgical technique, kyphoplasty *(124b,124c)*, have been shown to improve the back pain and quality of life of patients with MM *(124d,124e)*. The advantage of kyphoblasty is that it reverses the collapsed vertebral body, improving both back pain and mobility of the patient without significant surgical side effects *(124e)*. Large randomized trials are beginning in patients with MM with VCFS to further confirm the benefit of kyphoblasty.

4.3. Drug Therapy

Earlier attempts to reduce the incidence of skeletal complications of myeloma using sodium fluoride alone or in combination with calcium and androgenic steroids proved unsuccessful *(2,125,126)*. Gallium nitrate was evaluated in one published study, the findings of which suggested both a decrease in bone pain and loss of total body calcium with this treatment. However, this trial was open label and involved only 13 patients *(127)*.

4.3.1. BISPHOSPHONATES

In most of the recent studies evaluating oral or intravenous bisphosphonates, investigators have observed an impact on skeletal disease and its clinical manifestations. Bisphosphonates are specific inhibitors of osteoclastic activity and are effective in the treatment of hypercalcemia associated with malignancy *(9,128)*.

4.3.2. PHARMACOLOGY OF BISPHOSPHONATES

Pyrophosphates are natural compounds that contain two phosphonate groups bound to a common oxygen. They are potent inhibitors of bone resorption in

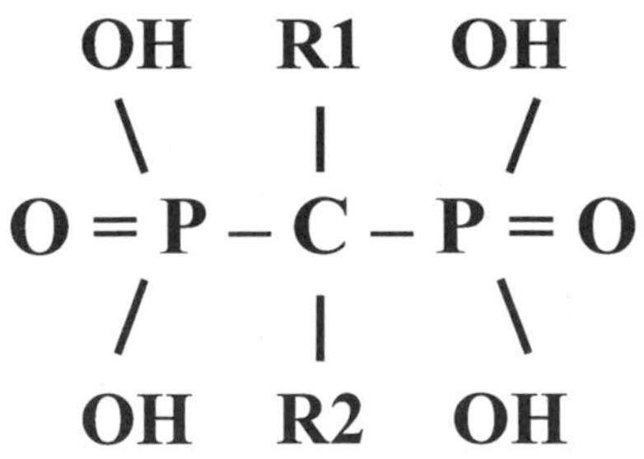

$$OH \quad R1 \quad OH$$
$$\diagdown \quad | \quad \diagup$$
$$O = P - C - P = O$$
$$\diagup \quad | \quad \diagdown$$
$$OH \quad R2 \quad OH$$

Fig. 1. Backbone chemical structure of a bisphosphonate.

Table 3
Relative Potency of Bisphosphonates
Evaluated in Patients With Multiple Myeloma

Drug	N-containing Agent?	Potency
Etidronate	No	1
Clodronate	No	10
Pamidronate	Yes	100
Ibandronate	Yes	1000–10,000
Zoledronic acid	Yes	10,000–100,000

vitro, but not in vivo, where they are readily hydrolyzed and ineffective at reducing bone resorption *(8,9)* Replacement of the oxygen with carbon renders this molecule resistant to hydrolysis without reducing its activity as an inhibitor of bone resorption. This synthetic compound, known as a bisphosphonate, contains two additional chains (R1 and R2) of variable structure that have given rise to a large number of drugs (Fig. 1). Most bisphosphonates contain a hydroxyl group on R1 that results in high affinity for calcium crystals and bone mineral. Marked differences in anti-resorptive potency result from differences in the R2 chain (Table 3). Most of the recently developed agents that are more potent than older agents are characterized by a nitrogen-containing moiety in R2 rather than the simple halide or methyl R2 side chains seen in earlier agents. The nitrogen-containing bisphosphonates also have different mechanisms of action than the older first-generation agents, which lack the nitrogen atom in the R2 chain (discussed later in this chapter).

When administered orally, these drugs are poorly absorbed (usually < 1%) and poorly tolerated, as indicated by significant gastrointestinal toxicity, particularly esophagitis and esophageal ulcers. The bisphosphonates are eliminated almost exclusively through renal excretion; consequently, patients taking these compounds are at significant risk for nephrotoxicity. Because bisphosphonates have

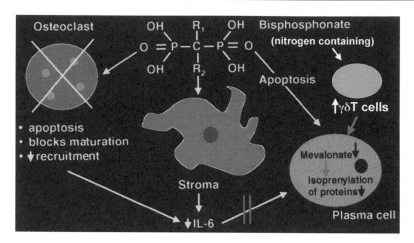

Fig. 2. Possible mechanisms of anti-tumor effect for bisphosphonates in myeloma bone marrow.

a high affinity for the mineral in bone, they become highly concentrated in bone. Once the drug becomes a part of the bone (which is not undergoing remodeling), it is biologically inactive. As a result, continued administration of bisphosphonates is required to achieve the desired lasting inhibition of bone resorption.

4.3.2. MECHANISMS OF ACTION OF BISPHOSPHONATES

The inhibition of bone resorption occurs as a result of the direct and indirect effects of bisphosphonates on osteoclasts. Emerging data suggest that these drugs also have direct and indirect effects in myeloma (Fig. 2). Initially, bisphosphonates were shown to reduce osteoclast development from their precursors, inhibit osteoclast movement to the bone surface to carry out bone resorption, and induce apoptosis in osteoclasts *(129)*. They can also induce apoptosis in myeloma tumor cells *(130)*. Interestingly, apoptosis is induced by inhibiting the mevalonic acid pathway both in myeloma cells and osteoclasts; this effect is particularly notable with nitrogen-containing bisphosphonates *(131,132)*. Statins, which lower cholesterol, also block enzymes in the mevalonic acid pathway. Both drug types prevent the prenylation of several proteins, including guanidine triphosphatases (e.g., *ras, rac,* and *rho*). The addition of geranylgeranylated derivatives rather than farnesylated compounds can overcome the apoptotic effects of aminobisphosphonates and statin derivatives *(129)*. A recent study shows that inhibition of geranylgeranylation of mcl-l, a recently identified anti-apoptotic growth factor for MM *(129a,129b)*, induces apoptosis of MM cells *(129c)*.

The nitrogen-containing bisphosphonates (e.g., pamidronate) have also been shown to enhance osteoclast differentiation and bone-resorbing activity *(133)*. However, they may also have an indirect resorption-blocking effect, because they reduce the production of IL-6 (which stimulates bone resorption) in myeloma bone marrow stromal cells exposed to bisphosphonates *(134,135)*. Recent study results indicated similar bisphosphonate effects in osteoblasts, *(136)* which are normally potent producers of IL-6. This cytokine is an important growth factor and anti-apoptosis factor in myeloma *(38)*. Reducing its availability in bone marrow may not only reduce bone loss but may also have an anti-myeloma effect.

The proteolytic activity of the MMPs involved in bone destruction is inhibited in the presence of nitrogen-containing bisphosphonates *(133)*. In recent animal studies, investigators found that the nitrogen-containing bisphosphonates also have potent anti-angiogenic activity *(135)*. Anti-angiogenesis agents such as thalidomide have recently been shown to be effective against myeloma tumors *(138)*. Thus, the bisphosphonates, which also have anti-angiogenic effects, may help destroy myeloma tumors. A potential anti-tumor mechanism was recently reported for intravenous pamidronate *(139)*, which was shown in vitro to induce the expansion and increase the cytotoxicity of $\gamma\delta T$ cells against malignant plasma cells in patients with myeloma. A recent clinical trial using intravenous pamidronate with IL-2 shows objective responses in the treatment of patients with MM, which correlates with expansion of $\gamma\delta T$ cells *(139a)*. Thus, the bisphosphonates, especially the nitrogen-containing compounds, may reduce bone loss and the tumor burden in myeloma. Using a murine 5T2 MM model, Radl and colleagues observed a reduced tumor burden in the bone marrow of pamidronate-treated mice *(140)*. Epstein and colleagues noted fewer lytic bone metastases and improved survival in pamidronate-treated SCID mice in which fresh human myeloma bone marrow and fetal bone tissue were implanted *(141)*. Zoledronic acid has recently been shown to have similar effects in this animal model *(62)*, but ibandronate only resulted in a reduction in lytic bone disease without an impact on tumor burden *(142)*.

4.3.3. BISPHOSPHONATES IN MYELOMA BONE DISEASE

These agents have been evaluated as monotherapy and as adjunctive therapy to primary anti-cancer treatment in patients with cancer involving the bone, including MM *(1,11–18,143)*. In large placebo-controlled clinical trials, investigators recently observed a reduction in skeletal complications in bisphosphonate-treated patients with myeloma, which suggests that these agents may alter the overall course of the disease.

Early bisphosphonate studies in myeloma suggested a reduction in bone pain and healing of lytic lesions, but involved relatively few patients *(12,13)*. The results of nine large randomized trials of long-term bisphosphonate therapy have now been published. These studies involved the use of either the first-generation bisphosphonates etidronate or clodronate or the second-generation aminobisphosphonate pamidronate or the more potent third-generation agents ibandronate or zoledronic acid *(1,11,15–18,141,143a–143d)*.

4.3.1.1. Etidronate. In a Canadian study *(2)*, 173 newly diagnosed patients received intermittent oral melphalan and prednisone as primary chemotherapy, then 166 were randomized to daily oral etidronate 5 mg/kg or placebo until death or discontinuation because of side effects. Both treated and placebo patients lost a significant amount of height, with no difference between the two arms. There was also no difference in outcome measures (new fractures, hypercalcemic episodes, and bone pain) between the two arms.

4.3.1.2. Clodronate. In a small study involving (N = 13), daily oral clodronate therapy was associated with a reduction in bone pain and lack of progression of bone lesions. In contrast, patients taking placebo demonstrated clinical deterioration *(144)*. Histomorphometric analysis of bone biopsies indicated a reduction in the number of osteoclasts in patients taking clodronate compared with a slight increase in patients taking placebo. Intravenously clodronate was evaluated in a randomized Italian study of 30 patients with active bone disease *(145)*. There was a reduction in new lytic lesions and pathological fractures with the bisphosphonate therapy.

The results of three large randomized trials of oral clodronate in myeloma have been published. A Finnish trial *(11)* enrolled 350 previously untreated patients, of whom 336 were randomized to clodronate 2.4 g/d or placebo for 2 yr. All patients in this study were also treated with intermittent oral melphalan and prednisolone. Radiographs were taken in slightly more than half of these patients at study entry and 2 yr later. Fewer patients in the clodronate group demonstrated progression of lytic lesions compared with the placebo group (12 vs 24%, respectively), but progression of all pathological fractures, as well as vertebral and nonvertebral fractures, and the development of hyperglycemia, and did not differ between groups. Change in pain index and use of analgesics were similar in both arms.

Clodronate was also evaluated in an open-label, randomized German trial involving 170 previously untreated patients who received intermittent intravenous melphalan and oral prednisone and were randomized to 1.6 g oral clodronate per day or no bisphosphonate for 1 yr. More than half of these patients dropped out of the study prematurely. The results showed no difference between the two arms in terms of the progression of bone disease, as indicated by plain radiographs. However, there was a trend toward a reduction in the number of new progressive sites in the clodronate-treated group after 6 and 12 mo; this reduction did not reach statistical significance. Although more patients in the clodronate group were without pain and were not using analgesics, the open-label design of this trial makes it difficult to interpret these findings.

The Medical Research Council recently published the results of a large randomized trial involving 536 patients recently diagnosed with myeloma who were randomized to 1.6 g oral clodronate per day or placebo plus alkylator-based chemotherapy *(16)*. The primary endpoints of the trial were unclear. However, after combining the proportion of patients who developed nonvertebral fractures or severe hypercalcemia—including those who dropped out because of severe hypercalcemia—investigators discovered that fewer clodronate-treated patients experienced this combination of events than patients taking placebo. The number of patients developing hypercalcemia was similar between the two arms. The number of patients with vertebral and nonvertebral fractures was lower in the clodronate group; it may be difficult to determine the significance of this finding, however, because post-baseline radiographs were taken in only half of these patients. Back pain and poor performance were not significantly different between the two groups, except at the 24-mo time point. The proportion of patients requiring radiotherapy was similar between the two arms, and there was no difference in time to first skeletal event or overall survival.

4.3.1.3. Pamidronate. In a double-blind randomized trial, a Danish-Swedish cooperative group evaluated oral pamidronate 300 mg/d compared with placebo in 300 patients newly diagnosed with myeloma who were also receiving intermittent melphalan and prednisone *(17)*. The primary endpoint was skeletal-related morbidity, indicated by bone fracture, surgery for impending fracture, vertebral collapse, or an increase in number or size of lytic lesions. After a median duration of 18 mo, no significant reduction in the incidence of the primary endpoint, hypercalcemia episodes, or survival was seen between the arms. Fewer episodes of severe pain and less height loss were observed in patients taking pamidronate, however.

The results of small open-label trials in patients with multiple myeloma lasting up to 24 mo suggested that infusional pamidronate disodium might be effective in reducing skeletal complications of MM *(13,14)*. This led to the development of a large, randomized, double-blind study to determine whether infusions of 90 mg of pamidronate per month reduced skeletal events in patients with multiple myeloma who were receiving chemotherapy compared with placebo for 21 mo *(18,19)*. This study included patients with Durie-Salmon stage III MM and at least one osteolytic lesion. Unlike the etidronate and clodronate trials, which involved untreated patients, patients were required to have received unchanged chemotherapy for at least 2 mo before enrollment. Patients were stratified according to anti-myeloma therapy at trial entry: stratum 1: first-line chemotherapy; stratum 2: second-line or greater chemotherapy. The primary endpoint—skeletal events (pathologic fractures, spinal cord compression associated with vertebral compression fracture, surgery to treat or prevent pathologic fracture or spinal cord compression associated with vertebral compression fracture, or radiation to bone)—and secondary endpoints (hypercalcemia, bone pain, analgesic drug use, performance status, and quality of life) were assessed monthly. Although the chemotherapeutic regimen was not uniform at study entry, the types and numbers of chemotherapeutic regimens were similar in the two groups at study entry and during the trial.

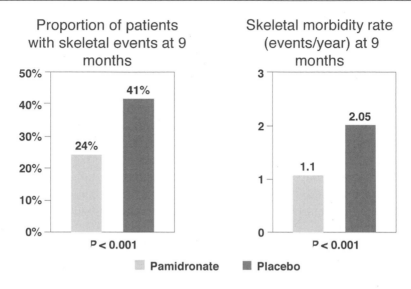

Fig. 3. Time to first skeletal-related event and mean number of skeletal events per year in patients with multiple myeloma treated with intravenous pamidronate or placebo (intent-to-treat patients).

After nine cycles of therapy *(18)*, 41% of patients in the placebo group exhibited any kind of skeletal event compared with 24% in the pamidronate group (Fig. 3). Half as many skeletal events were observed each year in the pamidronate group compared with the placebo group; this finding held for both stratum 1 and stratum 2 patients. The pamidronate group also exhibited a significant decrease in bone pain, no increase in analgesia use, and no deterioration in performance status and quality of life at the end of 9 mo. The skeletal morbidity rate continued to remain significantly lower in the pamidronate group than the placebo group throughout an additional 12 cycles of treatment *(19)*. However, no differences in the rate of healing or progression of osteolytic lesions was observed between groups. Overall survival was not significantly different between groups; however, in stratum 2 patients (patients who failed first-line chemotherapy), the median survival time was 21 mo in the pamidronate group compared with 14 mo in the placebo group (Fig. 4).

4.3.2. NEWER BISPHOSPHONATES

In vitro and animal in vivo studies have shown that the third-generation bisphosphonates zoledronic acid and ibandronate are more than 100 times more potent than second-generation aminobisphosphonates *(146,147)*. Clinical trials of the third-generation agents have now been completed. First, these trials have revealed that very small doses of these agents can effectively restore normocalcemia in patients with tumor-induced hypercalcemia *(148,149)*. Recently published results of a randomized study show the superiority of zoledronic acid

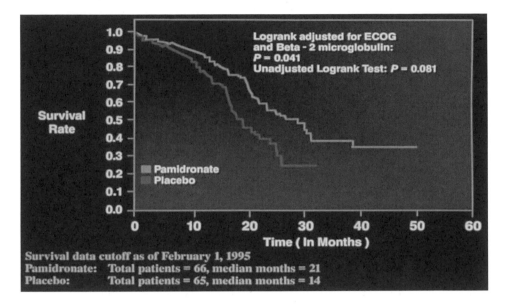

Fig. 4. Kaplan–Meier estimates of survival in stratum 2 patients with multiple myeloma treated with intravenous pamidronate or placebo. Survival was measured from randomization date to February 1, 1995. There was a median survival of 21 and 14 mo in pamidronate ($n = 66$) and placebo ($n = 65$) patients, respectively. Log-rank test was adjusted for Eastern Cooperative Oncology Group performance status and β_2 microglobulin that were the only two prognostic variables significantly influencing survival.

4 or 8 mg compared with 90 mg of pamidronate in reversing malignancy-related hypercalcemia in 287 patients *(127)*. Large, randomized studies of the effect of zoledronic acid and ibandronate on skeletal complications in patients with MM have recently been published *(143a–143d)*.

4.3.2.1. Zoledronic Acid. Zoledronic acid (1.5 mg) can be administered safely each month over several minutes to produce anti-resorptive effects similar to those observed with 90 mg pamidronate per month, as determined by bone resorption marker *(150,151)*. In a large, randomized phase II study of monthly infusions of zoledronic acid (0.4, 2.0, or 4.0 mg as a 5-min infusion) vs pamidronate (90 mg as a 2-h infusion) in 280 patients with lytic bone metastases (109 with myeloma) *(143b)*, fewer patients with any skeletal related events (SRE) (30–35%) were seen in the 2-mg and 4-mg zoledronic acid group and the pamidronate groups compared with the 0.4 mg zoledronic acid group (46%). These results are consistent with those of the 2 phase I trials in which doses of less than 1.5 mg did not effectively suppress bone resorption, as determined by marker.

A larger phase III randomized trial compared infusional zoledronic acid (4 or 8 mg) to 90 mg of pamidronate given every 3–4 wk for 24 mo in 1648 patients with MM or breast cancer with osteolytic bone disease *(143c,143d)*. The infusion time for the zoledronic acid was initially 5 min but was increased to 15 min because of rises in serum creatinine. Patients randomized to 8 mg were changed to 4 mg for similar reasons. The pamidronate was given over 120 min. The final results of this study showed that patients receiving zoledronic acid (4 mg) had skeletal events (47 vs 51%), delay in median time to first skeletal event (376 vs 356 d), and reduced number of median skeletal events per year (1.39 vs 1.04), although these differences did not reach statistical significance. However, the other pre-planned endpoint for the trial, multiple event analysis, showed a significan benefit for zoledronic acid compared to pamidronate treatment. This endpoint takes into account both the time to first skeletal event as well as to other subsequent events. Overall safety and renal tolerability were not different with the more rapid 15-min zoledronic acid infusion compared to 120 min of pamidronate.

4.3.2.2. Ibandronate. Ibandronate, administered as monthly bolus injections of 2 mg, was evaluated during a phase III placebo-controlled trial in 214 patients with myeloma with Durie Salmon stage II or III who were also receiving antineoplastic therapy *(143a)*. Ninety-nine patients in each group were evaluable for efficacy. The mean number of events per patient year was similar in both groups (ibandronate: 2.13; placebo: 2.05). However, patients taking ibandronate demonstrated a sustained reduction in bone resorption markers and fewer SREs per year. There was no difference in overall survival between groups. Thus, this dose of ibandronate is inadequate to achieve a significant effect in preventing skeletal complications in myeloma. Because studies of both zoledronic acid and ibandronate use higher doses, they may show that these drugs are not only more palliative in patients experiencing the devastating effects of bone disease but may also show that they are promising in terms of their ability to improve the overall survival of these patients while improving their quality of life.

These results show the added benefit of adjunctive bisphosphonate therapy in patients receiving chemotherapy compared with chemotherapy alone in patients with MM with respect to bone complications. Recently, the ASCO Guidelines for the Use of Bisphosphonates in patients with MM has been published *(143e)*. These drugs are recommended for treatment of patients with MM who have lytic bone disease and suggested for patients with demonstrated bone loss (ostepenia or osteoporosis). The three large randomized oral clodronate studies had inconsistent results *(11,15,141)*; curiously, the trial based on a larger dose *(12)* resulted in a lower effect *(16)*. In the latter trial *(16)*, clodronate did help reduce the incidence of fracture and severe hypercalcemia, but did not affect the time to first skeletal event or the need for radiotherapy. Similarly, oral pamidronate did not reduce the incidence of skeletal complications in myeloma *(17)*. Given these clinical results and the poor tolerability of oral agents, this route of administration for bisphosphonates is unlikely to be of much benefit. Intravenous zoledronic acid and pamidronate are associated with a reduced rate of skeletal complications and improved quality of life *(18,19,143b–143d)*. The recently completed phase III study suggests that zoledronic acid may be more effective than pamidronate, but further studies are needed to confirm this. Although 90 mg per month is efficacious, the optimal duration and dose of pamidronate remain unknown. Treatment should continue at least 24 mo, according to published trial results although patients are likely to benefit from ongoing treatment. Whether these drugs are effective during earlier stages of the disease or in patients without bone disease is unknown. A study evaluating zoledronic acid in this setting has begun. Furthermore, because of the enhanced bone loss and fracture risk in MGUS *(23,143f)*, studies are starting in these patients as well. Its role in myeloma may go beyond that of simply inhibiting bone resorption and preventing skeletal complications. Some preclinical studies suggest that it may have an anti-myeloma effect (Fig. 2), and the results of the large randomized clinical trial evaluating monthly intravenous pamidronate administration have shown that it improves survival in patients who failed first-line chemotherapy.

REFERENCES

1. Mundy GR, Bertoline DR. Bone destruction and hypercalcemia in plasma cell myeloma. Semin Oncology 1986; 13:291–299.
2. Belch AR, Bergsagel DE, Wilson K, et al. Effect of daily etidronate on the osteolysis of multiple myeloma. J Clin Oncol 1991; 9:1397–1402.
3. Kyle RA, Jowsey J, Kelly PJ, et al, Multiple myeloma bone disease: the comparative effect of sodium fluoride and calcium carbonate or placebo. N Eng J Med 1975; 293:1334–1338.
4. Kyle RA: Multiple myeloma: review of 869 cases. Mayo Clin Proc 1975; 50:29–40.
5. Stashenko P, Dewhirst FE, Peros WJ, et al. Synergistic interactions between interleukin 1, tumor necrosis factor, and lymphotoxin in bone resorption. J Immunol 1987; 138:1464–1468.
6. Mundy GR. Mechanisms of osteolytic bone destruction. Bone 1991; 12(Suppl 1):S1–S6.
7. Bataille R, Chappard D, Basle M. Excessive bone resorption in human plasmacytomas: direct induction by tumor cells in vivo. Brit J Haematol 1995; 90:721–724.
8. Berenson JR, Lipton A. Bisphosphonates in the treatment of malignant bone disease. Ann Rev Med 1999; 50:237–248.
9. Kanis JA, McCloskey EV, Taube T, et al. Rationale for the use of bisphosphonates in bone metastases. Bone 1991; 12 (suppl 1):S13–S18.
10. Fleisch H: Bisphosphonates: a new class of drugs in diseases of bone and calcium metabolism. In: Brunner KW, Fleisch H, Senn H-J, eds. Recent Results in Cancer Research. Vol. 116: Bisphosphonates and Tumor Osteolysis. Berlin-Heidelberg: Springer-Verlag; 1989:1–28.
11. Lahtinen R, Laakso M, Palva I, et al. Randomised, placebo-controlled multicentre trial of clodronate in multiple myeloma. Lancet 1992; 340:1049–1052.
12. Man Z, Otero AB, Rendo P, et al. Use of pamidronate for multiple myeloma osteolytic lesions. Lancet 1990; 335:663.
13. Thiebaud D, Leyuraz S, Von Fliedner V, et al. Treatment of bone metastases from breast cancer and myeloma with pamidronate. Eur J Cancer 1991; 27:37–41.
14. Purohit OP, Anthony C, Radstone CR, et al, High-dose intravenous pamidronate for metastatic bone pain. Brit J Cancer 1994; 70:554–558.

15. van Holten-Verzantvoort AATM, Kroon HM, Bijvoet OLM, et al. Palliative treatment in patients with bone metastases from breast cancer. J Clin Oncol 1993; 11:491–498.

16. McCloskey EV, MacLennan CM, Drayson MT, et al. A randomized trial of the effect of clodronate on skeletal morbidity in multiple myeloma. Brit J Haematol 1998; 101:317–325.

17. Brincker H, Westin J, Abildgaard, et al. Failure of oral pamidronate to reduce skeletal morbidity in multiple myeloma: a double-blind placebo-controlled trial. Brit J Haematol 1998;101:280–286.

18. Berenson JR, Lichtenstein A, Porter L, et al. Efficacy of pamidronate in reducing the skeletal events in patients with advanced multiple myeloma. N Eng J Med 1996; 334:488–493.

19. Berenson J, Lichtenstein A, Porter L, et al. Long-term pamidronate treatment of advanced multiple myeloma patients reduces skeletal events. J Clin Oncol 1998; 16:593–602.

19a. Menssen HD, Sakalova A, Fontana A, et al. Effects of long-term intravenous ibandronate therapy on skeletal-related events, survival, and bone resorption markers in patients with advanced multiple myeloma. J Clin Oncol 2002; 20:2353–2359.

19b. Rosen LS, Gordon D, Kaminski M, et al. Zoledronic acid versus pamidronate in the treatment of skeletal metastases in patients with breast cancer or osteolytic lesions of multiple myeloma: a phase III, double-blind, comparative trial. Cancer J 2001; 7:377–387.

19c. Rosen LS, Gordon D, Kaminski M, et al. Long-term efficacy and safety of zoledronic acid compared with pamidronate disodium in the treatment of skeletal complications in patients with advanced multiple myeloma or breast carcinoma: a randomized, double-blind, multicenter, comparative trial. Cancer 2003; 98:8:1735–1744.

20. Bataille R, Chappard D, Alexandre C, et al. Importance of quantitative histology of bone changes in monoclonal gammopathy. Br J Cancer 1986; 53:805–810.

21. Valentin-Opran A, Charhon SA , Meunier PJ, et al. Quantitative histology of myeloma-induced bone changes, Br J Haematol (1982) 52:601–610.

22. Taube T, Beneton MNC, McCloskey EV, et al. Abnormal bone remodelling in patients with myelomatosis and normal biochemical indices of bone resorption. Eur J Haematol 1992; 49:192–198.

23. Bataille R, Chappard D, Basle M. Quantifiable excess of bone resorption in monoclonal gammopathy is an early symptom of malignancy: a prospective study of 87 biopsies. Blood 1996; 87:4762–4769.

24. Chappard D, Rossi JF, Bataille R, et al. Cytomorphometry of osteoclasts demonstrates an abnormal population in B-cell malignancies but not in multiple myeloma. Calcif Tissue Int 1991; 48:13–17.

25. Bataille R, Chappard D, Marcelli C, et al, Mechanism of bone destruction in multiple myeloma: the importance of an unbalanced process in determining the severity of myeloma. J Clin Oncol 1989; 7:1909–1914.

26. Bataille R, Delmas PD, Chappard D, Sany J, Abnormal serum bone Gla protein levels in multiple myeloma. Cancer 1990; 66:167–172.

27. Carlson K, Ljunghall S, Simonsson B, et al. Serum osteocalcin concentrations in patients with multiple myeloma-correlation with disease stage and survival. J Intern Med 1992; 231:133–137.

28. Mundy GR, Raisz LG, Cooper RA, et al, Evidence for the secretion of an osteoclast stimulating factor in myeloma. New Eng J Med 1974; 291:1041–1046.

29. Lichtenstein A, Berenson J, Norman D, et al. Production of cytokines by bone marrow cells obtained from patients with multiple myeloma. Blood 1989; 74:1266–1273.

30. Cozzolino F, Torcia M, Aldinucci D, et al. Production of interleukin-1 by bone marrow myeloma cells. Blood 1989; 74:380–387.

31. Kawano M, Yamamoto I, Iwato K, et al. Interleukin-1 beta rather than lymphotoxin as the major bone resorbing activity in human multiple myeloma. Blood 1989; 73:1646–1649.

32. Yamamoto I, Kawano M, Sone T, et al. Production of interleukin-1β, a potent bone resorbing cytokine, by cultured human myeloma cells. Br J Haematol 1989; 49:4242–4246.

33. Bakkus MHC, Bakel-Van Peer KMJ, Adriaansen HJ, et al. Detection of interleukin-1β and interleukin-6 in human multiple myeloma by fluorescent *in situ* hybridisation. Leukemia Lymphoma 1991; 4:389–395.

34. Sati HIA, Greaves M, Apperley JF, et al. Expression of Il-1β and TNFα mRNA by neoplastic plasma cells, detected by dual colour fluorescence *in situ* hybridisation. Bone 1997; 20(Suppl):63S.

35. Torcia M, Lucibello M, Vannier E, et al. Modulation of osteoclast-activating factor activity of multiple myeloma bone marrow cells by different interleukin-1 inhibitors. Exper Hemat (1996) 24:868–874.

36. Alsina M, Boyce B, Devlin RD, et al. Development of an in vivo model of human multiple myeloma bone disease. Blood (1996) 87:1495–1501.

37. Garrett IR, Durie BGM, Nedwin GE, et al. Production of lymphotoxin, a bone-resorbing cytokine, by cultured human myeloma cells. New Eng J Med 1987; 317:526–532.

38. Iotsova V, Caamano J, Loy J, et al. Ostepetrosis in mice lacking NF-kappaB1 and NF-kappa B2. Nat Med 1997; 3:1285–1289.

39. Klein B, Zhang XG, Lu Z-Y, Bataille R. Interleukin-6 in multiple myeloma. Blood 1995; 85:863–872.

40. Kawano M, Hirano T, Matsuda T, et al. Autocrine generation and requirement of BSF-2/IL-6 for human multiple myelomas. Nature 1988; 332:83–85.

41. Uchiyama H, Barut BA, Mohrbacher A, et al. Adhesion of human myeloma-derived cell lines to bone marrow stroma stimulates IL-6 secretion. Blood 1993; 82:3712–3720.

42. Ishimi Y, Mijaura C, Jin CH, et al, IL-6 is produced by osteoblasts and induces bone resorption. J Immunol 1990; 145:3297–3303.

43. Hughes FJ, Howells GL. Interleukin-6 inhibits bone formation in vitro. Bone and Mineral 1993; 21:21–28.

44. Linkhart TA, Linkhart SG, McCharles DC, et al. Interleukin-6 messager RNA expression and interleukin-6 protein secretion in cells isolated from normal human bone: regulation by interleukin-1. J Bone Miner Res 1991; 6:1285–1294.

45. Bataille R, Barlogie B, Lu ZY, et al. Biologic effects of anti-interleukin-6 murine monoclonal antibody in advanced multiple myeloma Blood 1995; 86:685–691.

46. Dinarello CA. The biology of interleukin-1 and comparison to tumor necrosis factor. Immunol Lett 1987; 16:227–232.

47. Lacey DL, Grosso LE, Moser SA, et al. IL-1-induced murine osteoblast IL-6 production is mediated by the type 1 IL-1 receptor and is increased by 1,25 dihydroxyvitamin D$_3$. J Clin Invest 1993; 91:1731–1742.

48. Gaillard JP, Bataille R, Brailly H, et al. Increased and stable levels of functional soluble interleukin-6 receptor in sera of patients with monoclonal gammopathy. Eur J Immunol 1993; 23:820.

49. Tamura T, Udagawa N, Takahashi N, et al. Soluble interleukin-6 receptor triggers osteoclast formation by interleukin-6. Proc Natl Acad Sci USA 1993; 90:11924–11928.

50. Urashima M, Ogata A, Chauhan D, et al. Transforming growth factor-β1: Differential effects on multiple myeloma versus normal B cells. Blood 1996; 87:1928–1938.

51. Yoneda T. Cellular and molecular mechanisms of breast and prostate cancer metastasis to bone. Eur J Cancer 1998; 34:240–245.

52. Kaneda T, Nojima T, Nakagawa M, et al, Endogenous production of TGF-β is essential for osteoclastogenesis induced by a combination receptor activator of NF-κB ligand and macrophage-colony stimulating factor. J Immunol 2000; 165:4254–4263.

53. Rosen V, Thies RS. The BMP proteins in bone formation and repair. Trends Genet 1992; 8:97–102.

54. Kawamura C, Kizaki M, Yamato K, et al. Bone morphogenetic protein-2 induces apoptosis in human myeloma cells with modulation of STAT3. Blood 2000; 96:2005–2011.

55. Kaneko H, Arakawa T, Mano H, et al. Direct stimulation of osteoclastic bone resorption by bone morphogenetic protein (BMP)-2 and expression of BMP receptors in mature osteoclasts. Bone 2000; 27:479–486.

56. Hofbauer LC. Osteoprotegerin ligand and osteoprotegerin: novel implications for osteoclast biology and bone metabolism. Soc Eur J Endocrinol 1999; 141:195–210.

57. Kobayashi K, Takahashi N, Jimi E, et al. Tumor necrosis factor a stimulates osteoclast differentiation by a mechanism independent of the ODF/RANKL-RANK interaction. J Exp Med 2000; 191:275–285.

58. Altamirano CV, Ma HJ, Parker KM, et al. RANKL is expressed in malignant multiple myeloma (MM) cell lines. Blood 2000; 96:365a.

59. Shipman CM, Holen I, Lippitt JM, et al. Tumour cells isolated from patients wiuth multiple myeloma express the critical osteoclastogenic factor, RANKL. Blood 2000; 96:360a.

59a. Farrugia AN, Atkins GJ, To, LB, et al. Receptor activator of nuclear factor-kB ligand expression by human myeloma cells mediates osteoclast formation *in vitro* and correlates with bone destruction *in vivo*. Cancer Res 2003; 63:5438–5445.

60. Bucay N, Saroosi I, Dunstan CR, et al. Osteoprotegerin-deficient mice develop early onset osteoporosis and arterial calcification. Genes Dev 1998; 12:1260–1268.

61. Capparelli C, Kostenuik PJ, Morony S, et al. Osteoprotegerin prevents and reverses hypercalcemia in a murine model of humoral hypercacemia of malignancy. Cancer Res 2000; 60:783–787.

62. Honore P, Luger NM, Sabino MAC, et al. Osteoprotegerin blocks bone cancer-induced skeletal destruction, skeletal pain and pain-related neurochemical reorganization of the spinal cord, Nature Med 2000; 6:521–528.

63. Yaccoby S, Pearse R, Epstein J, et al. Reciprocal relationship between myeloma-induced changes in the bone marrow microenvironment and myeloma cell growth. Blood 2000; 96:549a.

64. Pearse RN, Sordillo EM, Yaccoby S, et al. Administration of the TRANCE-antagonist TR-Fc limits myeloma-induced bone destruction. Blood 2000; 96:549a.

64a. Terpos E, Szydlo R, Apperley JF, et al. A soluble receptor activator of nuclear factor κB ligand–osteoprotegrin ratio predicts survival in multiple myeloma: proposal for a novel prognostic index. Blood 2003; 102:3:1064–1069.

65. Nakamura M, Merchav S, Carter A, et al. Expression of a novel 3-5-kb macrophage colony-stimulating factor transcript in human myeloma cells. J Immunol 1989; 143:3543–3547.

66. Janowska-Wieczorek A, Belch AR, Jacobs A, et al. Increased circulating colony-stimulating factor-1 in patients with preleukemia, leukemia, and lymphoid malignancies. Blood 1991; 77:1796–1803.

67. MacDonald BR, Mundy GR, Clark S, et al. Effects of human recombinant CSF-GM and highly purified CSF-1 on the formation of multinucleated cells with osteoclast characteristics in long-term marrow cultures. J Bone Mineral Res 1986;1:227–233.

68. Sarma U, Flanagan AM. Macrophage colony-stimulating factor induces substantial osteoclast generation and bone resorption in human bone marrow cultures. Blood 1996; 88:2531–2540.

69. Fuller K, Owens JM, Jagger CJ, Wilson A, Moss R, Chambers TJ. Macrophage colony-stimulating factor stimulates survival and chemotactic behaviour in isolated osteoclasts. J Exp Med 1993; 189:1733–1744.

70. Girasole G, Passeri G, Jilka RL, et al. Interleukin-11: a new cytokine critical for osteoclast development. J Clin Invest 1994; 93:1516.

71. Hjertner O, Torgersen ML, Seidel C, et al. Hepatocyte growth factor (HGF) induces interleukin-11 secretion from osteoblasts: a possible role for HGF in myeloma-associated osteolytic bone disease. Blood 1999; 94:3883–3888.

72. Borset M, Hjorth-Hansen H, Seidel et al. Hepatocyte growth factor and its receptor c-Met in multiple myeloma. Blood 1996; 88:3998–4004.

73. Fuller K, Owens J, Chambers TJ. The effect of hepatocyte growth factor on the behaviour of osteoclasts. Biochem Biophys Res Comm 1995; 212:334–340.

74. Grano M, Galimi F, Zambonin G, et al. Hepatocyte growth factor is a coupling factor for osteoclasts and osteoblasts in vitro. Proc Nat Acad Sci USA 1996; 93:7644–7648.
75. Seidel C, Borset M, Turesson I, Abildgaard N, Sundan A, Waage A. Elevated serum concentrations of hepatocyte growth factor in patients with multiple myeloma. Blood 1998; 91:806–812.
76. Conway JG, Wakefield JA, Brown RH, et al. Inhibition of cartilage and bone destruction in adjuvant arthritis in the rat by a matrix metalloproteinase inhibitor. J Exp Med 1995; 182:449.
77. Hill PA, Docherty AJP, Bottomley KMK, et al. Inhibition of bone resorption in vitro by selective inhibitors of gelatinase and collagenase. Biochem J 1995; 308:167.
78. Yoneda T, Sasaki A, Dunstan C, et al. Inhibition of osteolytic bone metastasis of breast cancer by combined treatment with the bisphosphonate ibandronate and tissue inhibitor of the matrix metalloproteinase-2. J Clin Invest 1997; 99:2509–2517.
79. Barille S, Akhoundi C, Collette M, et al, Metalloproteinases in multiple myeloma: production of matrix metalloproteinase-9 (MMP-9), activation of proMMP-2, and induction of MMP-1 by myeloma cells. Blood 1997; 90:1649–1655.
80. Ray J, Stetler-Stevenson W. Gelatinase A activity directly modulates melanoma cell adhesion and spreading. EMBO J 1995; 14:908.
81. Vacca A, Ribatti D, Preta M, et al. Bone marrow neovascularization, plasma cell angiogenic potential, and matrix metalloproteinase-2 secretion parallel progression of human multiple myeloma. Blood 1999; 93:3064–3073.
82. Ridley RC, Xiao H, Hata H, et al. Expression of syndecan regulates human myeloma plasma cell adhesion to type I collagen. Blood 1993; 81:767–774.
83. Dhodapkar MV, Abe E, Theus A, et al. Syndecan-1 is a multifunctional regulator of myeloma pathobiology: Control of tumor cell survival, growth, and bone cell differentiation. Blood 1998; 91:2679–2688.
84. Choi SJ, Cruz JC, Craig F, et al. Macrophage inflammatory protein 1-alpha is a potential osteoclast stimulatory factor in multiple myeloma. Blood 2000; 96:671–675.
85. Choi SJ, Alsina M, Oba Y, et al. Antisense construct to MIP-1-alpha blocks bone destruction in an in vivo model of myeloma. Blood 2000; 96:549a.
85a. Oyajobi BO, Franchin G, Williams PJ, et al. Dual effects of macrophage inflammatory protein-1a on osteolysis and tumor burden in the murine 5TGM1 model of myeloma bone disease. Blood 2003; 102:1:311–319.
86. Vacca A, Ribatti D, Roncalli L, et al. Bone marrow angiogenesis and progression in multiple myeloma. Brit. J. Haematol. 1994; 87:505–508.
87. Bellamy WT, Richer L, Frutiger, et al. Expression of vascular endothelial crowty factor and ots receptors in hematopoietic malignancies. Cancer Res 1999; 59:728–733.
88. Dankbar B, Padro T, Leo R, et al. Vascular endothelial growth factor and interleukin-6 in paracrine tumor-stromal cell interactions in multiple myeloma. Blood 2000; 95:2630–2636.
89. Niida S, Kaku M, Amano H, et al. Vascular endothelial growth factor can substitue for macrophage colony-stimulating factor in the support of osteoclastic bone resorption. J Exp Med 1999; 190:293–298.
89a. Tian E, Zhan F, Walker R, et al. The role of the Wnt-signaling antagonist DKK1 in the development of osteolytic lesions in multiple myeloma. N Engl J Med 2003; 349:26: 2483–2494.
90. Smith DB, Scarffe JH, Eddleston B. The prognostic significance of x-ray changes at presentation and reassessment in patients with multiple myeloma. Hematol Oncol 1988; 6:1–6.
91. Bataille R, Chevalier J, Rossi M, et al. Bone scintigraphy in plasma-cell myeloma. Radiology 1982; 145:801–804.
92. Woolfenden JM, Pitt MJ, Durie BGM, et al. Comparison of bone scintigraphy and radiography in multiple myeloma. Radiology 1980; 134:723–728.
93. Agren B, Lonnqvist B, Bjorkstrand B, et al. Radiography and bone scintigraphy in bone marrow transplant multiple myeloma patients. Acta Radiologica 1997; 38:144–150.

94. Abildgaard N, Brixen K, Kristensen JE, et al. Assessment of bone involvement in patients with multiple myeloma using bone densitometry. Eur J Haematol 1996; 57:370–376.
95. Diamond T, Levy S, Day P, et al. Biochemical, histomorphometric and densitometric changes in patients with multiple myeloma: effects of glucocorticoid therapy and disease activity, Br J Haematol 1997; 97:641–648.
96. Cummings SR, Black DM, Thompson DE, et al. Effect of alendronate on risk of fracture in women with low bone density but without vertebral fractures. JAMA 1998; 280:2077–2082.
97. Berenson J, Webb I, et al. A phase II dose-ranging trial of single-agent pamidronate for relapsed/refractory multiple myeloma. Blood 1998; 92:107a.
98. Berenson J, Webb I, et al. A phase II dose-ranging trial of single-agent pamidronate for relapsed/refractory multiple myeloma. Blood 1998; 92:107a.
99. Berenson J, Rosen LS, Howell A, et al. Zoledronic acid reduces skeletal related events in patients with osteolytic metastases: a double-blind, randomized dose-response study. Cancer. In press.
100. Kusumoto S, Jinnai I, Itoh K. Magnetic resonance imaging patterns in patients with multiple myeloma. Br J Haematol 1997; 99:649–655.
101. Moulopoulos LA, Dimopoulos MA. Magnetic resonance imaging of the bone marrow in hematologic malignancies. Blood 1997; 90:2127–2147.
102. Moulopoulos LA, Dimopoulos MA, Smith TL, et al. Prognostic significance of magnetic resonance imaging in patients with asymptomatic multiple myeloma. J Clin Onc 1995; 13:251–256.
103. Frassica DA, Frassica FJ, Schray MF, et al. Solitary plasmacytoma of bone: Mayo Clinic experience. Int J Radiat Oncol Biol Phys 1989; 16:43–48.
104. Moulopoulos LA, Dimopoulos MA, Weber D, et al. Magnetic resonance imaging in the staging of solitary plasmacytoma of bone. J Clin Oncol 1993; 11:1311–1315.
105. Rahmouni A, Divine M, Mathieu D, et al. MR appearance of multiple myeloma of the spine before and after treatment. AJR 1993; 160:1053–1057.
106. Agren B, Rudberg U, Isberg B, et al. MR imaging of multiple myeloma patients with bone-marrow transplants. Acta Radiologica 1998; 39:36–42.
107. Lecouvet FE, Vande Berg BC, Michaux L. Development of vertebral fractures in patients with multiple myeloma: does MRI enable recognition of vertebrae that will collapse? Journal of Computer-assisted Tomography 1998; 22:430–436.
108. Moulopoulos LA, Dimopoulos MA, Alexanian R, et al. Multiple myeloma: MR patterns of response to treatment. Radiology 1994; 193:441–446.
109. Rahmouni A, Divine M, Mathieu D, et al. Appearance of multiple myeloma of the spine before and after treatment. AJR 1993; 160:1053–1057.
110. Tirovola EB, Biassoni L, Britton KE, et al The use of ^{99m}Tc-MIBI scanning in multiple myeloma. Br J Cancer 1996; 74:1815–1820.
111. Pace L, Catalano L, Pinto A, et al. Different patterns of technetium-99m sestamibi uptake in multiple myeloma. Eur J Nuclear Med 1998; 25:714–720.
112. Nawawi H, Samson D, Apperley J, et al. Biochemical bone markers in patients with multiple myeloma. Clinica Chimica Acta (1996) 253:61–77.
113. Abildgaard N, Bentzen, Nielsen et al. Serum markers of bone metabolism in multiple myeloma: prognostic significance of the carboxy-terminal telopeptide of type 1 collagen (ICTP) Br J Haematol 1997; 96:103–110.
114. Elomaa I, Risteli L, Laakso M, et al. Monitoring the action of clodronate with type I collagen metabolites in mutliple myeloma Eur J Cancer 1996; 32A:1166–1170.
115. Roux C, Ravaud P, Cohen-Solal M, et al. Biologic, histologic and densitometric effects of oral risedronate on bone in patients with multiple myeloma. Bone 1994; 15:41–49.
116. Clark RE, Flory AAJ, Ion EM, et al. Biochemical markers of bone turnover following high-dose chemotherapy and autografting in multiple myeloma. Blood 2000; 96:2697–2702.

117. Rowell NP, Tobias JS. The role of radiotherapy in the management of multiple myeloma. Blood Reviews 1991; 5:84–89.
118. Bosch A, Frias Z. Radiotherapy in the treatment of multiple myeloma. Int J Rad Onc Biol Phys 1988; 15:1363–1369.
119. Adamietz IA, Schober C, Schulte RWM, et al. Palliative radiotherapy in plasma cell myeloma. Radiotherapy and Oncology 1991; 20:111–116.
120. Rostom AY. A review of the place of radiotherapy in myeloma with emphasis on whole body irradiation. Hematol Oncol 1988; 6:193–198.
121. Giles FJ, McSweeney EN, Richards JDM, et al. Prospective randomised study of double hemibody irradiation with and without subsequent maintenance recombinant alpha 2b interferon on survival in patients with relapsed multiple myeloma. Eur J Cancer 1992; 28A:1392–1395.
122. Lecouvet F, Richard F, Vande Berg B, et al. Long-term effects of localized spinal radiation therapy on vertebral fractures and focal lesions appearance in patients with multiple myeloma. Br J Haematol 1997; 96:743–745.
123. Catell D, Kogen Z, Donahue B, et al. Multiple myeloma of an extremity: must the entire bone be treated? Int J Radiation Oncology Biol Phys 1998; 40:117–119.
124. Giralt S, Champlin R, Goodman M, et al. Preliminary results of a phase I/II study of multiple myeloma (MM) patients treated with [166]holmium-DOTMP in combination with high dose melphalan +/– total body irradiation (TBI) with autologous stem cell transplant (ASCT). Blood 2000; 96:558a.
124a. Martin JB, Jean B, Sugiu K, et al. Vertebroplasty: Clinical experience and follow-up results. Bone 1999; 25:11S–15S.
124b. Belkoff SM, Mathis JM, Fenton DC, et al. An ex vivo biomechanical evaluation of an inflatable bone tamp used in the treatment of compression fracture. Spine 2001; 26:151–156.
124c. Belkoff SM, Mathis JF, Deramond H, et al. An ex vivo biomechanical evaluation of a hydroxyapatite cement for use with kyphoplasty. Am J Neuroradiol 2001; 22:1212–1216.
124d. Cortet B, Cotton A, Boutry N, et al. Percutaneous vertebroplasty in patients with osteolytic metastases or multiple myeloma. Rev Rhum Engl Ed 1997; 64:177–183.
124e. Dudeney S, Lieberman IH, Reinhardt M-K, Hussein M. Kyphoplasty in the treatment of osteolytic vertebral compression fractures as a result of multiple myeloma. J Clin Oncol 2002; 20:9:2382–2387.
125. Cohen HJ, Silberman HR, Tornyos K, et al. Comparison of two long-term chemotherapy regimens, with or without agents to modify skeletal repair, in multiple myeloma. Blood 1984; 63:639–648.
126. Acute Leukemia Group B, Eastern Cooperative Oncology Group B. Ineffectiveness of fluoride therapy in multiple myeloma. N Eng J Med 1972; 286:1283–1288.
127. Warrell RP, Lovett D, Dilmanian A, et al. Low-dose gallium nitrate for prevention of osteolysis in myeloma: results of a pilot randomized study. J Clin Oncol 1993; 11:2443–2450.
128. Major P, Lortholary A, Hon J, et al. Zoledronic acid is superior to pamidronate in the treatment of hypercalcemia of malignancy. J Clin Oncol. In press.
129. Fleisch H. Bisphosphonates: mechanisms of action. Endocr Rev 1998; 19:80–100.
129a. Zhang B, Gojo I, Fenton RG. Myeloid cell factor-1 is a critical survival factor for multiple myeloma. Blood 2002; 99:6:1885–1893.
129b. Derenne S, Monia B, Dean NM, et al. Antisense strategy shows that Mcl-1 rather than Bcl-2 or Bcl-x$_L$ is an essential survival protein of human myeloma cells. Blood 2002; 100:1:194–199.
129c. van de Donk NWCJ, Kamphuis MMJ, van Kessel B, Lokhorst HM, Bloem AC. Inhibition of protein geranylgeranylation induces apoptosis in myeloma plasma cells by reducing Mcl-1 protein levels. Blood 2003; 102:9:3354–3362.
130. Aparicio A, Gardner A, Tu Y, et al. In vitro cytoreductive effects on multiple myeloma cells induced by bisphosphonates. Leukemia 1998; 12:220–229.

131. Shipman CM, Croucher PI, Russell GG, et al. The bisphosphonate incadronate (YM175) causes apoptosis of human myeloma cells in vitro by inhibiting the mevalonate pathway. Cancer Res 1998; 58:5294–5297.

132. Luckman SP, Hughes DE, Coxon FP, et al, Nitrogen-containing bisphosphonates inhibit the mevalonic pathway and prevent post-translational prenylation of GTP-binding proteins, including ras. J Bone Miner Res 1998; 13:581–589.

133. Reinholz GG, Getz B, Pederson L, et al. Bisphosphonates directly regulate cell proliferation, differentiation, and gene expression in human osteoblasts. Cancer Res 2000; 60:6001–6007.

134. Savage AD, Belson DJ, Vescio RA, et al. Pamidronate reduces IL-6 production by bone marrow stroma from myeloma patients. Blood 1996; 88:105a.

135. Derenne S, Amiot M, Barille S, et al. Zoledronate is a potent inhibitor of myeloma cell growth and secretion of IL-6 and MMp-1 by the tumoral environment. J Bone Mineral Res 1999; 14:2048–2056.

136. Giuliani N, Pedrazzoni M, Passeri G, et al. Bisphosphonates inhibit IL-6 production by human osteoblast-like cells. Scand J Rheumatol 1998; 27:38.

137. Wood J, Schnell C, Greeen J. Zoledronic acid (Zometa), a potent inhibitor of bone resorption, inhibits proliferation and induces apoptosis in human endothelial cells in vitro and is anti-angiogenic in a murine growth factor implant model. Proc Am Soc Clin Oncol 2000; 19:664a.

138. Singhal S, Mehta J, Desikan R, et al. Antitumor activity of thalidomide in refractory multiple myeloma. N Eng J Med 1999; 341:1565–1561.

139. Kunzmann V, Bauer E, Feurle J, et al, Stimulation of $\gamma\delta$T cells by aminobisphosphonates and induction of antiplasma cell activity in multiple myeloma. Blood 2000; 96:384–392.

139a. Wilhelm M, Kunzmann V, Eckstein S, et al. $\gamma\delta$ T cells for immune therapy of patients with lymphoid malignancies. Blood 2003; 102:1:200–206.

140. Radl J, Croese JW, Zurcher C, et al. Influence of treatment with APD-bisphosphonate on the bone lesions in the mouse 5T2 multiple myeloma. Cancer 1985; 55:1030–1040.

141. Heim ME, Clemens MR, Queisser W, et al. Prospective randomized trial of dichloro-methylene bisphosphonate (clodronate) in patietns with multiple myeloma requiring treatment: A multicenter study. Onkologie 1995; 18:439–448.

142. Dallas SL, Garrett IR, Oyajobi BO, et al. Ibandronate reduces osteolytic lesions but not tumor burden in a murine model of myeloma bone disease. Blood 1999; 93:1697–1706.

143. Heim ME, Clemens MR, Queisser W, et al. Prospective randomized trial of dichloro-methylene bisphosphonate (clodronate) in patients with multiple myeloma requiring treatment: a multicenter study. Onkologie 1995; 18:439–448.

143a. Menssen HD, Sakalova A, Fontana A, et al. for the Myeloma Ibandronate Study Group. Effects of long-term intravenous ibandronate therapy on skeletal-related events, survival, and bone resorption markers in patients with advanced multiple myeloma. J Clin Oncol 2002; 20:9:2353–2359.

143b. Berenson JR, Rosen LS, Howell A, et al. Zoledronic acid reduces skeletal-related events in patients with osteolytic metastases: A double-blind, randomized dose-response study. Cancer 2001; 91:7:1191–1200.

143c. Rosen LS, Gordon D, Kaminski M, et al. Zoledronic acid versus pamidronate in the treatment of skeletal metastases in patients with breast cancer or osteolytic lesions of multiple myeloma: A phase III, double-blind, comparative trial. Cancer J 2001; 7:5:377–387.

143d. Rosen LS, Gordon D, Kaminski M, et al. Long-term efficacy and safety of zoledronic acid compared with pamidronate disodium in the treatment of skeletal complications in patients with advanced multiple myeloma or breast carcinoma: A randomized, double-blind, multicenter, comparative trial. Cancer 2003; 98:8:1735–1744.

143e. Berenson JR, Hilner BE, Kyle RA, et al. for the American Society of Clinical Oncology Bisphosphonates Expert Panel. ASCO Special Article—American Society of Clinical

Oncology clinical practice guidelines: The role of bisphosphonates in multiple myeloma. J Clin Oncol 2002; 20:17:3719–3736.

143f. Melton JL, III, Rajkumar SV, Khosla S, Achenbach SJ, Oberg AL, Kyle RA. Fracture risk in monoclonal gammopathy of undetermined significance. J Bone Min Res 2004; 19:1:25–33.

144. Delmas PD, Charhon S, Chapuy MC, et al. Long-term effects of dichloromethylene diphosphonate (C12MDP) on skeletal lesions in multiple myeloma. Metabolic Bone Diseases and Related Research 1982; 4:163–168.

145. Merlini G, Parrinello GA, Piccinini L, et al. Long-term effects of parenteral dichloromethylene bisphosphonate (C12MDP) on bone disease of myeloma patients treated with chemotherapy. Hematol Oncol 1990; 90:2127–2147.

146. Muhlbacher RC, Bauss F, Schenk R, et al. BM.21.0955: a potent new bisphosphonate to inhibit bone resorption. J Bone Miner Res 1991; 6:1003.

147. Green JR, Muller K, Jaeggi KA. Preclinical pharmacology of CGP 42'446: a new, potent heterocyclic bisphosphonate compound. J Bone Miner Res 1994; 9:745–750.

148. Percherstorfer M, Hermann Z, Body, et al. Randomized phase II trial comparing different doses of the bisphosphonate idbandrone in the treatment of hypercacemia of malignancy J Clin Oncol 1996; 14:268–276.

149. Body JJ, Lortholary A, Romieu G, et al, A dose-finding study of zoledronate in hypercalcemic cancer patients. J Bone Miner Res 1999; 14:155–1661.

150. Berenson J, Vescio R, Henick K, et al. A phase I, open label, dose ranging trial of intravenous bolus zoledronic acid, a novel bisphosphonate, in cancer patients with metastatic bone disease. Cancer 2001; 91:144–154.

151. Berenson J, Vescio R, Rosen L, et al. A phase I dose-ranging trial of monthlyinfusions of zoledronic acid for the treatmentof osteolytic bone metastases. Clin Cancer Res. In press.

14 Renal Diseases Associated With Multiple Myeloma and Related Plasma Cell Dyscrasias

Alan Solomon, MD, Deborah T. Weiss, BS, and Guillermo A. Herrera, MD

CONTENTS

1. INTRODUCTION

Multiple myeloma (MM), light- or heavy-chain deposition disease (LCDD/HCDD), light- or heavy-chain-associated amyloidosis (AL/AH), and acquired Fanconi syndrome (AFS) represent a group of disorders characterized by the presence of monoclonal plasma cells in bone marrow and their homogeneous immunoglobulin products—i.e., M proteins—in serum, urine, or both (1–6). These immunoglobulin components can be nephrotoxic, as evidenced by their propensity to form pathologic deposits within the kidney (7–16). Furthermore, the relentless progression of this deposition eventually leads to organ failure and largely accounts for the poor prognoses of patients with these illnesses (17–21). Because of these factors, it is imperative that physicians are cognizant of the renal

From: *Current Clinical Oncology: Biology and Management of Multiple Myeloma*
Edited by: J. R. Berenson © Humana Press Inc., Totowa, NJ

diseases associated with MM and related plasma cell dyscrasias, so that they may institute appropriate therapeutic measures, especially those that can reduce the production of the toxic immunoglobulins responsible for the devastating and ultimately fatal nature of these disorders.

It has long been recognized that monoclonal light chains—i.e., Bence Jones proteins—are responsible for the nephropathology that results from their deposition as amorphous casts, basement membrane precipitates, fibrils, or crystals (as occurs in MM, LCDD, AL, and AFS, respectively) or from their inherently toxic effect on renal epithelial cells. Although it is now known that heavy chains, or even complete immunoglobulin molecules, also can form abnormal tissue deposits *(3–6,22–24)*, this chapter will focus primarily on the role of the light chain as the major causative factor in the pathologic ramifications of monoclonal immunoglobulin-related renal disease. The presentation is organized to include information germane to the pathogenesis and characteristic features of myeloma cast nephropathy (MCN), LCDD, AL, and AFS, as well as the currently available diagnostic and therapeutic strategies used in these disorders.

2. PATHOGENESIS

2.1. Light-Chain Structure

The two types of light chains, κ and λ, consist of a common structure composed of an approx 107- to 111-residue amino-terminal variable (V_L) region and an 107-residue carboxyl-terminal constant (C_L) domain. The V_L is the product of 2 genes, V and J, that encode the first approx 95 to 99 amino acids and the remaining approx 12 amino acids, respectively. Variation in the V_L sequence results from (a) the presence of approx 30 V_κ and V_λ germ-line genes that specify proteins divided, on the basis of homology, into four major V_κ (κ1, κ2, κ3, κ4) and five V_λ (λ1, λ2, λ3, λ6, λ8) subgroups or families; (b) somatic mutation; and (c) differences that result from recombination of the V- and J-gene encoded segments *(25–27)*. As will be discussed subsequently, this inherent variability accounts for the finding that certain light chains are pathologic, whereas others are apparently benign.

2.2. Light-Chain Synthesis and Catabolism

Circulating immunoglobulins are the products of terminally differentiated B cells, i.e., plasma cells. Light chains, both κ and λ, are synthesized in excess of heavy chains and are secreted from the cell in the "free" state *(28)*. κ molecules occur predominately as monomers or noncovalent dimers (Mrs approx 22,000 and 44,000 daltons, respectively), whereas λ proteins typically exist as covalent dimers *(29)*. Normally, these components are synthesized at a daily rate of approx 0.3 mg/kg/h and they are rapidly catabolized within the kidney ($T_{1/2}$: approx 1.5–2 h) *(30,31)*. Because of their relatively small size, they are readily filtered through the glomeruli; however, certain physicochemical properties determined by the V_L portion of the molecule (isoelectric point, hydrophobicity, etc.) may adversely affect glomerular clearance (32,33). After filtration, approx 90% of light chains are reabsorbed by endocytosis in the proximal tubules (29). Initially, these proteins bind to a low-affinity, high-capacity light-chain-specific receptor located on the tubular brush border (34) or to another glycoprotein, cubulin (Gp280), which is also involved in endocytosis and cell trafficking of other low-molecular-weight proteins such as lysozyme, insulin, cytochrome c, myoglobin, and β_2-microglobulin (35). Although light chains may undergo proteolysis at the brush border, the major site of degradation occurs intracellularly where, after endocytosis, these components are entrapped in vesicles that fuse with lysosomes; the proteins are then degraded enzymatically. Once the endocytic receptor(s) is saturated, unbound light chains pass into the distal nephron and are eventually excreted in the urine. These physiologic processes are altered in the plasma cell dyscrasias associated with excess synthesis of free monoclonal light chains. Although the proteinuric rate increases, the serum concentration of these components also rises as a result of their overproduction and also to decreased renal catabolism (30,31). Notably, certain Bence-Jones proteins may be inherently tubulopathic (36–39).

Under normal circumstances, free heavy chains are not found in the circulation. In patients who have heavy chain-related disease, such molecules can form amyloid fibrils (3–6,22–24) or basement membrane precipitates (1–6). However, there is no information currently available on how such proteins are processed by the kidney.

2.3. Molecular Features of Pathologic Light Chains

There is no evident relationship between the amount of Bence-Jones protein excreted daily and light-chain-related pathology (40). Thus, it has become increasingly evident that certain primary and/or tertiary structural features of light chains themselves enhance or diminish their pathologic potential.

Noteworthy is the fact that patients with MM, LCDD, and AFS predominately have κ-type monoclonal immunoglobulins, in contrast to individuals with AL, who have a prevalence of λ components (2,5,8,27). As discussed previously, this discordance may be related to differences in the quaternary structural properties of λ vs κ light chains that could affect their rate of glomerular filtration, as well as renal catabolism, and account for the finding that the ratio of κ to λ chains in urine is 2:1, whereas it is the opposite in serum (41). Additionally, λ Bence Jones proteins may possess certain features that render them more amyloidogenic, as evidenced by the discovery that proteins of 2 V_λ gene families—V_λ6a and V_λ3r—are typically associated with this process (42–46). Furthermore, patients with AL_λ6 amyloidosis most commonly have renal involvement (44,45). As for κ-type proteins, V_κ1 and V_κ4 products are seemingly over represented in LCDD and AFS *(47–50)*. In contrast to the hemoglobinopathies, no single, site-specific residue determines if a κ or λ light chain is pathologic or, conversely, benign *(50)*. Rather, it has become apparent that certain substitutions located at particular positions within the V_L domain affect the stability of these molecules and lead to their propensity to aggregate into fibrillar or other types of deposits *(50–67)*. Glycosylation or different posttranslational modifications of light chains, as well as their interaction with other molecules, also may potentiate nephrotoxicity *(68,69)*.

Chemical analyses of protein extracted from AL deposits have shown this material to consist predominately of light chain-related fragments containing the V_L or the V_L plus an additional approx 50 C_L residues; only rarely is the intact molecule or the C_L alone found *(27,70,71)*. Whether fibril formation is dependent on light-chain fragmentation or results from *in situ* digestion of the amyloid by proteolytic enzymes remains to be established. Foreshortened, presumably amyloidogenic light chains have been detected in some cases through biosynthetic studies utilizing plasma cells from patients with AL amyloidosis *(28,72)*. Additionally, immunohistochemical analyses of the deposits occurring in an individual with LCDD revealed them to be composed of a $V_\kappa 1$ fragment *(73)*.

3. PATHOPHYSIOLOGIC MANIFESTATIONS

3.1. Tubular Pathology

The most commonly occurring renal pathology is MCN where light chains precipitate predominantly in medullary tubules *(7,9)*. As shown in Figs. 1 and 2, casts exhibit certain characteristic features; namely, (a) they are eosinophilic when exposed to hematoxylin and eosin (H&E), but are not birefringent or fluorescent after staining with Congo red or thioflavin T, respectively; (b) they are amorphous in nature and lack defined structure, although fracture planes and, less commonly, needles can be visualized; and (c) they consist of monoclonal light chains, as demonstrated immunohistochemically using anti-κ and anti-λ antibodies. Cast formation is typically accompanied by an inflammatory reaction. Eventually, tubular basement membranes can rupture, creating gaps, and an adjacent multinucleated giant cell reaction may be evident. This type of pathology can result in renal tubular acidosis and, due to the inability of the kidney to concentrate urine, nephrogenic diabetes insipidus *(7,74)*.

Bence Jones proteins also can induce other forms of tubular pathology, e.g., tubular interstitial disease *(7,74,75)*. The resultant damage mimics that found in acute tubular necrosis, including vacuolation, fragmentation, desquamation, and, ultimately, total loss of the brush border. The lumens may be filled with cell nuclei and cytoplasmic fragments and, by immunoelectronmicroscopy, monotypic light chains can be visualized within lysosomal compartments and outer aspects of basement membranes *(74–80)*. Tubular interstitial disease adversely affects renal function, as evidenced by the failure of the kidney to concentrate or

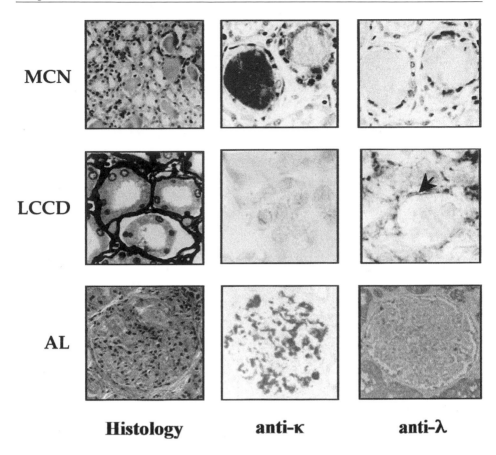

Histology **anti-κ** **anti-λ**

Fig. 1. Light microscopic and immunologic features of the light chain-associated renal diseases. Kidney biopsy specimens from patients with myeloma cast nephropathy (MCN), light chain deposition disease (LCDD), and AL amyloidosis (AL). (Left) MCN: hematoxylin and eosin stain (original magnification, ×250); LCDD: Jones stain (original magnification, ×400); AL: Congo red stain (original magnification, ×400). (Middle and right) The κ or λ nature of the pathologic immunoglobulin deposits was evidenced immunohistochemically using specific anti-light-chain monoclonal antibodies (alkaline phosphatase technique).

acidify urine. In the case of AFS, damage resulting from the presence of needle-shaped, light chain-containing intracellular crystals (Fig. 2) can induce similar morphologic abnormalities and result in glycosuria, phosphaturia, and aminoaciduria *(7,73)*.

A less commonly recognized form of monoclonal light chain-mediated tubular injury is associated with an inflammatory process that imitates acute interstitial nephritis. In such cases, cellular infiltrates consist primarily of lymphocytes or plasma cells and can be an early manifestation of LCDD *(9,79)*.

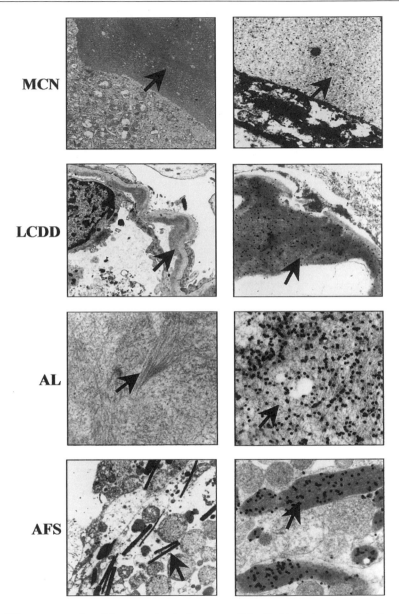

Fig. 2. Ultrastructural and immunologic features of the light chain-associated renal diseases. Kidney biopsy specimens from patients with myeloma cast nephropathy (MCN), light chain deposition disease (LCDD), AL amyloidosis (AL,) and acquired Fanconi syndrome (AFS). (*Left*) Electron photomicrographs, original magnifications: MCN, ×7500; LCDD, ×9000; AL, ×15500; AFS, ×8500. (*Right*) Immunoelectronmicrography. Reactivity of pathologic light-chain deposits with gold-labeled anti-κ or anti-λ antibodies (original magnifications: MCN, ×7500, LCDD, ×12,500; AL, ×15,500; AFS, ×22,500).

3.2. Glomerular Pathology

There are two predominant patterns of glomerular injury in the monoclonal immunoglobulin-related diseases, as exemplified by that found in LCDD and AL *(1–5,75,76,81,82)*. In LCDD (and HCDD), nodular glomerulosclerosis is characteristic (Fig. 2) and results from the co-deposition of monoclonal immunoglobulins and extracellular matrix proteins. The capillary walls appear thickened, and these components are present in subendothelial and mesangial areas, along tubular basement membranes, and in vessel walls, as evidenced immunohistochemically (Figs. 1 and 2) *(3–5)*. Ultrastructurally, this material appears punctate and electron dense (Fig. 2) and may extend into the lamina densa of glomerular basement membranes or even into subepithelial zones. Other manifestations of glomerular pathology have been noted in LCDD, particularly during the initial phase of the disease process. These alterations can mimic "minimal change" or other types of mesangial, membranoproliferative, and crescentic glomerulopathies. Owing to the focal and subtle nature of the deposits, especially during the early stages, the incidence of this disease is very likely underestimated *(79)*. Because HCDD and mixed LCDD/HCDD are the least common of the monoclonal immunoglobulin deposition diseases, relatively few cases have been reported *(3–6)*. However, the pathologic features found are similar to those occurring in LCDD.

In AL, the glomerular mesangium is replaced by eosinophilic material that has the characteristic tinctorial and ultrastructural features of amyloid; namely, after treatment with Congo red, a green to red birefringence is seen by polarizing light microscopy (Fig. 1) or fluorescence after staining with thioflavin T. The fibrillar nature of this material is evidenced by electron microscopy where 8- to 10-nm diameter, nonbranching fibrils of indeterminate length are found (Fig. 2). Although it may be possible to demonstrate immunohistochemically the κ or λ character of the amyloid *(82)*, definite proof of its composition only can be obtained by chemical analyses of the fibrillar protein extracted from these deposits *(83)*.

Due to the progressive nature of glomerular pathology, the kidney loses its ability to retain albumin and other serum proteins, a process that leads to the development of "nephrotic" syndrome. Furthermore, although LCDD and AL represent two distinct entities, pathologic deposits of both diseases have been noted in individual patients *(5,84–88)*.

3.3. Vascular Pathology

In LCDD, the characteristic punctate light-chain deposits are also present within renal blood vessel walls *(3–5,75,81)*. In some cases, these deposits result in a proliferative vasculopathy that may lead to hypoperfusion and contribute to the loss of renal function *(5)*. As for AL, amyloid fibrils typically are found within vasculature and may restrict blood flow *(11)*.

4. EXPERIMENTAL SYSTEMS

4.1. Protein (Light-Chain) Factors

The preeminent role of monoclonal light chains in the pathogenesis of the renal diseases in patients with MM and related monoclonal plasma cell dyscrasias has been demonstrated experimentally. For example, it has been shown that perfusion of rat tubules and incubation of tubular cells with human "tubulopathic" Bence-Jones proteins induced the typical morphologic changes associated with cellular injury, e.g., vacuolation, fragmentation, and desquamation, as well as physiologic abnormalities such as impairment of water, glucose, and chloride absorption (37,89–91). Furthermore, through size-exclusion chromatography, "toxic" and "nontoxic" light chains could be distinguished from one another on the basis of polymer formation (92).

Conclusive evidence that the protein itself is primarily responsible for the distinctive forms of light-chain-related renal disease has come from an in vivo experimental model involving mice injected with human Bence Jones proteins (40,93,94). The presence or absence of light-chain-related nephropathology in the animals correlated with that seen in the patients from whom the proteins were derived, i.e., light chains that were associated with tubular casts, basement membrane precipitates, or crystals in patient kidneys were deposited in similar fashion in the mouse (40). No pathology occurred when nonnephrotoxic components were used. Additionally, repeated injections into mice of Bence Jones proteins obtained from individuals with AL resulted in the deposition of these components in mouse organs as amyloid fibrils (95).

From in vitro studies using native proteins and recombinant or enzymatically derived V_L fragments (47,49–61), it has been shown that particular primary structural features of light chains can render these molecules pathologic. These experiments have revealed that certain amino acid substitutions may alter the tertiary conformation of the protein so that it becomes partially or completely unfolded (51,54,58,59). This intermediate form has been alleged to be the culprit in AL formation (56–66). When AFS is associated with proximal tubular damage and formation of crystalline inclusions, there frequently is an unusual hydrophobic residue at position 30 of the V domain that may account for resistance to cathepsin B proteolysis (96).

Computer modeling offers a powerful new tool for predicting the three-dimensional impact imparted on a protein by modification of and interactions between amino acids. Such information can have both prognostic and therapeutic relevance in the identification of pathologic light chains and development of drugs designed to stabilize these molecules.

4.2. Ancillary (Host) Factors

In addition to specific structural features that may render light chains toxic, accessory molecules and other factors are seemingly important in disease pathogenesis. Indeed, it has been shown experimentally that the precipitation of Bence Jones proteins as casts requires their interaction with Tam-Horsfall protein, a low-molecular-weight glycoprotein synthesized in the thick ascending limb of Henle's loop *(97,98)*. Using two different in vivo experimental models, cast formation was prevented by colchicine treatment owing presumably to its ability to inhibit Tam-Horsfall protein synthesis *(93,98)*. Additionally, the light chain-binding component BiP, a heat-shock protein found in the endoplasmic reticulum of B-lineage cells *(99)*, may have pathophysiologic relevance in the plasma cell-related monoclonal disorders. Because BiP has been shown to inhibit light-chain fibrillogenesis and aggregation by interacting with the V_L domain *(100–103)*, a deficiency in this molecular chaperone may lead to the formation of amyloid or other types of pathologic deposits.

A sudden and massive precipitation of Bence Jones proteins as casts within renal tubules is not uncommon and may lead to acute renal failure. Most often this occurs as a result of dehydration caused by limited fluid intake or excessive loss of liquid associated with vomiting, diarrhea, or the use of diuretics. In this state, the tubular concentration of light chains is effectively increased. Furthermore, an acidic pH and presence of other solutes in the distal nephron can render Bence Jones proteins less soluble and account for their predominant localization as casts in the renal medulla *(7)*. Although administration of radiographic contrast agents has been implicated in MCN, the pathology is more likely caused by water restriction or diarrhea resulting from use of the laxatives mandated for this procedure. The deleterious effects of dehydration on Bence Jones protein-induced nephropathology has also been demonstrated experimentally *(93)*.

In studies of LCDD- and AL-associated Bence Jones proteins cocultured with human mesangial cells, pathologic deposition was initiated by an interaction between light chains and putative, yet uncharacterized, mesangial cell surface receptors *(104–107)*. In the presence of "glomerulopathic" proteins obtained from patients with LCDD, it was noted initially that cellular proliferation occurred concomitantly with alteration in calcium homeostasis *(108)*, as well as activation of platelet-derived growth factor (PDGF)—β *(107)*. This cytokine has been localized to arterial walls and may play a role in the hyperplastic vasculopathy seen in some patients with LCDD *(9)*. Subsequently, transforming growth factor (TGF)-β activity also increased, whereas that of collagenase IV decreased *(104,107)*. These effects were associated with enhanced production of certain extracellular matrix proteins, e.g., tenascin, collagen IV, laminin, and fibronectin contained in the glomerular mesangial nodules of patients with LCDD and other disorders *(104,107,109,110)*. The alterations induced by LCDD-derived proteins did not occur when nonpathologic light chains were co-incubated with the mesangial cells. Early signaling events responsible for light-chain-mesangial-cell interactions have been delineated *(111)* and include activation of PDGF-β and its corresponding receptor, cytoplasmic-to-nuclear migration of c-fos and

NFκ-β signals, production of monocyte chemoattractant protein (MCI-1), and increased expression of Ki-67, a proliferation marker.

In similar experiments involving AL-associated Bence Jones proteins, a different response was noted; namely, mesangial cells were transformed from a normal smooth muscle phenotype to that of a CD68-positive macrophage *(105,106)*. Remarkably, the soluble light chains were converted into amyloid by a mechanism involving apparent clathrin-mediated endocytosis and subsequent lysosomal processing *(106)*. The addition of thrombospondin also potentiated amyloid formation. In contrast to LCDD *(107)*, AL extracellular matrix protein production was inhibited rather than stimulated, presumably as a result of the decreased expression of TGF-β and increased activity of collagenase IV *(106)*. These experimental findings could account for the destruction of normal mesangial tissue and its replacement with amyloid, as indicated in vivo trials *(9)*.

5. DIAGNOSIS

A kidney biopsy must be performed to diagnose a monoclonal immunoglobulin-associated renal disease definitively *(112)*. Because pathologic deposition is often subtle and not easily recognized, particularly during the earliest stages of LCDD and AL, it is essential that the specimen be examined by a nephropathologist who has special interest and expertise in these disorders. The procedure can be performed safely on an outpatient basis by a radiologist or nephrologist guided by computed tomography (CT), provided the patient has a normal coagulation profile (as indicated by platelet count, bleeding time, prothrombin levels, and partial thromboplastin time). Optimally, the amount of tissue obtained should be sufficient for light and electron microscopic examination, immunohistochemistry, and protein characterization. Two specimens are required: one is fixed in Carson Millonig's solution for routine staining (H&E, periodic acid Schiff, trichrome, Jones silver-methenamine, and Congo red or thioflavin T), immunoperoxidase analyses (if needed), and electron microscopy. The second is placed in Michel's or Zeus' transport medium for immunofluorescence studies.

There are pitfalls in diagnosing these disorders. The monotypic nature of pathologic deposits can be obscured by the presence of entrapped normal immunoglobulins. This problem can be obviated by using serially diluted antisera where reactivity of reagents with confounding proteins becomes diminished, whereas that of the pathologically deposited immunoglobulin is maintained. In this regard, more accurate results can be obtained with monoclonal rather than polyclonal anti-light-chain reagents *(113)*. Additionally, there is often less "background" staining when immunofluorescence vs immunoperoxidase is used to establish light-chain monoclonality. In LCDD, nodular glomerulosclerosis may be absent and, as previously discussed, other types of pathology can occur. Recognition of these forms of pathologic light-chain deposition often requires detailed analyses, including immunoelectronmicroscopy, that only can be performed in specialized laboratories *(79,117)*. For AL, deposits can be spotty and, thus, particular attention should be directed toward examination of the vasculature since such material is invariably present in this location. Congo red stains can be capricious unless properly performed, and small amounts of amyloid may remain undetected *(112,114–116)*. Freshly prepared solutions of the dye should be used, as well as appropriate controls and thicker (8–10 μm) sections. Thioflavin T stain, although more sensitive, can yield false-positive reactions. Proof that amyloid is indeed present is based on the finding by electron microscopy that the deposits are composed of nonbranching, randomly dispersed fibrils that are 8- to 10-nm in diameter. Additional tests can be used to substantiate the diagnosis of amyloid and include the immuno-histochemical demonstration that serum amyloid P component is codeposited *(118)*.

Because renal amyloid also can be composed of serum amyloid A-, apolipoprotein AI-, transthyretin-, fibrinogen-, or lysozyme-related molecules (i.e., AA, AApo-AI, ATTR, AFib, or ALys, respectively) *(119,120)*, it is imperative for therapeutic and prognostic reasons that the nature of this material be established *(121,122)*, preferably by chemical means *(83)*. In many cases, pathologic light- or heavy-chain renal deposits are detected unexpectedly in biopsies performed on patients with unexplained proteinuria or renal insufficiency. In these situations, the diagnosis of a monoclonal immunoglobulin-related nephropathy is made retrospectively through examination of bone marrow, blood, and urine, as well as other appropriate studies, e.g., skeletal X-rays.

The presence in bone marrow of plasma cells that are deemed monoclonal on the basis of a predominance of κ-positive or λ-positive cytoplasmic immunoglobulin is a characteristic feature of MM, as well as LCDD, AL, and AFS. In active ("nonsmoldering") MM, the percentage of plasma cells is usually high (>20%); thus, it is not difficult to document monoclonality. In contrast, that percentage is most often low (<5%) in LCDD, AFS, and AL; consequently, bone marrow in patients with these conditions is reported as "normal." To establish monoclonality in such cases, immunophenotyping analyses should be performed on cytospin preparations in which the number of plasma cells has been enriched by sedimentation through polysucrose/sodium diatrizoate (Histopaque-1077®, Sigma Diagnostics, St. Louis, MO). These studies require highly specific reagents, preferably those that distinguish free from bound light chains *(41)* or that recognize the major V_κ or V_λ subgroups or gene families *(113,123)*.

Another typical diagnostic feature of the monoclonal plasma cell disorders is the finding of homogeneous serum and/or urinary immunoglobulin-related M proteins. These can be identified using agarose gel and immunofixation electrophoreses (Paragon® Electrophoresis System, Beckman Instruments Inc.), techniques that are readily available in clinical laboratories. One caveat is that the kits do not contain antibodies against the two rare immunoglobulin (Ig) D and IgE heavy-chain classes; thus, serum specimens with "untypable" M-proteins should be subject to additional analyses using anti-IgD and anti-IgE antibodies. Furthermore, the serum is diluted 1:10, Bence Jones proteins may not be detected due to their often relatively low concentration (<0.5 mg/mL). This problem may be obviated by examining undiluted serum (A. Solomon, unpublished study). It should also be noted that Bence Jones proteinuria is frequently unrecognized when the amount excreted is low (<0.3 mg/mL) or when it is obscured by transferrin or other serum proteins, as occurs in nephrosis. In this situation, the urine sample must be concentrated at least 10- to 20-fold prior to analysis. The extreme sensitivity of immunofixation may allow free polyclonal light chains to be detected. These appear as multiple, closely spaced bands, most commonly of κ-type, and should not be mistaken for Bence Jones proteins. This pattern has been referred to as a "ladder" configuration and can be found in specimens obtained from presumably normal individuals (124).

The concentration of serum or urinary M-components can be determined by densitometric analyses of proteins separated by agarose gel electrophoresis or, alternatively, through nephelometry or serologic techniques utilizing specific anti-heavy- or -anti-light-chain antisera. Such measurements are necessary to document response to therapy or relapse. In this regard, monoclonal (41,125) and, more recently, polyclonal (126–129) anti-κ and anti-λ antibodies have been developed that can be used to distinguish free light chains from those bound to heavy chains. The availability of such reagents has provided a potentially useful clinical tool for the diagnosis and monitoring of patients with monoclonal plasma cell dyscrasias, particularly those with "nonsecretory" MM (130) or AL amyloidosis (131). The ability to quantitate by immunoassay free κ and λ light chains in serum and, especially, to determine the ratio of these components provides an objective means of establishing response to treatment or relapse. Reportedly, the data obtained using monoclonal rather than polyclonal reagents may be more reliable (125).

6. TREATMENT

Because of the preeminent role of monoclonal immunoglobulins in the pathogenesis of plasma cell-associated renal deposition diseases, major therapeutic efforts have been directed toward reducing or eliminating the synthesis of these components. Presently, this can be best achieved by antiplasma cell or other drug regimens, e.g., melphalan–prednisone (MP), vincristine, adriamycin, dexamethasone (VAD), high-dose dexamethasone, thalidomide and related compounds, proteosome inhibitors, arsenic trioxide, etc (2,132–140). A more complete and sustained suppression of monoclonal immunoglobulin synthesis and remission duration has been achieved through use of even larger doses of chemotherapy in conjunction with autologous/allogeneic transplants of peripheral blood-derived stem cells (141–148). Notably, this approach has been of benefit even in patients with impaired renal function *(149–153)*. Plasmapheresis can be an effective, albeit temporary, measure for individuals in whom rapid reduction in the concentration of circulating Bence Jones proteins is deemed essential, e.g., those with acute renal failure *(20)*. Because deposition of these components within the kidney as tubular casts is potentiated by dehydration, adequate fluid replacement can reduce this complication. The administration to tolerance of large amounts of hypotonic or physiologic solutions given intravenously and orally (1–4 L/d) can be beneficial. Sodium bicarbonate has also been recommended to render the urine alkaline, since certain Bence Jones proteins are less soluble at an acid pH.

Because factors other than pathologic M-components can adversely affect kidney function in patients with monoclonal plasma cell dyscrasias, treatment of hypercalcemia, electrolyte imbalance, anemia, and infection should be instituted, where applicable. Although it has been shown experimentally that cast formation can be prevented by colchicine *(93,98)*, presumably because of its effect on Tam-Horsfall protein synthesis *(97)*, the clinical benefit of this drug remains to be established.

Although cast nephropathy may be reversible, depending on the extent and duration of disease, the nephropathology found in patients with monoclonal immunoglobulin-associated glomerulopathies (i.e., LCDD and AL) rarely regresses, although a decrease in extent of glomerulosclerosis has been documented in several cases of LCDD after antiplasma cell therapy *(154,155)*. Additionally, improved renal function has been noted in persons with MM or AL amyloidosis who received high-dose chemotherapy and stem cell transplants *(141,149–153)*. However, in the great majority of cases, there is a progressive worsening of renal function that leads to oliguric kidney failure and institution of dialysis. Such individuals should be considered candidates for renal transplantation if, after 1 yr, they meet acceptable medical criteria, including disease stability and no clinically significant extrarenal deposition *(2,156,157)*. Recurrence of pathologic deposits in the transplanted kidney are less likely to occur in those in whom monoclonal immunoglobulin production has been suppressed by chemotherapy *(158)*. After transplantation, it is important to test urine specimens periodically (at approx 3- to 6-mo intervals) for the reappearance of such components and to reinstitute treatment, if necessary.

Other therapeutic strategies currently under study are those directed toward suppression of plasma cell proliferation by immune- or gene-mediated mechanisms *(159–160)*. New approaches will include agents that can block the binding of monoclonal immunoglobulins to basement membranes. For example, because TGF-β plays a role in mediating glomerulosclerosis in LCDD *(104)*, it could be a potential target *(161)*. The identification of compounds that can inhibit the formation or effect the resolution of pathologic protein aggregates also may prove beneficial *(162–164)*. One such drug, the iodinated anthracycline IDOX, has been found to bind and accelerate the removal of localized AL amyloid but, unfortunately, does not appear to affect renal or cardiac deposits *(165–167)*.

In the case of AL amyloidosis, other therapeutic options include the use of peptides to inhibit fibrillogenesis *(162)* or, alternatively, agents that could prevent the interaction of the molecules that codeposit with the fibrils, i.e., glycosoaminoglycans *(168)* or P-component *(169)*. Additionally, amyloid-reactive murine monoclonal antibodies have been obtained that accelerate removal of human light chain-containing fibrils injected into mice *(170)*. One such reagent has been chimerized and is under development for use in a phase I/II clinical trial *(171)*. Whether passive immunotherapy to effect amyloidolysis would benefit individuals with AL amyloidosis remains to be determined; however, if successful, it would represent a major therapeutic advance.

7. CONCLUSION

Over the past decade, progress has been made in advancing medical knowledge of the pathogenesis of plasma cell-associated monoclonal immunoglobulin renal deposition diseases. Although once considered rare, these entities now are recognized more frequently because of increased awareness of the disorders and the application of more sophisticated diagnostic techniques. Through further research, it is anticipated that more effective therapies will be developed and through these efforts, the prognosis of patients with these devastating diseases will be improved.

ACKNOWLEDGMENTS

We thank Ronda Reed for manuscript preparation. This work was supported in part by USPS Research Grant CA10056 from the National Cancer Institute (AS), the Aslan Foundation, and Grant 6198-98 from the Leukemia Society of America (GAH). AS is an American Cancer Society Clinical Research Professor.

REFERENCES

1. Gallo G, Picken M, Buxbaum J, Frangione B. The spectrum of monoclonal immunoglobulin deposition disease associated with immunocytic dyscrasias. Semin Hematol 1989; 26: 234–245.
2. Dhodapkar MV, Merlini G, Solomon A. Biology and therapy of immunoglobulin deposition diseases. Hematol Oncol Clin North Am 1997; 11:89–110.
3. Buxbaum JN, Chuba JV, Hellman GC, Solomon A, Gallo GR. Monoclonal immunoglobulin deposition disease: light chain and light and heavy chain deposition diseases and their relation to light chain amyloidosis. Clinical features, immunopathology, and molecular analysis. Am Intern Med 1990; 112:455–464.
4. Buxbaum J. Mechanisms of disease: monoclonal immunoglobulin deposition. Amyloidosis, light chain deposition disease, and light and heavy chain deposition disease. Hematol Oncol Clin North Am 1992; 6:323–346.

5. Buxbaum J, Gallo G. Nonamyloidotic monoclonal immunoglubulin deposition disease. Light-chain, heavy-chain, and light-and heavy-chain deposition diseases. Hematol Oncol Clin North Am 1999; 13:1235–1248.

6. Kambham N, Markowitz GS, Appel GB, Kleiner MJ, Aucouturier P, D'Agati VD. Heavy chain deposition disease: the disease spectrum. Am J Kidney Dis 1999; 33:954–962.

7. Misatti L, D'Amico G, Ponticelli C, eds. The Kidney in Plasma Cell Dyscrasias. Dordrecht, The Netherlands: Kluwer Academic Publishers, 1988.

8. Kyle RA. Monoclonal gammopathies and the kidney. Ann Rev Med 1989; 40:53–60.

9. Sanders PW, Herrera GA. Monoclonal immunoglobulin light chain-related renal diseases. Semin Nephrol 1993; 13:324–341.

10. Cohen AH. The kidney in plasma cell dyscrasias: Bence-Jones cast nephropathy and light chain deposit disease. Am J Kidney Dis 1998; 32:529–532.

11. Herrera GA. Renal manifestations of plasma cell dyscrasias: an appraisal from the patient's bedside to the research laboratory. Ann Diagn Pathol 2000; 4:174–200.

12. Lin J, Markowitz GS, Valeri AM, et al. Renal monoclonal immunoglobulin deposition disease: the disease spectrum. J Am Soc Nephrol 2001; 12:1482–1492.

13. Pozzi C, Locatelli F. Kidney and liver involvement in monoclonal light chain disorders. Semin Nephrol 2002; 22:319–330.

14. Shaver-Lewis MJ, Shah SV. The kidney in plasma cell disorders. In: Mehta J, Singhal, eds. Myeloma. London: Martin Dunitz, 2002:203–221.

15. Solomon A, Weiss DT, Herrera GA. Light-chain deposition disease. In: Mehta J, Singhal, eds. Myeloma. London: Martin Dunitz, 2002:507–518.

16. Gertz MA, Lacy MQ, Dispenzieri A. Immunoglobulin light chain amyloidosis and the kidney. Kidney Int 2002; 61:1–9.

17. Rota S, Mougenot B, Baudouin B, et al. Multiple myeloma and severe renal failure: a clinico-pathologic study of outcome and prognosis in 34 patients. Medicine 1987; 66:126–137.

18. Alexanian R, Barlogie B, Dixon D. Renal failure in multiple myeloma: pathogenesis and prognostic implications. Arch Intern Med 1990; 150:1693–1695.

19. Pozzi C, Fogazzi GB, Banfi G, Strom EH, Ponticelli C, Locatelli F. Renal disease and patient survival in light chain deposition disease. Clin Nephrol 1995; 43:281–287.

20. Blade J, Fernández-Llama P, Bosch F, et al. Renal failure in multiple myeloma: presenting features and predictors of outcome in 94 patients from a single institution. Arch Intern Med 1998; 158:1889–1893.

21. Gertz MA, Kyle RA, Greipp PR. Response rates and survival in primary systemic amyloidosis. Blood 1991; 77:257–262.

22. Eulitz M, Weiss DT, Solomon A. Immunoglobulin heavy-chain-associated amyloidosis. Proc Natl Acad Sci USA 1990; 87:6542–6546.

23. Solomon A, Weiss DT, Murphy C. Primary amyloidosis associated with a novel heavy-chain fragment (AH amyloidosis). Am J Hematol 1994; 45:171–176.

24. Mai HL, Sheikh-Hamad D, Herrera GA, Gu X, Truong LD. Immunoglobulin heavy chain can be amyloidogenic: morphologic characterization including immunoelectron microscopy Am J Surg Pathol 2003; 27:541–545.

25. Klein R, Jaenichen R, Zachau HG. Expressed human immunoglobulin kappa genes and their hypermutation. Eur J Immunol 1993; 23:3248–3262.

26. Kawasaki K, Minoshima S, Nakato E, et al. One-megabase sequence analysis of the human immunoglobulin lambda gene locus. Genome Res 1997; 7:250–261.

27. Solomon A, Weiss DT. Protein and host factors implicated in the pathogenesis of light-chain amyloidosis (AL amyloidosis). Amyloid: Int J Exp Clin Invest 1995; 2:269–279.

28. Buxbaum J. Aberrant immunoglobulin synthesis in light chain amyloidosis. Free light chain and light chain fragment production by human bone marrow cells in short-term tissue culture. J Clin Invest 1986; 78:798–806.

29. Stevens FJ, Solomon A, Schiffer M. Bence-Jones proteins: a powerful tool for the fundamental study of protein chemistry and pathophysiology. Biochemistry 1991; 30:6803–6805.
30. Solomon A, Waldmann TA, Fahey JL, McFarlane AS. Metabolism of Bence-Jones proteins. J Clin Invest 1964; 43:103–117.
31. Waldmann TA, Strober W, Mogielnicki RP. The renal handling of low molecular weight proteins. II. Disorders of serum protein catabolism in patients with tubular proteinuria, the nephrotic syndrome, or uremia. J Clin Invest 1972; 51:2162–2174.
32. Coward RA, DeLamore IW, Mallick NP, Robinson EL. The importance of urinary immunoglobulin light chain isoelectric point (pI) in nephrotoxicity in multiple myeloma. Clin Sci (Lond) 1984; 66:229–232.
33. Bellotti V, Merlini G, Bucciarelli E, Perfetti V, Quaglini S, Ascari E. Relevance of class, molecular weight and isoelectric point in predicting human light chain amyloidogenicity. Br J Haematol 1990; 74:65–69.
34. Batuman V, Guan S. Receptor-mediated endocytosis of immunoglobulin light chains by renal proximal tubule cells. Am J Physiol 1997; 272:521–530.
35. Batuman V, Verroust PJ, Navar GL, et al. Myeloma light chains are ligands for cubilin (gp 280). Am J Physiol 1998; 275:246–254.
36. Sanders PW, Herrera GA, Galla JH. Human Bence-Jones protein toxicity in rat proximal tubule epithelium in vivo. Kidney Int 1987; 32:851–861.
37. Batuman V, Guan S, O'Donovan R, Puschett JB. Effect of myeloma light chains on phosphate and glucose transport in renal proximal tubule cells. Ren Physiol Biochem 1994; 17:294–300.
38. Guan S, el-Dahr S, Dipp S, Batuman V. Inhibition of Na-K-ATPase activity and gene expression by a myeloma light chain in proximal tubule cells. J Invest Med 1999; 47:496–501.
39. Pote A, Zwizinski C, Simon EE, Meleg-Smith S, Batuman V. Cytotoxicity of myeloma light chains in cultured human kidney proximal tubule cells. Am J Kidney Dis 2000; 36:735–744.
40. Solomon A, Weiss DT, Kattine AA. Nephrotoxic potential of Bence-Jones proteins. N Engl J Med 1991; 324:1845–1851.
41. Abe M, Goto T, Kosaka M, Wolfenbarger D, Weiss DT, Solomon A. Differences in kappa to lambda ((:() ratio of serum and urinary free light chains. Clin Exp Immunol 1998; 111: 457–462.
42. Solomon A, Frangione B, Franklin EC. Bence-Jones proteins and light chains of immunoglobulins. Preferential association of the V(VI subgroup of human light chains with amyloidosis AL. J Clin Invest 1982; 70:453–460.
43. Ozaki S, Abe M, Wolfenbarger D, Weiss DT, Solomon A. Preferential expression of human (-light-chain variable-region subgroups in multiple myeloma, AL amyloidosis, and Waldenström's macroglobulinemia. Clin Immunol Immunopathol 1994; 71:183–189.
44. Comenzo RL, Wally J, Kica G, et al. Clonal immunoglobulin light chain variable region germline gene use in AL amyloidosis: association with dominant amyloid-related organ involvement and survival after stem cell transplantation. Br J Haematol 1999; 106:744–751.
45. Comenzo RL, Zhang Y, Martinez C, Osman K, Herrera GA. The tropisim of organ involvement in primary systemic amyloidosis: contributions of Ig VL germ line gene use and clonal plasma cell burden. Blood 2001; 98:714–720.
46. Perfetti V, Casarini S, Palladini G, et al. Analysis of V (lambda)-J(lambda) expression in plasma cells from primary (AL) amyloidosis and normal bone marrow identifies 3r (lambdaIII) as an amyloid-associated germline gene segment. Blood 2002; 100:948–953.
47. Cogne M, Preud'homme JL, Bauwens M, Touchard G, Aucouturier P. Structure of a monoclonal kappa chain of the V kappa IV subgroup in the kidney and plasma cells in light chain deposition disease. J Clin Invest 1991; 87:2186–2190.
48. Denoroy L, Deret S, Aucouturier P. Overrepresentation of the V(IV subgroup in light chain deposition disease. Immunol Lett 1994; 42:63–66.

49. Rocca A, Khamlichi AA, Touchard G, et al. Sequences of V(I subgroup light chains in Fanconi's syndrome. Light chain V region gene usage restriction and peculiarities in myeloma-associated Fanconi's syndrome. J Immunol 1995; 155:3245–3252.

50. Stevens FJ, Weiss DT, Solomon A. Structural bases of light chain-related pathology. In: Zanetti M, Capra JD, eds. The Antibodies. Vol. 5. Amsterdam: Harwood Academic Publishers, 1999; 175–208.

51. Hurle MR, Helms LR, Li L, Chan W, Wetzel R. A role for destabilizing amino acid replacements in light-chain amyloidosis. Proc Natl Acad Sci USA. 1994; 91:5446–5450.

52. Preud'homme JL, Aucouturier P, Touchard G, et al. Monoclonal immunoglobulin deposition disease (Randall type). Relationship with structural abnormalities of immunoglobulin chains. Kidney Int 1994; 46:965–972.

53. Stevens PW, Raffen R, Hanson DK, et al. Recombinant immunoglobulin variable domains generated from synthetic genes provide a system for in vitro characterization of light-chain amyloid proteins. Protein Sci 1995; 4:421–432.

54. Helms LR, Wetzel R. Specificity of abnormal assembly in immunoglobulin light chain deposition disease and amyloidosis. J Mol Biol 1996; 257:77–86.

55. Gallo G, Goñi F, Boctor F, et al. Light chain cardiomyopathy. Structural analysis of the light chain tissue deposits. Am J Pathol 1996; 148:1397–1406.

56. Bellotti V, Stoppini M, Mangione PP, et al. Structural and functional characterization of 3 human immunoglobulin kappa light chains with different pathological implications. Biochim Biophys Acta 1996; 1317:161–167.

57. Deret S, Chomilier J, Huang DB, Preud'homme JL, Stevens FJ, Aucouturier P. Molecular modeling of immunoglobulin light chains implicates hydrophobic residues in non-amyloid light chain deposition disease. Protein Eng 1997; 10:1191–1197.

58. Wetzel R. Domain stability in immunoglobulin light chain deposition disorders. Adv Protein Chem 1997; 50:183–242.

59. Raffen R, Dieckman LJ, Szpunar M, et al. Physicochemical consequences of amino acid variations that contribute to fibril formation by immunoglobulin light chains. Protein Sci 1999; 8:509–517.

60. Pokkuluri PR, Solomon A, Weiss DT, Stevens FJ, Schiffer M. Tertiary structure of human λ6 light chains. Amyloid: Int J Exp Clin Invest 1999; 6:165–171.

61. Vidal R, Goñi F, Stevens F, et al. Somatic mutations of the L12a gene in V-kappa (1) light chain deposition disease: potential effects on aberrant protein conformation and deposition. Am J Pathol 1999; 155:2009–2017.

62. Wall J, Schell M, Murphy CL, Hrncic R, Stevens FJ, Solomon A. Thermodynamic instability of human λ6 light chains: correlation with fibrillogenicity. Biochemistry 1999; 38: 14101–14106.

63. Ionescu-Zanetti C, Khurana R, Gillespie JR, et al. Monitoring the assembly of Ig light-chain amyloid fibrils by atomic force microscopy. Proc Natl Acad Sci USA 1999; 96: 13175–13179.

64. Bellotti V, Mangione P, Merlini G. Review: immunoglobulin light chain amyloidosis—the archetype of structural and pathogenic variability. J Struct Biol 2000; 130:280–289.

65. Davis DP, Gallo G, Vogen SM, et al. Both the environment and somatic mutations govern the aggregation pathway of pathogenic immunoglobulin light chain. J Mol Biol 2001; 313:1021–1034.

66. Khurana R, Gillespie JR, Talapatra A, et al. Partially folded intermediates as critical precursors of light chain amyloid fibrils and amorphous aggregates. Biochemistry 2001; 40:3525–3535.

67. Stevens FJ. Four structural risk factors identify most fibril-forming kappa light chains. Amyloid: Int J Exp Clin Invest 2000; 7:200–211.

68. Omtvedt LA, Bailey D, Renouf DV, et al. Glycosylation of immunoglobulin light chains associated with amyloidosis. Amyloid: Int J Protein Folding Disord 2000; 7:227–244.

69. Stevens FJ, Kisilevsky R. Immunoglobulin light chains, glycosaminoglycans, and amyloid. Cell Mol Life Sci 2000; 57:441–449.
70. Solomon A, Weiss DT, Murphy CL, Hrncic R, Wall JS, Schell M. Light chain-associated amyloid deposits comprised of a novel kappa constant domain. Proc Natl Acad Sci USA. 1998; 95:9547–9551.
71. Engvig JP, Olson KE, Gislefoss RE, Sletten K, Wahlstrom O, Westermark P. Constant region of a kappa III immunoglobulin light chain as a major AL-amyloid protein. Scand J Immunol 1998; 48:92–98.
72. Buxbaum JN. Abnormal immunoglobulin synthesis in monoclonal immunoglobulin light chain and light and heavy chain deposition disease. Amyloid: Int J Protein Folding Disord 2001; 8:84–93.
73. Takeda S, Takazakura E, Haratake J, Hoshii Y. Light chain deposition disease detected by antisera to a variable region of the kappa l light chain subgroup. Nephron 1998; 80:162–165.
74. Herrera GA. Low molecular weight proteins and the kidney: physiologic and pathologic considerations. Ultrastruct Pathol 1994; 18:89–98.
75. Sanders PW, Herrera GA, Kirk KA, Old CW, Galla JH. Spectrum of glomerular and tubulointerstitial renal lesions associated with monotypical immunoglobulin light chain deposition. Lab Invest 1991; 64:527–537.
76. Picken MM, Shen S. Immunoglobulin light chains and the kidney: an overview. Ultrastruct Pathol 1994; 18:105–112.
77. Herrera GA, Paul R, Turbat-Herrera EA, et al. Ultrastructural immunolabeling in the diagnosis of light chain-related renal disease. Pathol Immunopathol Res 1986; 5:170–187.
78. Silver MM, Hearn SA, Walton JC, Lines LA, Walley VM. Immunogold quantitation of immunoglobulin light chains in renal amyloidosis and kappa light chain nephropathy. Am J Pathol 1990; 136:997–1007.
79. Herrera GA, Sanders PW, Reddy BV, Hasbargen JA, Hammond WS, Brooke JD. Ultrastructural immunolabeling: a unique diagnostic tool in monoclonal light chain-related renal diseases. Ultrastruct Pathol 1994; 18:401–416.
80. Sanders PW, Herrera GA, Lott RL, Galla JH. Morphologic alterations of the proximal tubules in light chain-related renal disease. Kidney Int 1988; 33:881–889.
81. Strom EH, Fogazzi GB, Banfi G, Pozzi C, Mihatsch MJ. Light chain deposition disease of the kidney. Morphological aspects in 24 patients. Virchows Arch 1994; 425:271–280.
82. Gallo GR, Feiner HD, Chuba JV, Beneck D, Marion P, Cohen DH. Characterization of tissue amyloid by immunofluorescence microscopy. Clin Immunol Immunopathol 1986; 39: 479–490.
83. Murphy CL, Eulitz M, Hrncic R, et al. Chemical typing of amyloid protein contained in formalin-fixed paraffin-embedded biopsy specimens. Am J Clin Pathol 2001; 116:135–142.
84. Ganeval D, Noël L-H, Preud'homme JL, Droz D, Grunfeld JP. Light-chain deposition disease: its relation with AL-type amyloidosis. Kidney Int 1984; 26:1–9.
85. Jacquot C, Saint-Andre JP, Touchard G, et al. Association of systemic light-chain deposition disease and amyloidosis: a report of three patients with renal involvement. Clin Nephrol 1985; 24:93–98.
86. Smith NM, Malcom AJ. Simultaneous AL-type amyloid and light chain deposition disease in a liver biopsy: a case report. Histopathology 1986; 10:1057–1064.
87. Kaplan B, Vidal R, Kumar A, Ghiso J, Frangione B, Gallo G. Amino-terminal identity of co-existent amyloid and non-amyloid immunoglobulin kappa light chain deposits. A human disease to study alterations of protein conformation. Clin Exp Immunol 1997; 110:472–478.
88. Casiraghi MA, De Paoli A, Assi A, et al. Hepatic amyloidosis with light chain deposition disease. A rare association. Dig Liver Dis 2000; 32:795–798.
89. Clyne DH, Pollak VE. Renal handling and pathophysiology of Bence-Jones proteins. Contrib Nephrol 1981; 24:78–87.

90. Smolens P, Venkatachalam M, Stein JH. Myeloma kidney cast nephropathy in a rat model of multiple myeloma. Kidney Int 1983; 24:192–204.

91. Smolens P, Barnes JL, Stein JH. Effect of chronic administration of different Bence-Jones proteins on rat kidney. Kidney Int 1986; 30:874–882.

92. Myatt EA, Westholm FA, Weiss DT, Solomon A, Schiffer M, Stevens FJ. Pathogenic potential of human monoclonal immunoglobulin light chains: relationship of in vitro aggregation to in vivo organ deposition. Proc Natl Acad Sci USA 1994; 91:3034–3038.

93. Solomon A, Weiss DT, Williams TK. Experimental model of human light-chain-associated disease. Curr Top Microbiol Immunol 1992; 182:261–267.

94. Khamlichi AA, Rocca A, Touchard G, Aucouturier P, Preud'homme JL, Cogne M. Role of light chain variable region in myeloma with light chain deposition disease: evidence from an experimental model. Blood 1995; 86:3655–3659.

95. Solomon A, Weiss DT, Pepys MB. Induction in mice of human light-chain-associated amyloidosis. Am J Pathol 1992; 140:629–637.

96. Leboulleux M, Lelong B, Mougenot B, et al. Protease resistance and binding of Ig light chains in myeloma-associated tubulopathies. Kidney Int 1995; 48:72–79.

97. Sanders PW, Booker BB. Pathobiology of cast nephropathy from human Bence-Jones proteins. J Clin Invest 1992; 89:630–639.

98. Huang ZQ, Sanders PW. Biochemical interaction between Tamm–Horsfall glycoprotein and Ig light chains in the pathogenesis of cast nephropathy. Lab Invest 1995; 73:810–817.

99. Stevens FJ, Argon Y. Protein folding in the ER. Semin Cell Dev Biol 1999; 10:443–454.

100. Hendershot L, Wei J, Gaut J, Melnick J, Aviel S, Argon Y. Inhibition of immunoglobulin folding and secretion by dominant negative BiP ATPase mutants. Proc Natl Acad Sci USA 1996; 93:5269–5274.

101. Skowronek MH, Hendershot LM, Haas IG. The variable domain of nonassembled Ig light chains determines both their half-life and binding to the chaperone BiP. Proc Natl Acad Sci USA 1998; 95:1574–1578.

102. Davis DP, Khurana R, Meredith S, Stevens FJ, Argon Y. Mapping the major interaction between binding protein and Ig light chains to sites within the variable domain. J Immunol 1999; 163:3842–3850.

103. Davis PD, Raffen R, Dul JL, et al. Inhibition of amyloid fiber assembly by both BiP and its target peptide. Immunity 2000; 13:433–442.

104. Zhu L, Herrera GA, Murphy-Ullrich JE, Huang ZQ, Sanders PW. Pathogenesis of glomerulosclerosis in light chain deposition disease. Role for transforming growth factor-β. Am J Pathol 1995; 147:375–385.

105. Tagouri YM, Sanders PW, Picken MM, Siegal GP, Kerby JD, Herrera GA. In vitro AL-amyloid formation by rat and human mesangial cells. Lab Invest 1996; 74:290–302.

106. Isaac J, Kerby JD, Russel WJ, Dempsey SC, Sanders PW, Herrera GA. In vitro modulation of AL-amyloid formation by human mesangial cells exposed to amyloidogenic light chains. Amyloid: Int J Exp Clin Invest 1998; 5:238–246.

107. Herrera GA, Russell WJ, Isaac J, et al. Glomerulopathic light chain-mesangial cell interactions modulate in vitro extracellular matrix remodeling and reproduce mesangiopathic effects documented in vivo. Ultrastruct Pathol 1999; 23:107–126.

108. Zhu L, Herrera GA, White CR, Sanders PW. Immunoglobulin light chain alters mesangial cell calcium homeostasis. Am J Physiol 1997; 272:F319–F324.

109. Turbat-Herrera EA, Isaac J, Sanders PW, Truong LD, Herrera GA. Integrated expression of glomerular extracellular matrix proteins and beta 1 integrins in monoclonal light chain related renal diseases. Mod Pathol 1997; 10:485–495.

110. Bruneval P, Foidart JM, Nochy D, Camilleri JP, Bariety J. Glomerular matrix proteins in nodular glomerulosclerosis in association with light chain deposition disease and diabetes mellitus. Hum Pathol 1985; 16:477–484.

111. Russell WJ, Cardelli J, Harris E, Baier RJ, Herrera GA. Monoclonal light chain-mesangial cell interactions: early signaling events and subsequent pathologic effects Lab Invest 2001; 81:689–703.
112. Isaac J, Herrera GA. Renal biopsy as a primary diagnostic tool in plasma cell dyscrasias. Pathol Case Rev 1998; 3:183–189.
113. Abe M, Goto T, Kennel SJ, et al. Production and immunodiagnostic applications of anti-human light chain monoclonal antibodies. Am J Clin Pathol 1993; 100:67–74.
114. Klastskin G. Non-specific green birefringence in Congo-red stained tissues. Am J Pathol 1969; 56:1–13.
115. Carson FL, Kingsley WB. Non-amyloid green birefringence following Congo red staining. Arch Pathol Lab Med 1980; 104:333–335.
116. Puchtler H, Waldrop FS, McLoan SN. A review of light, polarization and fluorescence microscopic methods for amyloid. Appl Pathol 1985; 3:5–17.
117. Arbustini E, Morbini P, Verga L, et al. Light and election microscopy immunohistochemical characterization of amyloid deposits. Amyloid: Int J Exp Clin Med 1997; 4:157–170.
118. Pepys MB, Rademacher TW, Amatayakul-Chantler S, et al. Human serum amyloid P component is an invariant constituent of amyloid deposits and has a uniquely homogeneous glycostructure. Proc Natl Acad Sci USA 1994; 91:5602–5606.
119. Röcken C, Schwotzer EB, Linke RP, Saeger W. The classification of amyloid deposits in clinicopathological practice. Histopathology 1996; 29:325–335.
120. Benson MD. The metabolic and molecular bases of inherited disease. In: Scriver CR, Beaudet AL, Sly WS, Valle D, eds. Amyloidosis 8th ed. New York: McGraw Hill, 2001:5345–5378.
121. Anesi E, Palladini G, Perfetti V, Arbustini E, Obici L, Merlini G. Therapeutic advances demand accurate typing of amyloid deposits. Am J Med 2001; 111:243–244.
122. Lachmann HJ, Booth DR, Booth SE, et al. Misdiagnosis of hereditary amyloidosis as AL (primary) amyloidosis. N Engl J Med 2002; 346:1786–1791.
123. Solomon A, Weiss DT, Macy SD, Antonucci RA. Immunocytochemical detection of kappa and lambda light chain V region subgroups in human B-cell malignancies. Am J Pathol 1990; 137:855–862.
124. Harrison HH. The "ladder light chain" or "pseudo-oligoclonal" protein in urinary immunofixation electrophoresis (IFE) studies: a distinctive IFE pattern and an explanatory hypothesis relating it to free polyclonal light chains. Clin Chem 1991; 37:1559–1564.
125. Nakano T, Nagata A. ELISAs for free light chains of human immunoglobulins using monoclonal antibodies: comparison of their specificity with available polyclonal antibodies. J Immunol Methods 2003; 275:9–17.
126. Bradwell AR, Carr-Smith HD, Mead GP, et al. Highly sensitive, automated immunoassay for immunoglobulin free light chains in serum and urine. Clin Chem 2001; 47:673–680.
127. Katzmann JA, Clark RJ, Abraham RS, et al. Serum reference intervals and diagnostic ranges for free κ and free λ immunoglobulin light chains: relative sensitivity for detection of monoclonal light chains. Clin Chem 2002; 48:1437–1444.
128. Abraham RS, Clark RJ, Bryant SC, et al. Correlation of serum immunoglobulin free light chain quantification with urinary Bence-Jones protein in light chain myeloma. Clin Chem 2002; 48:655–657.
129. Le Bricon TL, Bengoufa D, Benlakehal M, Bousquet B, Erlich D. Urinary free light chain analysis by the Freelite(r) immunoassay: a preliminary study in multiple myeloma. Clin Biochem 2002; 35:565–567.
130. Drayson M, Tang LX, Drew R, Mead GP, Carr-Smith H, Bradwell AR. Serum free light-chain measurements for identifying and monitoring patients with nonsecretory multiple myeloma. Blood 2001; 97:2900–2902.
131. Abraham RS, Katzmann JA, Clark RJ, Bradwell AR, Kyle RA, Gertz MA. Quantitative analysis of serum free light chains. A new marker for the diagnostic evaluation of primary systemic amyloidosis. Am J Clin Pathol 2003; 119:274–278.

132. Heilman RL, Velosa JA, Holley KE, Offord KP, Kyle RA. Long-term follow-up and response to chemotherapy in patients with light-chain deposition disease. Am J Kidney Dis 1992; 20:34–41.

133. Kyle RA, Gertz MA, Greipp PR, et al. A trial of three regimens for primary amyloidosis: colchicine alone, melphalan and prednisone, and melphalan, prednisone, and colchicine. N Engl J Med 1997; 336:1202–1207.

134. Zomas A, Dimopoulos MA. Conventional treatment of myeloma. In: Mehta J, Singhal S, eds. Myeloma. London: Martin Dunitz, 2002:313–326.

135. Dhodapkar MV, Jagannath S, Vesole D, et al. Treatment of AL-amyloidosis with dexamethasone plus alpha interferon. Leuk Lymphoma 1997; 27:351–356.

136. Palladini G, Anesi E, Perfetti V, et al. A modified high-dose dexamethasone regimen for primary systemic (AL) amyloidosis. Br J Haematol 2001; 113:1044–1046.

137. Singhal S, Mehta J, Desikan R, et al. Anti-tumor activity of thalidomide in refractory multiple myeloma. N Engl J Med 1999; 341:1565–1571.

138. Barlogie B, Tricot G, Anaissie E. Thalidomide in the management of multiple myeloma. Semin Oncol 2001; 28:577–582.

139. Richardson PG, Schlossman RL, Weller E, et al. Immunomodulatory drug CC-5013 overcomes drug resistance and is well tolerated in patients with relapsed multiple myeloma. Blood 2002; 3063–3067.

140. Munshi NC, Tricot G, Desikan R, et al. Clinical activity of arsenic trioxide for the treatment of multiple myeloma. Leukemia 2002; 16:1835–1837.

141. Barlogie B, Shaughnessy J, Zangari M, Tricot G. High-dose therapy and immunomodulatory drug in multiple myeloma. Semin Oncol 2002; 29:26–33.

142. Kyle RA. High-dose therapy in multiple myeloma and primary amyloidosis: an overview. Semin Oncol 1999; 26:74–83.

143. Desikan R, Barlogie B, Sawyer J, et al. Results of high-dose therapy for 1000 patients with multiple myeloma: durable complete remissions and superior survival in the absence of chromosome 13 abnormalities. Blood 2000; 95:4008–4010.

144. Moreau P, Facon T, Attal M, et al. Comparison of 200 mg/m2 melphalan and 8 Gy total body irradiation plus 140 mg/m2 melphalan as conditioning regimens for peripheral blood stem cell transplantation in patients with newly diagnosed multiple myeloma: final analysis of the Intergroupe Francophone du Myelome 9502 randomized trial. Blood 2002; 99:731–735.

145. Singhal S. High-dose therapy and autologous transplantation. In: Mehta J, Singhal S, eds. Myeloma. London: Martin Dunitz, 2002:327–347.

146. Mehta J. Allogeneic hematopoietic stem cell transplantation in myeloma. In: Mehta J, Singhal S, eds. Myeloma. London: Martin Dunitz, 2002:349–365.

147. Comenzo RL, Gertz MA. Autologous stem cell transplantation for primary systemic amyloidosis. Blood 2002; 99:4276–4282.

148. Child JA, Morgan GJ, Davies FE, et al. High-dose chemotherapy with hematopoietic stem-cell rescue for multiple myeloma. N Engl J Med 2003; 348:175–183.

149. Sezer O, Schmid P, Shweigert M, et al. Rapid reversal of nephrotic syndrome due to primary systemic AL amyloidosis after VAD and subsequent high-dose chemotherapy with autologous stem cell support. Bone Marrow Transplant 1999; 23:967–969.

150. San Miguel JF, Lahuerta JJ, Garcia-Sanz R, et al. Are myeloma patients with renal failure candidates for autologous stem cell transplantation? Hematol J 2000; 1:28–36.

151. Badros A, Barlogie B, Siegel E, et al. Results of autologous stem cell transplant in multiple myeloma patients with renal failure. Br J Haematol 2001; 114:822–829.

152. Sirohi B, Powles R, Mehta J, et al. The implication of compromised renal function at presentation in myeloma: similar outcome in patients who receive high-dose therapy: a single-center study of 251 previously untreated patients. Med Oncol 2001; 18:39–50.

153. Casserly LF, Fadia A, Sanchorawala V, et al. High-dose intravenous melphalan with autologous stem cell transplantation in AL amyloidosis-associated end-stage renal disease. Kidney Int 2003; 63:1051–1057.

154. Komatsuda A, Wakui H, Ohtani H, et al. Disappearance of nodular mesangial lesions in a patient with light chain nephropathy after long-term chemotherapy. Am J Kidney Dis 2000; 35:E9.

155. Hotta O, Taguma Y. Resolution of nodular glomerular lesions in a patient with light-chain nephropathy. Nephron 2002; 91:504–505.

156. Gerlag PG, Koene AK, Berden JH. Renal transplantation in light chain nephropathy: case report and review of the literature. Clin Nephrol 1986; 25:101–104.

157. Pasternack A, Ahonen J, Kuhlback B. Renal transplantation in 45 patients with amyloidosis. Transplantation 1986; 42:598–601.

158. Short AK, O'Donoghue DJ, Riad HN, Short CD, Roberts IS. Recurrence of light chain nephropathy in a renal allograft. A case report and review of the literature. Am J Nephrol 2001; 21:237–240.

159. Teoh G, Chen L, Urashima M, et al. Adenovirus vector-based purging of multiple myeloma cells. Blood 1998; 92:4591–4601.

160. Anderson KC. Multiple myeloma. Advances in disease biology: therapeutic implications. Semin Hematol 2001; 38:6–10.

161. Border WA, Nobel NA. TGF-beta in kidney fibrosis: a target for gene therapy. Kidney Int 1997; 51:1388–1396.

162. Dul JL, Davis DP, Williamson EK, Stevens FJ, Argon Y. Hsp 70 and antifibrillogenic peptides promote degradation and inhibit intracellular aggregation of amyloidogenic light chains. J Cell Biol 2001; 152:705–716.

163. Kim Y, Wall JS, Meyer J, et al. Thermodynamic modulation of light chain amyloid fibril formation. J Biol Chem 2000; 275:1570–1574.

164. Kim YS, Cape SP, Chi E, et al. Counteracting effects of renal solutes on amyloid fibril formation by immunoglobulin light chains. J Biol Chem 2001; 276:1626–1633.

165. Gianni L, Bellotti V, Gianni AM, Merlini G. New drug therapy of amyloidosis: resorption of AL-type deposits with 4(-iodo-4(-deoxydoxorubicin. Blood 1995; 86:855–861.

166. Merlini G, Anesi E, Garini P, et al. Treatment of AL amyloidosis with 4'-iodo-4'-deoxydoxorubicin: an update. Blood 1999; 93:1112–1113.

167. Gertz MA, Lacy MQ, Dispenzieri A, et al. A multicenter phase II trial of 4'-iodo-4'-deoxydoxorubicin (IDOX) in primary amyloidosis (AL) Amyloid: J Protein Folding Disord 2002; 9:24–30.

168. Kisilevsky R, Lemieux LJ, Fraser PE, Kong X, Hultin PG, Szarek WA. Arresting amyloidosis in vivo using small-molecule anionic sulphonates or sulphates: implications for Alzheimer's disease. Nat Med 1995; 1:143–148.

169. Pepys MP, Herbert J, Hutchinson WL, et al. Targeted pharmacological depletion of serum amyloid P component for treatment of human amyloidosis. Nature 2002; 417:254–259.

170. Hrncic R, Wall J, Wolfenbarger DA, et al. Antibody-mediated resolution of light chain-associated amyloid deposits. Am J Pathol 2000; 157:1239–1246.

171. Solomon A, Weiss DT, Wall JS. Therapeutic potential of chimeric amyloid-reactive monoclonal antibody 11-1F4. Clin Cancer Res 2003; 9:3831S–3838S.

15 Pathogenesis and Treatment of Anemia

Heinz Ludwig, MD and Anders Österborg, MD, PhD

1. INTRODUCTION

Anemia is a common complication of myeloma that may already be manifest at the time of diagnosis. A high proportion of patients with myeloma presenting with anemia were reported in early publications: Kyle and colleagues *(1)* found hemoglobin (Hb) levels of less than 12.0 g/dL in 62% of patients diagnosed from 1960 to 1976; the authors of the third Medical Research Council trial, conducted between 1975 and 1978, reported Hb values of less than 10.0 g/dL in 49% of patients and severe anemia (Hb < 7.5 g/dL) in 19% of patients at the time of diagnosis *(2)*. In a recent study—the European Cancer Anemia Survey (ECAS)—investigators identified 2316 patients with myeloma or non-Hodgkin's lymphoma (NHL) among 15,370 cancer patients who were followed for 6 mo to determine the distribution of most tumor types seen in clinical settings in Europe. The prevalence of anemia (Hb < 12 g/dL) among the patients with myeloma or NHL in this study was 52% at enrollment, and 73% of these patients had an Hb level of less than 12 g/dL at at least one observation point during the survey *(3)*. Anemia usually (but not always) normalizes in patients who achieve complete remission after high-dose chemotherapy. However, it persists in patients who are unresponsive to myeloma treatment and recurs with a relapse or disease progression. Anemia frequently accompanies long-standing disease, when toxicity of

From: *Current Clinical Oncology: Biology and Management of Multiple Myeloma*
Edited by: J. R. Berenson © Humana Press Inc., Totowa, NJ

long-term treatment, impairment of renal function, and a heavy tumor load contribute to its induction and aggravation.

2. PATHOGENESIS OF ANEMIA

Anemia in multiple myeloma (MM) can be caused by several factors, including a decreased number of erythroid precursor cells, reduced responsiveness of the erythron to proliferative signals, shortened life span of red blood cells (RBCs), dilutional anemia as a result of paraprotein-induced expansion of the plasma volume, and impaired iron utilization. Among them, inadequate erythropoietin (EPO) production seems to be of major pathogenic importance *(4)*. It is found in practically all patients with impaired kidney function and in approx 25% of those with normal creatinine levels *(5)*.

Many of these pathogenetic processes are mediated by inflammatory cytokines, such as interleukin (IL)-1, tumor necrosis factor (TNF), and interferon-γ, which have been shown to inhibit erythropoiesis in vitro as well as in vivo *(6,7)*. The effects of these cytokines are synergistic, and they mutually enhance each other's release *(8)*. Their inhibitory effect on erythropoietic precursor cells can be overcome in vitro by erythropoietic agents *(9)*. IL-1 and TNF also suppress EPO synthesis *(10)*.

Recently, a novel pathogenetic mechanism for anemia has been described that implicates direct killing of erythroid precursors by myeloma cells *(11)*. Myeloma cells in patients with aggressive disease express a very high level of apoptogenic receptors, including both the Fas ligand and TNF-related apoptosis-inducing ligand, which trigger apoptosis in immature erythroblasts by stimulating specific death receptors, namely Fas and the DR4/DR5 complex. Persistence of such myeloma-cell-mediated erythroblast cytotoxicity probably accounts for the progressive destruction of the erythroid matrix seen in patients with an aggressive disease course.

Another factor contributing to a blunted EPO response to the anemic condition is the increased plasma viscosity associated with hypergammaglobulinemia. Singh and colleagues *(12)* reported an inverse correlation between EPO formation in response to anemia and plasma viscosity in patients with myeloma and an almost complete blunting of the EPO response at extremely high gammaglobulin concentrations in an animal model.

Functional iron deficiency can be attributed to the inappropriate release of iron from macrophages, i.e., normal or overloaded iron stores concurrent with low serum iron levels. Activated macrophages are also partly responsible for the shortened life span of RBCs, because they tend to remove and degrade minimally damaged but still fully functional RBCs from circulation.

A further cause of shortened red cell survival has been ascribed to an anemia-inducing substance—a 50-kD protein that reduces the osmotic resistance of erythrocytes *(13)*. Up to now, data on its possible relevance in anemia associated with MM have not been reported.

The impact of the mechanical displacement of erythropoiesis in the bone marrow by myeloma-cell infiltration was probably overestimated in the past, because normal blood counts are seen even in patients with heavy myeloma cell infiltration of the bone marrow.

Anemic conditions may also be induced in myeloma by anti-tumor therapy. A variety of cytostatic drugs as well as irradiation directly impair erythropoietic precursor cells in the bone marrow and, thus, inhibit their proliferation. Endogenous EPO production may also be reduced by some cytostatic drugs, leading to inadequate serum EPO levels.

3. INDICATIONS FOR TREATMENT

For decades, a substantially decreased Hb level was the only indication of a need for treatment of anemia; however, no specific cut-off value for anemia has ever been generally accepted. If a blood transfusion is the only treatment available, many physicians will order one for patients with Hb levels between 8 and 10 g/dL. With the introduction of recombinant human erythropoietin (rhEPO) for clinical use, this policy has considerably changed. Nowadays, it has become as important to maintain an optimal quality of life (QOL) as it is to carry out intensive attempts to control the tumor. This change in the treatment paradigm is partly associated with the safety and relative ease of rhEPO therapy, but mainly it is a consequence of a better understanding of the clinical role of anemia in cancer patients.

The manifestation of symptoms caused by the anemic condition depends not only on the degree of anemia but also very much on the patient's individual situation. Myeloma is a disease of the elderly, and many patients with myeloma experience a decline in cardiovascular function and impairment of other organs. Antitumor therapy may cause further deterioration of organ function, and myeloma-related complications such as amyloidosis, pulmonary and other infections, and deformities in the thoracic cage may enhance the patient's vulnerability to the sequelae of anemia.

Thus, almost all anemic patients with myeloma experience fatigue *(14)*, often in combination with emotional disturbances, depression, and decreased cognitive function. Moderate to severe anemia leads to peripheral hypoxia and vasodilation, with consecutive hyperactive heart syndrome manifested as tachycardia, left ventricular hypertrophy, and decreased exercise capacity. Patients with severe anemia may develop congestive heart disease with pulmonary edema which, in extreme cases, may be fatal.

The negative impact of low hematocrit (Hct) values is still often underestimated. However, the beneficial effects of treating cancer patients with symptomatic mild or moderate anemia with rhEPO have been clearly shown *(15,16)* and need to be stressed. During EPO therapy, quality-of-life parameters and exercise capacity improve with increasing Hb levels. Thus, rhEPO therapy seems to be indicated whenever anemia leads to a decreased QOL, and improving QOL should be generally accepted as a major treatment goal in patients with myeloma.

3.1. Blood Transfusions: Pro and Con

The major advantage of the allogeneic RBC transfusion is its rapid effect in practically all patients. For this reason, it is always used in patients with severe or life-threatening anemia. In patients with cancer-related anemia, transfusions are frequently not used until the anemia is severe and the anemia is seldom completely corrected with a transfusion alone (17). Even if the risk of infection associated with allogeneic RBC transfusions has been reduced by the use of screening tests, other negative aspects of transfusions need to be taken into account. Despite all precautions, life-threatening immediate hemolytic transfusion reactions caused by the transfusion of ABO- and Rhesus-incompatible blood cannot be completely avoided. Febrile reactions to human lymphocyte antigens (HLA), leukocyte, platelet, and plasma antigens and pyrogens and bacterial toxins lead to much more frequent and immediate complications. The transfusion of HLA antibodies may lead to noncardiogenic pulmonary edema, and the development of alloantibodies in the transfused host may cause delayed hemolytic reactions, posttransfusion purpura, or both (18). Allogeneic RBC transfusions may induce or worsen immunosuppression, which introduces a significant risk for infectious complications, (19,20) and the transfusion of allogeneic leukocytes into an immunocompromised patient may be complicated by the evolution of graft-vs-host disease. Iron overload can occur in patients with a history of long-term transfusion treatments. RBC transfusions may also inhibit endogenous EPO production, which can result in further impairment of erythropoiesis and, thus, an even higher dependence on allogeneic transfusions (21). Repeated RBC transfusions are associated with a highly variable, unstable Hb concentration, which often leads to periods of overt anemic symptoms. The fluctuating Hct may negatively influence physiological compensatory mechanisms, e.g., increased cardiac output and production of red cell 2,3-diphosphoglycerate.

Considering the effectiveness and tolerability of rhEPO in patients with myeloma (discussed later in this chapter), the main obstacle to treatment is cost. However, the actual financial cost of RBC transfusions is not insignificant. A recent publication from the United Kingdom estimated the cost of a single RBC transfusion to the National Health Service to be as high as 635 £, and this estimate did not include the cost of lost productivity (22).

3.2. rhEPO Treatment

The development of rhEPO provided a new therapeutic modality for patients with symptomatic anemia. Its beneficial effects on erythropoiesis have been shown both in patients with chronic renal failure and in patients with different types of malignancy, including MM. Results from major phase II and III studies in MM are summarized in the following subsections.

3.2.1. PHASE II STUDIES

The first pilot study was carried out by Ludwig and colleagues *(23)*, who observed an increase in Hb concentration of at least 2 g/dL in 11 of 13 patients with myeloma receiving rhEPO 150 to 300 IU/kg. Symptoms of anemia subsided and no adverse side effects were reported. These results were confirmed in a later study by the same group *(24)* and in a study by Barlogie and Beck *(25)*, in which 21 of 28 patients responded to rhEPO therapy with a rise in Hb concentration. In all three studies, the patients had stable disease when cytotoxic therapy began. The effects of rhEPO therapy on erythropoiesis were thus attributable to rhEPO and not regression of myeloma tumor cell infiltration in the bone marrow or a change in the dose intensity for concomitant chemotherapy.

A slightly lower response (48%) was reported by Bessho and colleagues in 29 patients with myeloma *(26)*. Musto and colleagues *(27)* conducted a phase II trial in 37 patients with advanced, transfusion-dependent, chemotherapy-refractory multiple myeloma. The rhEPO dose was 10,000 IU three times a week for 2 mo. Thirty-five percent of these poor-prognosis patients responded with a rise in Hb concentration and elimination of the need for further transfusions. Mittelman and colleagues *(28)* reported a significant rise in Hb concentration in 12 of 17 chemotherapy-treated patients; 6 of 11 transfused patients became transfusion-independent.

In these trials, the average weekly rhEPO dose was 450 IU/kg, which was usually given as a thrice weekly subcutaneous (SC) injection of 150 IU/kg each (corresponding to 10,000 IU per injection for an individual with a body weight of 70 kg). The overall response rate in these trials, which was usually defined as a rise in Hb of at least 2 g/dL, was 60% among 142 patients (Table 1).

3.2.2. RANDOMIZED STUDIES

Factors other than rhEPO therapy—including concomitant chemotherapy and regression or progression of myeloma cell infiltration into bone marrow—may also influence the Hb concentration and need for transfusion. Several randomized studies have been carried out to verify and extend the results obtained from the phase II trials (Table 2).

Garton and colleagues *(29)* conducted a prospective, randomized, placebo-controlled trial of rhEPO in 25 anemic patients with myeloma. RhEPO 150 IU/kg was administered three times per week. The dose was doubled in nonresponders after 6 wk. After 12 wk, nonresponders in the placebo arm were switched to rhEPO for 6 wk. Twenty patients were evaluable for response. Of the 10 patients who received rhEPO, 6 developed a normalized Hct, whereas no responses were

Table 1
Phase II Clinical Trials of rhEPO in Anemic Patients With Multiple Myeloma

Reference	Patients, N	Response Rate, %	Predictor for Response
Ludwig et al., 1990 (23)	13	85[a]	Serum EPO concentration
Ludwig et al., 1993 (24)	18	78[a]	—
Barlogie and Beck, 1993 (28)	28	75[a]	Serum EPO concentration
Bessho et al., 1994 (26)	29	48[b]	—
Musto et al., 1997 (27)	37	35[c]	• Serum EPO concentration • High-fluorescence reticulocytes • Soluble transferrin receptor
Mittelman et al., 1997 (28)	17	71[a]	—
Total	262	60	

[a] increase in Hb concentration by 2 g/dL
[b] increase in Hb concentration by 1.5 g/dL
[c] abolition of RBC transfusions
EPO, erythropoietin; Hb, hemoglobin; RBC, red blood cell.

observed in the 10 patients in the control arm. During the open-label phase, 4 of these patients responded to subsequent rhEPO treatment.

In a study by Silvestris and colleagues (30), 54 patients received rhEPO therapy ($n = 30$) or no rhEPO therapy ($n = 24$) over a total treatment period of 24 wk. Of the rhEPO-treated patients, 78% responded with at least a 2 g/dL rise in Hb concentration, but the difference compared with controls was statistically significant only for those who had not received RBC transfusions previously.

In the three-arm study carried out by Österborg and colleagues (31), 121 anemic transfusion-dependent patients with myeloma ($n = 65$) or low-grade NHL ($n = 56$) were randomized to rhEPO 10,000 IU/d, 7 d/wk (fixed-dose group; $n = 38$) or rhEPO 2000 IU/d for 8 wk, followed by step-wise escalation in rhEPO dose in nonresponders (titration group; $n = 44$); or to no rhEPO treatment (control group; $n = 39$). The total treatment time was 24 wk, and response was defined as elimination of the need for transfusion in combination with an increase in the Hb concentration by at least 2 g/dL. At the end of the study, 60% of the patients in each rhEPO group and 24% in the control group fulfilled the response criteria. The difference between each rhEPO group and the control group was statistically significant ($p < 0.02$). No relevant differences between the rhEPO treatment groups and the control group were observed during the first 8 wk. Thereafter, the cumulative response rate differed markedly between the rhEPO treatment groups and the control group. Of patients in the titration group, 14% responded to rhEPO therapy at the first dose level (2000 IU/d). After step-wise escalation to 5000 and 10,000 IU daily, the cumulative response rate increased to 42 and 60%, respectively.

This trial shows that there is a lag time of at least 4 wk before the emerging clinical effects of rhEPO can be detected and that the first dose level (2000 IU/d) used in the titration group was clearly inferior.

Cazzola and colleagues *(32)* conducted a randomized dose-finding trial in anemic but nontransfusion-dependent patients with MM or NHL, in which the efficacy of four different dose levels of rhEPO (1000 IU/d n = 31, 2000 IU/d n = 29, 5000 IU/d n = 31, and 10,000 IU/d n = 26, daily for 8 wk) were compared in these patients vs an untreated control group (n = 29). Response was defined as an increase in Hb level of at least 2 g/dL. The response rate was significantly higher with 5000 IU/d (61%) and 10,000 IU/d (62%) than with 2000 IU/d (31%). However, patients with a normal platelet count achieved an acceptable response rate (50%) on 2000 IU/d of rhEPO. The results indicated that rhEPO 1000 IU/d was clearly inferior, because the results were not different from those observed in the untreated control group.

In both of these trials *(31,32)*, the effect of rhEPO appeared to be more striking in patients with myeloma than in those with NHL.

Dammacco *(33)* conducted a 12-wk, double-blind, placebo-controlled study in 145 anemic (Hb <11 g/dL) patients with MM. Patients received 150 IU/kg epoetin or placebo thrice weekly; this dose was doubled if the Hb response at week 4 was inadequate. Epoetin treatment significantly reduced the need for transfusions compared with placebo (28 vs 47%) regardless of the patient's transfusion history, and increased mean Hb concentration by 1.8 g/dL vs 0.0 g/dL compared with controls. QOL was significantly improved with rhEPO vs placebo in univariate but not multivariate analysis. Performance status was significantly better in the rhEPO-treated patients. At the end of the blinded treatment phase, patients continued rhEPO or were switched from placebo to rhEPO. Patients in the former group maintained their Hb concentrations and in the latter achieved a mean Hb increase of 2.4 g/dL.

Österborg and colleagues *(34)* randomized 117 patients with transfusion-dependent multiple myeloma and low endogenous EPO levels to either rhEPO 150 IU/kg or placebo thrice weekly. Also included in the study were 106 patients with NHL and 126 with chronic lymphocytic leukemia (CLL). The response rate was 76% in patients taking epoetin vs 29% in those taking placebo. In the entire patient population, transfusion-free survival and severe anemia-free survival were significantly greater in the rhEPO group compared with the placebo group (relative risk reduction [RRR]: 43 vs 51%). Cox's multivariate regression analysis revealed that treatment with rhEPO (hazard ratio [HR]: 0.55), a platelet count of at least 100×10^9 (HR: 0.416), a Hb level of up to 9 g/dL (HR: 0.589) and low pretreatment transfusion requirement of no more than 2 units within 3 mo before

Table 2
Randomized Trials of rhEPO in Anemic Patients With Multiple Myeloma

Reference	Clinical Condition			Patients, N	Response Rate	Response Predictor
	MM	CLL	NHL			
Garton et al., 1995 (29)	20			20	• rhEPO: 6/10(60%)[a] • Control: 0/10(0%)	
Silvestris et al., 1995 (30)	54			54	• rhEPO: 21/27(78%)[b,c] • Control: not given	
Cazzola et al., 1995 (32)	84	62		146	• rhEPO • 10,000 IU: 62%[b] • 5000 IU: 61%[b] • 2000 IU: 31%[b] • 1000 IU: 6%[b] • Control: 7%[b]	• Serum EPO concentration • Platelet count
Österborg et al., 1996 (31)	65	26	30	121	rhEPO: 60%[d]	• Serum EPO concentration • Platelet count

Study					Response	
Dammacco et al., 2001 (33)[f]	145			145	• rhEPO: 58%[d] • Control: 24%[d]	
Österborg et al., 2002 (34)[f]	117	126	106	349[e]	• rhEPO: 76% • Control: 29%	• Platelet count • Hb baseline • Pretreatment transfusion requirement
Cazzola et al., 2003 (35)[f]	158	47	51[e]	244[e]	30,000 IU/wk: 72% 10,000 IU/TIW: 75%	Serum EPO concentration
Hedenus et al., 2003 (42)[f]	173	55	192	344	• Darbepoetin 2.25µg/kg: 60%[b] • Control: 18%[b]	Serum EPO concentration.

[a] normalization of Hct
[b] increase in Hb ≥ 2g/dL
[c] significantly superior in transfusion-dependent patients only
[d] increase in Hb ≥ 2g/dL plus elimination of transfusion need
[e] only patients with low EPO serum concentration (≤ 100 mU/mL) enrolled
[f] double-blind, placebo-controlled trial

MM, multiple myeloma; CLL, chronic lymphocytic leukemia; NHL, non-Hodgkin's lymphoma; EPO, erythropoietin; TIW, three times a week; Hct, hematocrit; Hb, hemoglobin.

enrollment (HR: 0.645) were characteristics predictive of a low risk for transfusion need.

Recently, Cazzola *(35)* showed in a prospective randomized trial that 30,000 IU rhEPO given once weekly subcutaneously produces response rates similar to those seen with 10,000 IU thrice weekly subcutaneously in 241 anemic (Hb 9–11 g/dL) patients with MM ($n = 158$) and other lymphoproliferative disorders, including CLL ($n = 47$), NHL ($n = 32$), and Hodgkin's disease ($n = 19$). Response rates were 72% in the once-weekly group and 75% in the thrice-weekly group, and correlated inversely with baseline endogenous EPO levels.

The efficacy of darbepoetin, a hyperglycosylated EPO molecule, was given at a dose of 2.25 µg/kg once weekly for 12 wk and compared with the effect of placebo in 344 anemic (Hb 11 g/dL) patients with MM ($n = 173$), CLL ($n = 55$), Hodgkin's disease ($n = 21$), or NHL ($n = 171$). Sixty percent of the patients in the darbepoetin group and 18% of those in the placebo group demonstrated a Hb response, regardless of baseline EPO level *(36)*. Darbepoetin resulted in a higher mean change in Hb compared with placebo (2.66 g/dL vs 0.69 g/dL) and in a significantly lower need for RBC transfusions ($p < 0.001$). The efficacy of darbopoetin was consistent for patients with myeloma or lymphoma.

The results of these randomized multicenter studies showed that patients with myeloma who were treated with rhEPO had a significantly higher response rate, indicated by the rise in Hb level and transfusion independence, than patients in the control group. The difference could be attributed to the rhEPO administration, because (a) no between-group differences were observed with regard to reduction or progression of the underlying malignant disease during the study period, and (b) the intensity of concomitant chemotherapy was similar in all groups. These studies have thus proved the efficacy of rhEPO in ameliorating anemia and transfusion dependence in patients with MM.

3.2.3. INDICATION FOR TREATMENT AND DOSING OF rhEPO

Guidelines for the use of rhEPO in cancer patients with anemia have been issued by the American Society of Hematology/American Society of Clinical Oncology (ASH/ASCO) *(37)* and by an international group of experts *(38)* specifically for the use in patients with myeloma and lymphoma. Both groups recommend initiation of treatment in all patients with Hb of up to 10 g/dL and in those with a Hb level between 10 and 12 g/dL, provided the patient has symptoms of anemia, meets the criteria established by the international experts guidelines, or both, if the patient is being treated by chemotherapy. The target Hb level is 12 g/dL, according to the international experts' recommendation, and the ASH/ASCO guidelines. Good clinical practice always orients itself according to the specific needs of an individual patient and much less on simple laboratory levels. Hence, treatment with rhEPO seems to be indicated whenever a patient with MM has symptoms of anemia. This may, in some individual patients, lead to the initiation of rhEPO therapy at a higher Hb level than is suggested by the guidelines. Treatment with rhEPO may be withheld in young patients with slowly developing anemia without overt clinical symptoms.

To reduce costs, it is important to identify the optimal rhEPO dose. A high dose (10,000 IU/d, 7 d/wk) seems to be only marginally better than 5000 IU/d in transfusion-dependent patients *(31)* and not better at all in nontransfused patients with anemia *(32)*. In two studies *(31,32)*, rhEPO 1000 or 2000 IU/d was clearly suboptimal. Thus, a starting dose of 10,000 IU three times a week may be recommended in those patients. For patients with well-preserved bone marrow function—indicated by a normal platelet count—lower doses (5000 IU, three times a week) may be considered, because the response rate in such patients may still be as high as 50% *(32)*. Alternatively, a once-weekly regimen may be used. Recommended doses are 30,000 IU or 40,000 IU once weekly. The dose may be increased to either 20,000 IU thrice weekly or 60,000 IU once weekly in patients who do not respond within 4 wk. The half-life for darbepoetin is more than twice that of epoetin α and epoetin β and allows less frequent dosing. Presently, studies using 2-, 3-, or 4-wk dosing intervals are ongoing.

3.2.4. QUALITY OF LIFE

Health-related QOL is a highly complex, multidimensional concept. The importance of these dimensions may vary between individuals. It is subjective— i.e., evaluated by the patient—and dynamic, i.e., it may change over time. Thus, it should be possible to use QOL instruments used in rhEPO trials to analyze patient-reported functional outcomes, as well as physical, emotional, and social parameters. Unfortunately, most investigators of rhEPO and its effect on QOL in cancer patients in general *(39,40)* and MM in particular *(28)* have analyzed only the functional aspects of QOL (e.g., the performance status) or made within-group comparisons; such methodological limitations may have seriously hampered the interpretation of data *(41)*. Despite this limitation, it is noteworthy that practically all published reports on rhEPO, anemia and QOL in cancer patients showed a positive relationship between rhEPO-induced correction of anemia and QOL-related parameters.

The Functional Assessment of Cancer Therapy Anemia scale (FACT-An) is a recently developed validated, sensible instrument that measures general QOL along with specific items that assess the impact of fatigue and other anemia-related symptoms on QOL *(42)*. In a phase IV study by Demetri and colleagues *(15)*, the QOL (FACT-An) benefit in cancer patients with anemia who respond to rhEPO was found to be independent of tumor response or tumor type. The most pronounced effects on QOL parameters were seen in patients who had the highest increment change in Hb concentration (>2 g/dL), irrespective of tumor response to concomitant chemotherapy (complete/partial remissions or stable disease). Although patients with progressive disease showed an overall decline in QOL, patients who responded to rhEPO experienced a stable QOL compared with the decline observed in rhEPO-resistant patients. This trial provides substantial evidence that there are quantifiable QOL benefits that can be derived from the use of rhEPO in anemic patients with various types of cancer, including MM.

Recent studies have carefully investigated the impact of treatment with erythropoietic agents on QOL in patients with cancer, including MM. The most comprehensive analysis of patients with MM, NHL, or CLL used the FACT-An questionnaire filled out blindly (with regard to current Hb concentration) and under strict, predefined conditions *(34)*. Scores in both groups had a tendency to rise, but with a significantly higher benefit in patients taking rhEPO. Notably, the effect on QOL became apparent only after 12 wk of therapy. The comparison of the gain in QOL between responders and nonresponders (independent on which group they were from) yielded a more pronounced and highly significant improvement in total FACT-An and most FACT-An subscales in the patients with a Hb response >2 g/dL, already after few weeks of treatment.

Hedenus and colleagues *(36)* used the Functional Assessment of Fatigue (FACT-F) subscale (13 items) in a similar patient population on either darbepoetin or placebo. Patients on darbepoetin showed a greater (but statistically not significant) improvement in their FACT-F score compared with placebo. Patients with the lowest QOL score at baseline reported the biggest gain at the end of treatment.

3.3. Adverse Effects

Most patients with myeloma-associated anemia tolerate rhEPO treatment well. Approximately 15% of patients complain about pain or a mild erythema at the injection site. Severe adverse effects, reported in the first studies of rhEPO therapy for chronic anemia associated with renal insufficiency, were not observed in patients with cancer-related anemia.

Recently, an increased risk of developing anti-EPO antibodies and the subsequent development of pure red cell aplasia (PRCA) was described for patients with chronic renal failure *(43)*. Most cases described so far have been attributable to the preparation of epoetin-α in non-US markets, and no cases have yet been reported in patients with myeloma.

3.4. Predictors of Response

Identification of prognostic factors would be valuable in clinical decision making regarding rhEPO therapy. Several models have been published that allow a prediction of response to rhEPO treatment in individual patients. All of them are based on two fundamental criteria, namely whether the endogenous EPO response to the anemic condition is blunted *(44)*, and whether first signs of therapeutic benefits can be detected during the early phase of rhEPO therapy. Recently, Österborg and colleagues *(31,34)* identified the bone marrow reserve as an additional important factor for predicting the outcome of erythropoietin treatment.

Cazzola and colleagues *(32)* proposed a predictive model based on the first criterion. Blunted EPO response is quantified using the O:P ratio, in which O stands for the observed serum EPO level and P for the hypothetical elevated EPO level that would be expected based on the degree of anemia detected in the patient. An O:P ratio of more than 0.9 can be used to predict a highly probable failure to respond to rhEPO treatment. A model of the second criterion, developed by Henry and colleagues, *(45)* evaluates increases in the patient's reticulocyte counts during the first few weeks of rhEPO therapy. A response to rhEPO therapy is considered very likely if the reticulocyte count increases by at least 40,000/µL after 2 wk of treatment (after 4 wk in patients receiving concomitant chemotherapy). This prediction can be further improved by combining it with the criterion of an increase in Hb level of at least 1 g/dL within the first 4 wk of rhEPO treatment.

The most precise prediction models involve two criteria. A substantial increase in the serum concentration of soluble transferrin receptor, for instance, indicates responsiveness to rhEPO treatment *(35)*. By combining this predictive factor with the patient's baseline EPO level, treatment response can be predicted with an accuracy of 88% *(46)*. Henry and Glaspy *(47)* combined the O:P ratio with the change in Hb level during the first 4 wk of treatment to achieve a predictive accuracy of 85%. Ludwig and colleagues *(48)* conducted a thorough analysis of possible predictive factors and found that an increase in Hb by more than 0.5 g/dL combined with a baseline EPO level below 100 mU/mL predicts a response to rhEPO therapy with an accuracy of more than 95%. If data on EPO levels are unavailable, the combination of early Hb increases with baseline serum ferritin levels below 400 ng/mL allows predictions of similarly high accuracy. More recent data confirm the validity of the two-criteria concept. Cazzola *(35)* identified early treatment induced increase in Hb (in weeks 1–3) as strongest predictor of response, followed by low baseline serum EPO levels. The latter finding is noteworthy, because only patients with endogenous EPO levels of less than 100 mU/mL have been enrolled in this trial. This shows even in patients with defective endogenous EPO production, an inverse correlation between serum EPO concentration and response to therapy. Österborg and colleagues *(34)* performed a multivariate Cox proportional hazard analysis to determine baseline parameters that predict transfusion-free survival during weeks 5 to 16. Only patients with inadequate endogenous serum EPO levels were enrolled. Baseline platelet counts of at least 100×10^9 and Hb levels of at least 9 g/dL as well as a lower pre-study transfusion requirement (2 units) were the factors most strongly associated with a low risk for rhEPO failure. Other parameters—such as type of underlying malignancy (e.g., MM, NHL, or CLL), performance status and QOL score—had no effect on the analysis. These findings are interesting because they underline the importance of the bone marrow reserve to treatment outcome and reflect the realities of clinical practice.

Although these predictive models may aid clinical decision-making, a short induction phase for rhEPO treatment will reveal the chance of response with great accuracy. Recent investigations were designed to determine whether increased rhEPO doses at the beginning therapy (the front-loading concept) will allow clinicians to obtain information about the outcome of rhEPO therapy and make a decision to continue or terminate treatment even earlier. Thus, costly, inefficient therapy may be avoided in patients with a very low likelihood of a response.

3.4.1. COST–BENEFIT RATIO FOR RHEPO

Considering the effectiveness and tolerability of rhEPO, it is obvious that the main obstacle to its use is cost (49). As discussed above, increasing knowledge of prognostic factors at baseline or after a short (2-wk) treatment period may result in a considerably better cost–benefit relationship. A further cost reduction may be achieved by the use of iron supplementation, which is mandatory to compensate rhEPO-induced iron deficiency. Intravenous iron supplementation has been found to reduce the weekly rhEPO requirement by 30 to 70% in patients with renal anemia (50) and is ongoing in hematology/oncology practice. In addition, individual titration of the lowest effective rhEPO maintenance dose (51) may further reduce the total rhEPO treatment cost.

ACKNOWLEDGMENT

This research is supported by the Wilhelminen Cancer Research Institute of the Austrian Forum Against Cancer.

REFERENCES

1. Kyle RA, Beard CM, O'Fallon WM, Kurland LT. Incidence of multiple myeloma in Olmsted County, Minnesota: 1978 through 1990, with a review of the trend since 1945. J Clin Oncol 1994; 12:1577–1583.
2. Medical Research Council's Working Party on Leukaemia in Adults. Prognostic features in the third MRC myelomatosis trial. Medical Research Council's Working Party on Leukaemia in Adults. Br J Cancer 1980; 42:831–840.
3. Ludwig H, Barrett-Lee P, Birgegård G, et al. The European Cancer Anaemia Survey (ECAS): The first large, multinational, prospective survey defining the prevalence, incidence, and treatment of anaemia in cancer patients. Eur J Cancer. Submitted for publication.
4. Musto P. The role of recombinant erythropoietin for the treatment of anemia in multiple myeloma. Leuk Lymphoma 1998; 29:283–291.
5. Beguin Y, Yerna M, Loo M, Weber M, Fillet G. Erythropoiesis in multiple myeloma: defective red cell production due to inappropriate erythropoietin production. Br J Haematol 1992; 82:648–653.
6. Balkwill F, Osborne R, Burke F, et al. Evidence for tumour necrosis factor/cachectin production in cancer. Lancet 1987; ii:1229–1232.
7. Denz H, Fuchs D, Huber H, et al. Correlation between neopterin, interferon-gamma and haemoglobin in patients with haematological disorders. Eur J Haematol 1990; 44:186–189.

8. Means RT. Pathogenesis of the anemia of chronic disease: a cytokine-mediated anemia. Stem Cells 1995; 13:32–37.

9. Means RT, Krantz SB. Inhibition of human erythroid colony-forming units by gamma interferon can be corrected by recombinant human erythropoietin. Blood 1991; 78:2564–2567.

10. Faquin WC, Schneider TJ, Goldberg MA. Effect of inflammatory cytokines on hypoxia-induced erythropoietin production. Blood 1992; 79:1987–1994.

11. Silvestris F, Tucci M, Quatraro C, Dammacco F. Recent advances in understanding the pathogenesis of anemia in multiple myeloma. Int J Hematol. 2003; 78:121–125.

12. Singh A, Eckardt KU, Zimmermann A, et al. Increased plasma viscosity as a reason for inappropriate erythropoietin formation. J Clin Invest 1993; 91:251–256.

13. Honda KI, Ishiko O, Yoshida H, Ogita S. Mouse erythroblast formation is inhibited by anemia-inducing substance from the plasma of a patient with a malignant neoplasm. Int J Mol Med. 2001 Sep; 8:257–260.

14. Maxwell MB. When the cancer patient becomes anemic. Cancer Nurs 1984; 7:321–326.

15. Demetri GD, Kris M, Wade J, Degos L, Cella D. Quality-of-life benefit in chemotherapy patients treated with epoetin alfa is independent of disease response or tumor type: results from a prospective community oncology study. J Clin Oncol 1998; 16:3412–3425.

16. Leitgeb C, Pecherstorfer M, Fritz E, Ludwig H. Quality of life in chronic anemia of cancer during treatment with recombinant human erythropoietin. Cancer 1994; 73:2535–2542.

17. Glaspy J. The impact of epoetin alfa on quality of life during cancer chemotherapy: A fresh look at an old problem. Semin Hematol 1997; 34 (3, suppl 2):20–26.

18. Ludwig H. Anemia of hematologic malignancies: what are the treatment options? Semin Oncol. 2002 Jun; 29 (3 Suppl 8):45–54.

19. George CD, Morella PJ. Immunologic effects of blood transfusion upon renal transplantation, tumor operations, and bacterial infections. Am. J. Surg 1986; 152:329–337.

20. Heiss MM, Mempel W, Jauch KW, et al. Beneficial effect of autologous blood transfusion on infectious complications after colorectal cancer surgery. Lancet 1993; 342:1328–1333.

21. Stockman JA. III. Anemia of prematurity. Current concepts in the issue of when to transfuse. Pediatr Clin North Am 1996; 33:111–128.

22. Varney SJ, Guest JF. The annual cost of blood transfusions in the UK. Transfus Med. 2003; 13:205–218.

23. Ludwig H, Fritz E, Kotzmann H, et al. Erythropoietin treatment of anemia associated with multiple myeloma. N Engl J Med 1990; 322:1693–1699.

24. Ludwig H, Leitgeb C, Fritz E, et al. Erythropoietin treatment of chronic anemia of cancer. Eur J Cancer 1993; 29A (suppl. 2):8–12.

25. Barlogie B, Beck T. Recombinant human erythropoietin and the anemia of multiple myeloma. Stem Cells 1993; 11:88–94.

26. Bessho M, Hirashima K, Tsuchiya J. Improvement of anemia in patients with multiple myeloma by recombinant erythropoietin: a multicenter study. Exp Hematol 1994; 22:705.

27. Musto P, Falcone A, D'Arena G, et al. Clinical results of recombinant erythropoietin in transfusion-dependent patients with refractory multiple myeloma; role of cytokines and monitoring of erythropoiesis. Eur J Haematol 1997; 58:314–319.

28. Mittelman M, Zeidman A, Fradin Z, et al. Recombinant human erythropoietin in the treatment multiple myeloma-associated anemia. Acta Hamaetol 1997; 98:204–210.

29. Garton JP, Gerz MA, Witzig TE. et al. Epoetin alfa for the treatment of the anemia of multiple myeloma. A prospective, randomized, placebo-controlled, double-blind trial. Arch Intern Med 1995; 155:2069–2074.

30. Silvestris F, Romito A, Fanelli P, et al. Long-term therapy with recombinant human erythropoietin (rHu-EPO) in progressing multiple myeloma. Ann Hematol 1995; 70:313–318.

31. Österborg A, Boogaerts M, Cimino R, et al. Recombinant human erythropoietin in transfusion-dependent anemic patients with multiple myeloma and non-Hodgkin's lymphoma: a randomized multicenter study. Blood 1996; 87: 2675–2682.

32. Cazzola M, Messinger D, Battistel V, et al. Recombinant human erythropoietin in the anemia associated with multiple myeloma or non-Hodgkin's lymphoma: dose finding and identification of predictors of response. Blood 1995; 86:4446–4453.

33. Dammacco F, Castoldi G, Rödjer S. Efficacy of epoetin alfa in the treatment of anaemia of multiple myeloma. Br J Haematol 2001; 113:172–179.

34. Österborg A, Brandberg Y, Molostova V, et al. Randomized, double-blind, placebo-controlled trial of recombinant human erythropoietin, epoetin beta, in hematologic malignancies. J Clin Oncol 2002; 20:2486–2494.

35. Cazzola M, Beguin Y, Kloczko J, Spicka I, Coiffier B. Once-weekly epoetin beta is highly effective in treating anaemic patients with lymphoproliferative malignancy and defective endogenous erythropoietin production. Br J Haematol. 2003; 122:386–393.

36. Hedenus M, Adriansson M, San Miguel J, et al, for the Darbepoetin Alfa 20000161 Study Group. Efficacy and safety of darbepoetin alfa in anaemic patients with lymphoproliferative malignancies: a randomized, double-blind, placebo-controlled study. Br J Haematol. 2003; 122:394–403.

37. Rizzo JD, Lichtin AE, Woolf SH, et al, for the American Society of Clinical Oncology; American Society of Hematology. Use of epoetin in patients with cancer: evidence-based clinical practice guidelines of the American Society of Clinical Oncology and the American Society of Hematology. Blood. 2002; 100:2303–2320.

38. Ludwig H, Rai K, Blade J, et al. Management of disease-related anemia in patients with multiple myeloma or chronic lymphocytic leukemia: epoetin treatment recommendations. Hematol J. 2002; 3:121–130.

39. Brandberg Y. Quality of life in clinical trials: assessment and utility with special reference to rHuEPO. Med Oncol 1998; 15(suppl. 1):8–12.

40. Thomas ML. Anemia and quality of life in cancer patients: impact of transfusion and erythropoietin. Med Oncol 1998; 15(suppl 1):13–18.

41. Bottomley A, Thomas R, van Steen V, Flechtner H, Djulbegovic B: Human recombinant erythropoietin and quality of life: a wonder drug or something to wonder about? Lancet Oncol 2002; 3:145–153.

42. Cella D. The functional assessment of cancer therapy-anemia (FACT-An) scale: a new tool for the assessment of outcomes in cancer anemia and fatigue. Semin Hematol 1997; 34(suppl. 2):13–19.

43. Casadevall N, Nataf J, Viron B, et al. Pure red cell aplasia and antierythropoietin antibodies in patients treated with recombinant erythropoietin. N Engl J Med 2002; 346:469–475.

44. Miller CB, Jones RJ, Piantadose S, Abeloff MD, Spivak JL. Decreased erythropoietin response in patients with the anemia of cancer. N Engl J Med 1990; 322:1689–1692.

45. Henry D, Abels R, Larholt K. Prediction of response to recombinant human erythropoietin (r-HuEPO/epoetin-alpha) therapy in cancer patients. Blood 1995; 85:1676–1678.

46. Cazzola M, Ponchio L, Pedrotti C, et al. Prediction of response to recombinant human erythropoietin (rHuEpo) in anemia of malignancy. Haematologica 1996; 81:434–441.

47. Henry D, Glaspy J. Predicting response to epoetin alfa in anemic cancer patients receiving chemotherapy. J Clin Oncol 1997; 16:49a.

48. Ludwig H, Fritz E, Leitgeb C, Pecherstorfer M, Samonigg H, Schuster J. Prediction of response to erythropoietin treatment in chronic anemia of cancer. Blood 1994; 84:1056–1063.

49. Sheffield RE, Sullivan SD, Saltiel E, Nishimura L. Cost comparison of recombinant human erythropoietin and blood transfusion in cancer chemotherapy-induced anemia. Ann Pharmacother 1997; 31:15–22.

50. Sunder-Plassmann G, Hörl WH. Importance of iron supply for erythropoietin therapy. Nephrol Dial Transplant 1995; 10:2070–2076.

51. Österborg A. Recombinant human erythropoietin (rHuEPO) therapy in patients with cancer-related anaemia: what have we learned? Med Oncol 1998; 15(suppl 1):47–49.

16 New Therapeutic Approaches to Myeloma

Terry H. Landowski, PhD,
William S. Dalton, PhD, MD,
and Sydney E. Salmon, MD

CONTENTS

INTRODUCTION
OVERCOMING DRUG RESISTANCE
NEW AGENTS
NEW TARGETS
THE TUMOR MICROENVIRONMENT AS A TARGET FOR
    NOVEL THERAPY
ESSENTIALS FOR DEVELOPING NEW THERAPEUTIC APPROACHES
REFERENCES

1. INTRODUCTION

Effective treatment for myeloma began in the early 1960s with the introduction of melphalan and cyclophosphamide *(1)*. During the past four decades, clinicians have found that the most effective drugs for the treatment of myeloma belong to the following pharmacologic classes: alkylating agents (melphalan, cyclophosphamide, 1,3-bis-[2-chloroethyl]-1-nitrosurea [BCNU]), topoisomerase II inhibitors (doxorubicin and etoposide), glucocorticoids (prednisone and dexamethasone) and the antitubulin agent, vincristine. With the exception of the glucocorticoids, most of these agents are relatively ineffective as monotherapy and need to be combined with other drugs. The combination of oral melphalan and prednisone is considered the mainstay of myeloma therapy, producing responses in approx 50 to 60% of patients, compared with 30% in patients who receive melphalan alone. Since the introduction of melphalan–prednisone (MP) combination therapy, a

From: *Current Clinical Oncology: Biology and Management of Multiple Myeloma*
Edited by: J. R. Berenson © Humana Press Inc., Totowa, NJ

number of cytotoxic drug combinations have been investigated. A popular example is the M2 protocol, consisting of vincristine, carmustine, melphalan, cyclophosphamide, and prednisone (VBMCP) *(2)*.

Although a higher percentage of patients responds to combination chemotherapy, the improvement in overall survival is marginal and appears to occur chiefly in patients with a poor prognosis *(3)*. Similar observations have been made for vincristine + melphalan + cyclophosphamide + prednisone (VMCP) alternating with vincristine + carmustine + doxorubicin [Adriamycin] + prednisone (VBAP) *(4)*. Generally speaking, MP appears to be effective as combination chemotherapy in patients who are elderly or patients who have good prognosis, but inferior in patients with a poor prognosis. Because melphalan has variable oral bioavailability, it is important to induce some myelosuppression in the patient when melphalan is used to be sure that the dose being given is adequate.

Essentially, all patients who respond to combination chemotherapy will eventually relapse, developing drug-resistant disease *(5)*. The combination of vincristine + doxorubicin [Adriamycin] + dexamethasone (VAD) produces responses in 60 to 70% of patients who develop resistance to alkylating agents; unfortunately, these patients will ultimately also develop drug resistance *(6)*.

Substantial progress has been made in the last decade to identify cellular mechanisms that confer clinical drug resistance. Research has chiefly focused on mechanisms that reduce the intracellular concentration of drugs. Recent evidence has shown that clinical drug resistance is multifactorial, however; therefore, overcoming a single mechanism of drug resistance is not likely to result in long-standing remission *(7)*. In all probability, substantial progress in the treatment of myeloma will require new therapeutic approaches to this disease.

Today, at least three different approaches to improving the therapeutic outcome for patients with myeloma are being investigated: (1) enhancing the efficacy of currently available drugs by identifying and overcoming drug-resistance mechanisms, (2) identifying new cellular targets that regulate cell survival and growth, and (3) developing a means of enhancing the host immune response against myeloma cells. This chapter focuses on the development of small molecules that can target unique cellular structures or pathways to improve the therapeutic outcome for patients with myeloma. It will begin with a discussion of several means of improving the efficacy of currently available drugs by addressing the issue of drug resistance, the two major approaches being high-dose chemotherapy with stem cell rescue and combination therapy using chemosensitizers with chemotherapy to block individual mechanisms of cellular resistance. Because Chapter 12 covers high-dose chemotherapy and stem cell rescue in depth, this chapter will focus primarily on the use of combination therapy to overcome individual mechanisms of drug resistance.

Identifying new cellular targets or pathways that regulate myeloma cell growth and survival is another approach that in the long run may be more rewarding. Developing small molecules that inhibit or interrupt pathways should allow us to target myeloma cells and spare normal cells. These pathways may be intrinsic to the myeloma cell itself, such as signal transduction pathways altered by mutations, or they may involve communication between the bone marrow microenvironment and the myeloma cell. We know, for example, that the primary source of interleukin (IL)-6 is the bone marrow stroma and not the myeloma cell itself *(8)*. Inhibiting IL-6 production, binding to myeloma cells, or downstream signaling may block myeloma cell proliferation and result in apoptosis. We also know that myeloma cells express cell adhesion molecules that allow attachment and communication between myeloma cells and the bone marrow microenvironment; interrupting this cellular adhesion may induce apoptosis and enhance the efficacy of standard treatments *(9)*. In addition, it has recently been reported that myeloma cell growth and dissemination may depend on angiogenesis *(10,11)*, which may be regulated by interactions between the microenvironment and the myeloma cells and, as a result, stimulate myeloma growth and progression. Blocking these interactions may represent a new approach for treating myeloma.

Finally, stimulating the immune system to recognize and eliminate myeloma cells is an attractive approach to the treatment of myeloma. Mellstedt, Bendani, Österborg, and Kwak present this approach in depth in Chapter 14. Theoretically, this treatment should be more tumor-specific and result in less morbidity compared with chemotherapy. Recently, however, evidence has been reported that drugs used in the treatment of myeloma, including cytotoxic drugs and glucocorticoids, may mediate their anti-myeloma activity by using programmed cell death pathways that are normally associated with immune-mediated cell death *(12)*. Specifically, drugs may induce apoptosis in tumor cells by activating programmed cell death pathways, including components of the fas/fas ligand pathway *(13)*. If cytotoxic drugs and effectors of the immune system share programmed cell death pathways to eliminate myeloma cells, it is possible that drug resistance may also confer resistance to immune effectors of apoptosis, thereby potentially reducing the efficacy of the immune therapies proposed for myeloma *(14)*. Preclinical studies have been performed to address this question and will be reviewed in this chapter.

2. OVERCOMING DRUG RESISTANCE

A great deal of attention has been devoted to elucidating the mechanisms responsible for drug resistance that develop during the treatment of myeloma *(14a)*. Once they are identified, the ultimate goal will be to reverse their activity or prevent their activation in myeloma cells. Because most of the agents used in the treatment of myeloma are alkylating agents (including melphalan, cyclophosphamide, and carmustine), topoisomerase inhibitors (doxorubicin and etoposide), or glucocorticoids (prednisone and dexamethasone), research efforts have been focused on cellular mechanisms that confer resistance to these agents.

Melphalan is the primary alkylating agent used in myeloma. Cellular mechanisms associated with resistance to melphalan include decreased intracellular uptake, DNA damage repair, and enhanced detoxification *(5)*. Melphalan is a bifunctional nitrogen mustard derivative of the amino acid L-phenylalanine that forms inter- or intrastrand crosslinks, as well as DNA–protein crosslinks by alkylation via its two chloroethyl groups. Intracellular uptake of melphalan utilizes the L-type amino acid transporter. Resistance to melphalan has been reported to correlate with reduced expression or activity of the L-phenylalanine transporter CD98 in freshly purified myeloma cells and in a mutant myeloma cell line that once displayed resistance to melphalan *(15)*. Investigations into the mechanism of substrate recognition and transport may reveal characteristics that allow investigators to develop strategies that can be used to enhance drug uptake. Such strategies may also affect the permeability of the blood–brain barrier, however, thereby increasing the systemic toxicity of the drug.

Enhanced repair of DNA damage has also been identified as a mechanism of resistance to melphalan *(16)*. In a study comparing interstrand cross-link formation and repair in plasma cells obtained from patients who relapsed following a melphalan-conditioned autograft vs patients who had never been exposed to melphalan, investigators found that myeloma cells from previously treated patients had a higher intrinisic interstrand crosslink repair rate *(17)*. However, the specific mechanism of DNA repair was not fully defined.

The most common mechanism associated with melphalan resistance involves enhanced drug detoxification using the glutathione/glutathione-*S*-transferase (GSH/GST) system. Glutathione is an intracellular antioxidant that is essential for the formation of GSH-S conjugates, which are catalyzed by GST. Glutathione levels are increased in melphalan-resistant myeloma cells *(18)*. Melphalan resistance was reversed in this cell line by using the agent buthionine sulfoximine (BSO) to reduce intracellular pools of glutathione. The prevailing presumption is that GST catalyzes the formation of GSH–melphalan conjugates that are inactive in alkylating DNA and are more efficiently exported from the cell. However, GSH plays a central role in reduction-oxidation (redox) activity in the cell; thus, additional cellular processes are probably influenced by intracellular GSH. BSO might be useful for overcoming this form of drug resistance, although its effects are probably not specific to myeloma cells, and its toxic effects on normal tissue— including the liver, kidney, and bone marrow—may prevent its use in clinical settings.

Carmustine (BCNU) is a nitrosourea that is commonly used in myeloma. A major documented form of resistance to this drug is seen with the repair of O-6-methylguanine, which is formed by BCNU *(19)*. Methylguanine DNA methyl-

Table 1
Chemotherapeutic Drugs Exhibiting
Cross-Resistance in Multidrug Resistance

Doxorubicin	Taxol
Daunorubicin	Trimetrexate
Vincristine	Mitomycin C
Vinblastine	Dactinomycin
Etoposide	Mitoxantrone
Dexamethasone	

transferase (MGMT) is responsible for catalyzing this repair. Cells that are relatively resistant to BCNU have elevated levels of MGMT (19). One strategy for improving the response to BCNU is to deplete the cell of MGMT using agents such as streptozocin or O-6-benzylguanine prior to administering BCNU. Recently completed phase I studies of these agents in combination with BCNU have provided toxicity data that suggest that phase II trials of O-6-benzylguanine may be appropriate in patients with tumors that are refractory to alkylating agents (20).

Multidrug resistance (MDR) describes cross-resistance among numerous anti-cancer drugs, especially natural products (including vincristine, doxorubicin, and etoposide), as well as glucocorticoids (e.g., dexamethasone) (21). Clinically, this phenomenon is characterized by an initial response to cytotoxic drugs, eventually followed by a relapse characterized by the presence of tumors that are frequently resistant not only to the drug initially used, but to a variety of structurally and functionally unrelated chemotherapeutic agents as well (Table 1). Overexpression of P-glycoprotein (P-gp) has been identified as a major mechanism in MDR. P-gp is an adenosine 5'-triphosphate (ATP)-dependent efflux pump that actively transports cytotoxic agents out of the cell, resulting in reduced intracellular accumulation of the drug (22,23). More recent studies have demonstrated that P-gp may also be expressed on the surface of intracellular vesicles with an "inside-out" orientation (24) that allows substances in the cytosol to be transported into the intravesicular space. As a result, drugs become sequestered and unable to reach their intracellular targets. Generally, higher levels of P-gp expression correlate directly with cellular drug resistance. Therefore, agents that block P-gp allow the intracellular concentration of cytotoxic drugs to increase. These agents, known as "chemosensitizers," (7) have no anti-cancer activity, but can potentiate anti-cancer drug the activity in cells that overexpress P-gp.

During the past decade, chemosensitizing agents have been studied in clinical settings for their ability to reverse P-gp-mediated MDR (Table 2). Initial studies using the calcium channel-blocking agents verapamil and cyclosporine A as chemosensitizers showed some promise in eliminating P-gp-positive myeloma cells, (25,26) but the quality and duration of the responses were modest and

Table 2
Chemosensitizers Known to
Modulate P-Glycoprotein Function

Chemical Class	Example
Calcium channel blockers	Verapamil
Calmodulin inhibitors	Trifluoperazine
Indole alkaloids	Reserpine
Lysosomotropic agents	chloroquine
Steroids	Progesterone
Triparanol analogs	Tamoxifen
Detergents	Cremophor EL
Cyclic peptide antibiotics	Cyclosporines

cardiotoxicity was dose-limiting. Similarly, a large randomized trial adding oral quinine to a VAD-like regimen showed no efficacy in a randomized Southwest Oncology Group study as initial treatment for patients with MM *(26a)*. It was concluded that more effective and less toxic chemosensitizers are needed to reverse MDR in myeloma. Second-generation P-gp modulators include valspodar (PSC 833), a cyclosporine derivative that has shown 10 to 20 times the activity in reversing MDR than had been seen with cyclosporine *A (26)*. Although phase I/II trials demonstrated that P-gp inhibition could be achieved at clinically tolerable doses, patient responses in phase III trials have been largely disappointing, owing perhaps to cross-reactivity between valspodar and the P450 isoenzyme 3A4 that resulted in unpredictable pharmacokinetic interactions and made it difficult to determine a safe and effective dose for the chemotherapeutic agent *(27)*. Third-generation P-gp inhibitors have been developed that recognize the ATP hydrolysis domain of the molecule, rather than the substrate-binding domain *(28)*. One of the most promising third-generation P-gp inhibitors is the anthanilamide derivative XR9576/tariquidar, which binds P-gp with high affinity and inhibits the ATPase activity required for transport. XR9576/tarquidar is not a substrate; thus, standard doses of cytotoxic drugs do not have to be reduced when it is used. Phase I clinical trials demonstrate that this agent is well tolerated in healthy volunteers and highly effective at inhibiting P-gp-mediated transport at clinically achievable levels *(29)*.

Although P-gp is considered the prototype drug-resistant protein responsible for MDR, recent evidence suggests that other proteins may confer a similar phenotype. P-gp is a member of the ATP-binding-cassette (ABC) transport family of proteins. ABC transport proteins are characterized by two conserved halves, each containing six highly hydrophobic regions that are characteristic of transmembrane segments and a large hydrophilic domain containing a classical con-

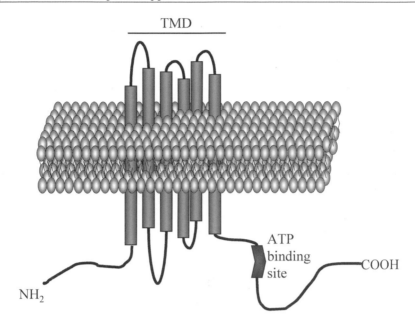

Fig. 1. Prototypical structure of the adenosine 5'-triphosphate (ATP)-binding-cassette (ABC) transport family of proteins. The simplest of the transport family members, BCRP is composed of one ABC. P-glycoprotein and MRP4 and MRP5 contain two identical units of six transmembrane domains and one ATP-binding site each, whereas the atypical MRPs 1, 2, 3, and 6 contain three transmembrane units and two ATP binding sites.

sensus sequence for nucleotide binding (Fig. 1). These proteins are highly conserved throughout evolution and have been shown to transport a wide variety of substrates *(21)*. They generally require ATP to remove the drug from the cell. Two candidate ABC proteins that may confer clinical drug resistance include the *m*ultidrug *r*esistance-associated *p*rotein (MRP) and the *b*reast *c*ancer *r*esistance *p*rotein (BCRP) *(30,31)*. Investigators studying myeloma patients report low levels of MRP in myeloma cells; thus, this protein probably does not play a significant role in conferring drug resistance in patients with myeloma *(32)*. The BCRP protein is apparently expressed in myeloma cell lines that are resistant to doxorubicin and mitoxantrone; future studies are needed to determine if this protein is expressed in patients with drug resistance *(33,34)*. If it is expressed in myeloma cells, it may be important to develop agents that inhibit its function, because P-gp inhibitors do not affect the function of BCRP *(31,34)*. Another protein that may alter drug distribution and result in an MDR phenotype is the major vault protein (also known as LRP) *(35)*. In two recent studies, investigators found that myeloma patients who overexpress this protein may have a drug-resistant phenotype that includes resistance to melphalan *(36,37)*. Chemosensitizing agents that reverse P-gp activity are ineffective against LRP-associated resistance. A combination of chemosensitizing agents may be necessary to prevent or overcome transport-mediated drug resistance in myeloma.

The cause of clinical drug resistance in myeloma is probably multifactorial; the use of chemosensitizers to eliminate MDR1/P-gp-mediated drug resistance may be beneficial, but could potentially result in selection for non-P-gp-mediated mechanisms of resistance. This possibility has been investigated in human myeloma cell lines *(38)* using the chemosensitizer verapamil to co-select for doxorubicin resistance. Investigators found that MDR1 expression was prevented and a non-P-gp mechanism accounted for the acquired drug resistance. Resistance in this selected cell line was limited to topoisomerase II inhibitors; cells remained sensitive to other natural agents, including vincristine. Not surprisingly, the non-P-gp mechanism was determined to be a decrease in topoisomerase II expression and activity. It was concluded that the use of chemosensitizers early in the course of disease to prevent MDR1/P-gp expression might be more effective than using them later in the course of disease to reverse P-gp-mediated drug resistance.

3. NEW AGENTS

As mentioned in the introduction, the vast majority of drugs used in the treatment of myeloma today are alkylating agents, topoisomerase II inhibitors, glucocorticoids, or tubulin inhibitors. New agents with different mechanisms of activity are now being studied and have either entered phase I/II clinical trials or have shown promise in preclinical studies. These agents may target the myeloma cell itself or the tumor bone marrow microenvironment. These new agents may also act synergistically with currently available drugs used for myeloma.

3.1. Topoisomerase I Inhibitors

Topoisomerase I and II govern the topological state of DNA and, thus, effect DNA replication and RNA transcription *(39)*. They transiently introduce either single-strand (topoisomerase I) or double-strand (topoisomerase II) DNA breaks. Drugs that stabilize the transient covalent DNA–protein complexes (also known as "cleavable complexes") are thought to interfere with DNA replication and transcription, which ultimately leads to apoptosis. Topoisomerase II inhibitors include the anti-myeloma drugs doxorubicin and etoposide. Although these agents are considered to be active in the treatment of myeloma (especially doxorubicin), resistance eventually develops. P-gp may mediate this type of resistance; other mechanisms include reduced topoisomerase II levels and activity *(39)*. In a recent Southwest Oncology Group study, investigators found that the topoisomerase I agent topotecan has moderate activity in patients with myeloma who develop resistance or experience a relapse *(40,41)*. The overall response rate was 16%, and the median progression-free survival was 13 mo. These results are encouraging enough to pursue further studies of topotecan in combination with other drugs. One possible combination to consider is that of topotecan with an alkylating agent (e.g., melphalan or cyclophosphamide), because topoisomerase I inhibitors may inhibit the repair of DNA damage induced by alkylating agents.

3.2. Arsenic Trioxide

Arsenic has been used as a therapeutic agent and a poison for more than 2400 yr, as far back as the ancient Roman and Greek empires, where it was used to treat a wide spectrum of ailments, ranging from ulcers to convulsions. One of the earliest anti-cancer formulations was a 1% solution of arsenic trioxide (ATO) in potassium bicarbonate, known as Fowler's solution. First described in 1878, Fowler's solution was used to treat leukemia until the advent of radiation therapy in the early 1900s. Concerns about its toxicity and reports of chronic arsenic poisoning led to its general discontinuance in cancer therapy until the late 1990s, when ATO was reported to be highly effective for inducing remission in patients with acute promyelocytic leukemia (42). Recent reports of studies in myeloma cell lines and myeloma cells from patients indicate that ATO is capable of inducing apoptosis at concentrations that can be achieved clinically (43,43a). Zhang and colleagues reported that in the myeloma cell line NOP-1, proliferation and viability were inhibited at an ATO concentration of 1 µM (44). Furthermore, Chen and colleagues reported that ATO induced apoptosis in the myeloma cell lines RPMI 8226 and U266 by activating caspase-3 and possibly by inducing mitochondrial transmembrane collapse (45). ATO also inhibits IK kinase, preventing degradation of IKB ultimately inhibiting NF-KB DNA-binding activity (43a). ATO appears to directly perturb mitochondrial function by several mechanisms that involve the generation of reactive oxygen species (ROS) and the inhibition of the cellular redox system (46). This combined activity induces oxidative stress and leads to mitochondrial-dependent apoptosis. Reduction of the intracellular defense system against oxidative stress would effectively lower the threshold and enhance drug activity. Indeed, two independent groups reported that depletion of GSH by BSO or ascorbic acid enhanced ATO activity in myeloma cell lines through a wide variety of drug-resistance mechanisms (46,47). Furthermore, in a limited phase I/II clinical trial, Bahlis and colleagues demonstrated that coadministration of ascorbic acid and ATO was clinically tolerable and resulted in a partial response in one-third of the patients and stable disease in two-thirds of the patients in the study ($N = 6$) (48). All six patients in this study had stage IIIA myeloma, which suggests that ATO, with modulation of cellular redox status, has therapeutic potential in patients with relapsed or refractory myeloma.

ATO has been evaluated in three recent clinical trials as a single agent (48a). Munshi and colleagues treated 14 patients with relapsing myeloma with 0.15 mg/kg daily for 60 d. Three patients showed a reduction in paraprotein levels of more than 25%. A multicenter trial used 0.25 mg/kg ATO daily × 5 for 2 wk, followed by a 2-wk rest *(48b)*. Eight of 24 (33%) patients showed paraprotein reductions of at least 25%. Recently, the schedule was changed to twice weekly with 3 out of 13 evaluable patients showing a response *(48c)*.

Because ATO inhibits NF-KB activity and this transcription factor's DNA binding is associated with drug resistance *(48d,48e)*, a recent study evaluated a combination of low-dose melphalan (0.1 mg/kg) orally for 4 d, 0.25 mg/kg ATO twice weekly, followed by 1 g intravenous ascorbic acid in 10 heavily pretreated relapsing multiple myeloma (MM) patients, including 5 with renal dysfunction. All 10 patients showed significant decreases in M-protein levels and marked sustained improvement in renal dysfunction in all 5 azotemic patients. Based on these promising results, a large multicenter trial is currently evaluating this regimen. In addition, ATO is also being evaluated with steroids and Velcade.

3.3. Imexon

Imexon is a cyanoaziridine molecule that was initially developed in Europe as a "cancer immunomodulator" during the late 1970s. The trials were incomplete, but showed that imexon was well tolerated in cancer patients at cumulative doses of up to 1.2 g. Although a few objective responses were observed in the phase I study, corporate interest in immunomodulation declined and the drug was abandoned without being advanced to phase II trials *(49)*. More recently, investigators demonstrated that imexon had selective toxicity in B-cell neoplasms, including human MM, in preclinical in vitro and in vivo systems in severe combined immunodeficiency (SCID) mice. Among 10 human tumor types examined in the human tumor cloning assay, myeloma was the most sensitive cell type, with an IC_{50} of 0.2 μg/mL *(50)*. Imexon is nonmyelosuppressive in all species studied to date, including humans, dogs, and rodents; however the formal maximum tolerated dose (MTD) and dose-limiting toxicities for this agent have not yet been established. Its unique structure suggests it may function as an alkylating agent, although preclinical investigations have demonstrated that it does not directly lead to DNA alkylation. Rather, it appears to interact with the sulfur moieties on physiologic thiols, such as cysteine and glutathione, which leads to the depletion of reduced thiols, the inhibition of sulfhydryl-dependent enzymes, and a net change in the cellular oxidation state. As a result, reactive oxygen species accumulate in the cytoplasm, particularly in the mitochondria, which leads to a reduction in the mitochondrial membrane potential *(51,52)*. Myeloma cells selected because of their resistance to imexon demonstrate partial cross-resistance to ATO, which further supports the hypothesis that these drugs may have a similar mechanism of action. Their intracellular targets do not appear to be identical, however. Accelerated phase I/II clinical trials of imexon have been initiated in a number of advanced tumors, including myeloma *(53)*.

3.4. Paclitaxel

The taxanes are antitubulin agents that were recently found to have a broad spectrum of antitumor activity in human cancers, including ovarian, breast, and lung cancer. The Eastern Cooperative Oncology Group treated 18 previously untreated patients with four cycles of paclitaxel 250 mg/m^2 by a continuous intravenous infusion for 24 h every 21 d *(54)*. All patients received granulocyte colony-stimulating factor (G-CSF) daily at standard doses until the neutrophil count reached 10,000/mm^3. Four of the 14 eligible patients (29%) did not have a complete response and 3 died of toxicity (sepsis was identified in 2 of these patients). The median survival was 2.8 yr, which was quite consistent with historical data for MP. An additional study conducted at M.D. Anderson using a lower dose of paclitaxel yielded less severe toxic effects but an objective response rate of only 15% *(55)*. In summary, paclitaxel has some activity in myeloma and may be useful in combination chemotherapy. Other taxanes such as docetaxel might also be evaluated.

3.5. Hexamethylene Bisacetamide

Hexamethylene bisacetamide (HMBA) is a hybrid polar compound reported to be effective in patients with myeloid leukemia and myelodysplastic syndrome *(56)*. Its mechanism of action is generally believed to involve the terminal differentiation of tumor cells, although Siegel and colleagues recently reported that HMBA induced apoptosis in myeloma cell lines, as well as freshly isolated human myeloma cells *(57)*. Its effect was associated with down-regulation of the anti-apoptotic protein bcl-2. HMBA activity was also observed in human myeloma cell lines that had been selected for their resistance to doxorubicin and overexpression of P-gp (8226/Dox). A more recent report showed that HMBA-mediated differentiation was associated with the induction of the cyclin-dependent kinase inhibitor p27 *(58)*. Inhibition of p27 by antisense oligonucleotides in combination with reduction of bcl-2 led to massive apoptosis; this suggests that the combination of HMBA with bcl-2 antisense, cell-cycle inhibitors, or both may prove useful in the treatment of patients with myeloma.

3.6. Bisphosphonates

Bisphosphonates are simple chemical compounds that have a phosphorous-carbon-phosphorous backbone with specific side chains attached to the central carbon moiety. First-generation bisphosphonates have simple hydroxyl (Etidronate) or chloride (Clodronate) side chains; second-generation bisphosphonates (pamidronate, ibandronate, and zoledronic acid) have an additional nitrogen-containing aliphatic side chain. Zoledronic acid was approved by the US Food and Drug Administration (FDA) on February 22, 2002, in conjunction with standard antineoplastic therapy for patients with MM and documented bone metastases from solid tumors. The recommended dosing schedule is 4 mg infused over 15 min every 3 to 4 wk. Renal toxicity, which also occurs with pamidronate treatment with a similar frequency, was the only serious adverse effect observed during zoledronic acid therapy, with toxicity related to dose, infusion duration, and the total number of infusions (59).

Recent clinical trials have shown that other bisphosphonates, primarily pamidronate (Aredia), can protect patients from complications resulting from osteolytic bone lesions (60). Furthermore, in a double-blind randomized trial, pamidronate was associated with prolonged survival in a patient subgroup being treated with salvage chemotherapy (60). The reason for this prolonged survival is unknown, although it is possible that pamidronate has a direct anti-tumor effect or may accentuate the activity of chemotherapy. Aparicio and associates performed in vitro studies in myeloma cell lines and found that bisphosphonates (specifically, zoledronic acid and pamidronate) exerted a direct antitumor effect by inducing apoptosis in some cell lines (61). The apoptotic effect of bisphosphonates could be blocked by forced expression of bcl-2. In another report of a study of the direct effects of bisphosphonates on myeloma cells, Shipman and colleagues found that incadronate (YM175) caused apoptosis in human myeloma cells by inhibiting the mevalonate pathway (62). This pathway is essential for the biosynthesis of sterols and long-chain isoprenoid lipids, including farnesyl PPi and geranylgeranyl PPi. These two compounds serve as substrates for farnesyltransferase and geranylgeranyl transferase, respectively, and are transferred to small guanosine 5'-triphosphate-binding proteins, such as ras. Inhibition of the isoprenylation of these critical proteins may induce apoptosis in myeloma cells.

It is also possible that bisphosphonates act indirectly to inhibit myeloma cell growth. For example, they reduce IL-6 production or release from bone marrow stromal cells, or both (63). Another possibility may involve the antiadhesive effect of bisphosphonates. Several investigators have shown that bisphosphonates prevent the adhesion of tumor cells to bone marrow matrices (64). They selectively concentrate at the interface of the active osteoclast and the bone resorption surface, where they have been shown to inhibit osteoclast activity. Inhibition of the interaction of tumor cells with components of the bone marrow microenvironment may block the signal transduction pathway that is initiated by the receptor activator NF-KB (RANK)/RANK ligand (RANKL) system of osteoclastogenesis. In normal bone, homeostasis is maintained by the bone resorbing effects of RANK/RANKL and is antagonized by the soluble decoy receptor osteoprotegerin (OPG). Recent evidence indicates that RANKL is highly expressed on the surface of bone marrow plasma cells and that the level of expression correlates with formation of osteolytic bone lesions in myeloma patients (65). Bisphosphonates have been shown to reduce osteoclast activity in mouse models of myeloma (66). It is possible that the bisphosphonates inhibit

RANK/RANKL osteoclastogenesis either by physically interrupting the receptor/ligand interaction or by inhibiting an intracellular signal transduction pathway initiated by this interaction.

3.7. Tamoxifen

It has been reported that myeloma cells often express estrogen receptors *(67)*. Treon and colleagues recently studied the effects of anti-estrogens on myeloma cell lines and patient-derived specimens *(68)*. They found that tamoxifen (and other anti-estrogens) inhibit proliferation in all myeloma cell lines studied, in addition to myeloma cells from two patients. Tamoxifen was also capable of inducing apoptosis that could not be blocked by exogenous estrogen or IL-6. Importantly, tamoxifen-induced apoptosis occurred at physiologically achievable concentrations and did not affect normal hematopoietic progenitor cells. More recently, the estrogen metabolite 2-methoxyestradiol (2-ME2) has been shown to induce low levels of apoptosis in myeloma cell lines and freshly isolated plasma cells obtained from patients with myeloma *(69)*. Perhaps more significant, however, is the observation that 2-ME2 appears to prevent tumor cell engraftment in a SCID mouse model. This suggests that it may have anti-angiogenic activity as well, perhaps mediated by interference with IL-6-mediated interactions of myeloma tumor cells and the bone marrow stroma *(69–71)*. Using IL-6-dependent cell lines, Wang and coworkers demonstrated that steroid-activated estrogen receptor blocks the IL-6 signal transduction pathway by inhibiting the transcription of STAT3 *(72,73)*. Together, these studies suggest that estrogens and anti-estrogens may comprise a novel therapeutic strategy for myeloma.

3.8. 8-Chloro-cyclic Adenosine-3′,5′-Diphosphate

Work by Halgren and colleagues has shown that 8-chloro adenosine diphosphate (8Cl-AD), is the active metabolite of 8Cl-cAMP *(74)*. Although the exact mode of action for this agent is unknown, its ability to kill steroid-sensitive and steroid-insensitive myeloma cells in the absence of IL makes this compound attractive for future myeloma therapy *(74)*. Additionally, recent studies from the same investigators showed that 8Cl-AD was equally effective against doxorubicin- and melphalan-resistant myeloma cells *(75)*. Clinical studies pursuing 8Cl-AD as a novel therapeutic approach to myeloma should be considered.

4. NEW TARGETS

The emergence of molecular genetics has provided an opportunity to systematically identify novel therapeutic targets within the myeloma cell itself or within the tumor cell environment. Agents that activate these targets or disrupt key signaling pathways required for myeloma cell survival may comprise a new therapeutic approach to myeloma.

4.1. Farnesyltransferase Inhibitors

Mutations of the *ras* gene are among the most commonly identified transforming events in multiple myeloma. Examination of myeloma patient tumor cells for oncogenic *ras* mutations has revealed activating mutations in 30 to 47% of either K- or N-*ras (76–78)*. More importantly, the incidence of *ras* mutations suggested a direct correlation among a number of critical clinical parameters. Median survival of patients with a K-ras mutation was approx 2 yr, compared with 3.7 yr for patients without K-*ras* mutations. Based on these observations, agents that inhibit *ras* activity have been proposed as molecular therapeutic agents for myeloma. The enzyme farnesyltransferase is responsible for transferring the farnesyl group from farnesyl diphosphate (a cellular chemical used in the synthesis of cholesterol) to certain proteins such as ras. This process, called prenylation of proteins, facilitates *ras* activation by allowing it to attach to the inner plasma cell membrane *(79)*. Preventing *ras* from going to the plasma membrane by blocking its farnesylation short circuits oncogenic growth signals to the nucleus. Inhibition of the farnesylation process is a prime target for drugs aimed at preventing ras activity. Recently, several drugs known as farnesyl transferase inhibitors (FTIs) were created to block protein farnesylation *(80)*. Preclinical studies have shown FTIs to be effective in myeloma cell lines with *ras* mutations *(81,82)*.

In phase I clinical trials of FTI monotherapy, plasma FTI concentrations that could inhibit FTase activity were achieved by both oral and intravenous administration. Alsina and associates reported phase II clinical findings from a study of FTI (R11577/Zarnestra) in heavily pretreated patients with myeloma that indicated disease stabilization (defined by less than 25% reduction in monoclonal proteins) in 50% of patients *(83)*. Treatment with R115777 suppressed FTase, but not GGTase I activity in bone marrow and peripheral blood mononuclear cells in patients with MM. Similarly, R115777 inhibited prenylation of the exclusively farnesylated protein HDJ-2 in all patients. Similarly, Cortes and colleagues reported a response in only 1 of 10 patients with relapsed or refractory myeloma *(84)*. However, the 600-mg twice-daily dosing schedule utilized in their study allowed a median treatment period of only 7 wk before it had to be interrupted because of toxicity. Alsina and associates initiated treatment with 300 mg twice daily for 3 wk and repeated this protocol every 4 wk. At the time of publication, four of six responding patients had completed four cycles of therapy without significant toxicity.

Preclinical studies have demonstrated the greatest inhibition of growth in myeloma tumor cells with N-*ras* mutations, whereas clinical studies in myeloma and other malignancies have shown no correlation between *ras* mutation status and response to FTIs *(85)*. These studies suggest that the ras protein may not be the primary target of these agents in vivo. Many laboratories are actively attempting to define the molecular activity of FTIs. Other proposed farnesylated targets include the ras-related family of rho proteins, particularly rhoB, and the mitotic spindle segregation proteins CENP-E and CENP-F, although these targets have not been validated in all cell types *(86,87)*. More importantly, in studies using myeloma cells that have acquired mechanisms of resistance to standard chemotherapeutic drugs, investigators have demonstrated that FTIs are equally active in drug-sensitive and drug-resistant cells. This finding supports the use of these agents in refractory disease either as monotherapy or in combination therapy and suggest further that myeloma patients may benefit from prolonged treatment at lower doses. However, additional studies are needed to identify the optimum scheduling for FTI efficacy in myeloma.

Recent studies suggest that the major target in the mevalonic acid biosynethesis pathway for inducing an anti-MM effect may not be farnesylated compounds. Although inhibition of myeloma growth and of apoptosis can be induced by inhibitors of this pathway (statins or bisphosphonates) *(87a–87c)*, these effects can be reversed by geranylgeranylated derivatives but not farnesylated ones *(87b,87c)*. Several key B-cell and myeloma growth and survival proteins, including mcl-1 and rac have been shown to require geranylgeranylation for their activity *(87c–87e)*.

4.2. IL-6 Inhibitors

IL-6 is a critical factor for B-cell growth and differentiation *(88)*. Although it participates in the normal process of B-cell development, overproduction of this cytokine may play a vital role in the pathogenesis of myeloma *(8)*. The most common source of IL-6 is the bone marrow stromal cell, which suggests that IL-6 is a paracrine rather than autocrine growth factor in myeloma *(89)*. In light of these findings, it is generally believed that antagonizing the effects of IL-6 would be a valuable asset in the treatment of myeloma. Theoretically, this could be accomplished by inhibiting IL-6 production, inhibiting the binding of IL-6 to its receptor, or blocking IL-6 signal transduction pathways in the myeloma cell. Initial attempts at blocking the binding of IL-6 to its receptor involved the use of monoclonal antibodies against IL-6 *(89)*. However, anti-IL-6 antibodies stabilize IL-6 in the form of circulating complexes. They only inhibit IL-6 bioactivity in patients who produce fewer than 16 µg/d of IL-6 *(90)*. Conversely, strategies designed to inhibit IL-6 activity at its receptor may result in more specific agents with higher anti-myeloma activity. One approach to IL-6 receptor inhibition involves the use of humanized monoclonal anti-IL-6 receptor antibodies *(91)*. Another approach involves the generation of IL-6 variants that block activation of the IL-6 receptor *(92)*. Ciliberto and colleagues used molecular modeling to generate IL-6 variants that behave like potent cytokine receptor super-antagonists *(93)*. One super-antagonist in particular, sant7, was found to be effective at blocking IL-6 because it combines potency with a wide spectrum of efficacy. This agent varies from IL-6 at two locations (sites 2 and 3), and these substitutions abolish its ability to interact with gp130. Preclinical testing of sant7 suggest that this super-antagonist may be most effective in combination therapy, because it blocks cell proliferation but is not highly cytotoxic as a single agent *(94–96)*.

Recently, IL-1 expression in monoclonal plasma cells has been suggested to differentiate MGUS from overt myeloma *(96a)*. Inhibition of IL-1 signaling by an IL-1 receptor antagonist is now being evaluated in a clinical trial involving early stage myeloma patients.

4.3. JAK/STAT Pathway Inhibitors

Another approach to inhibiting IL-6 activity is to interrupt the intracellular signaling necessary for cytokine-receptor activation. IL-6 induces intracellular signaling through the signal transducers and activators of transcription (STAT) family of proteins *(97)*. Engagement of cell-surface cytokine receptors activates the Janus kinase (JAK) family of tyrosine kinases, which phosphorylate and activate cytoplasmic STAT proteins *(98)*. STATs dimerize when activated by JAKs, then translocate to the nucleus, where they bind with specific DNA response elements and induce STAT-regulated gene expression. Constitutive activation of STATs has been associated with oncogenesis; the critical STAT-regulated genes involved in this process have not been identified. Jove and colleagues recently reported that one STAT family member, Stat3, is constitutively activated in bone marrow mononuclear cells obtained from patients with myeloma *(99)*. Using specific inhibitors of the IL-6 receptor (sant7), JAK family kinases (AG490) and Stat3 protein (Stat3β), Jove and coworkers were able to delineate an IL-6 signaling pathway from the JAKs through Stat3 to the *bcl-xl* gene promoter in myeloma cells. Using these inhibitors to block the activation of Stat3 in U266 cells resulted in the inhibition of *bcl-xl* expression and induced apoptosis; it also overcame resistance to fas-mediated apoptosis. However, the cytotoxic response to standard chemotherapeutic drugs was found to be highly drug-dependent, which suggests that additional Stat3-responsive genes—e.g., *cyclin D1*—are involved *(100)*. These findings support the use of JAK/Stat3 inhibitors after cytoreduction with chemotherapy to prolong in vivo responses and enhance immune surveillance. The data also suggest that a thorough understanding of the mechanism by which specific signal transduction pathways regulate downstream gene expression is necessary to design strategies for using targeted therapy to enhance the activity of cytotoxic agents.

4.4. Antisense Inhibition of Gene Expression

Therapy that is targeted to block proto-oncogenic activity is generally most effective in malignancies that rely on those gene products for tumor growth. Multiple myeloma is largely a latent disease, however, and it has been suggested that the primary transforming events are those that dysregulate apoptosis *(101)*. Therefore, strategies that block the expression of anti-apoptotic molecules or the expression of gene products that confer drug resistance may comprise one of the most promising approaches for myeloma therapy.

Bcl-2 was one of the first proto-oncogenes with antiapoptotic activity to be identified *(102,103)*. Originally isolated from follicular *B*-cell *l*ymphoma, the *bcl-2* gene was found to be translocated into the *IgH* locus in more than 80% of follicular B-cell malignancies, resulting in highly constitutive expression of the protein product. The frequency of *bcl-2* translocations is much lower in myeloma than in other B-cell malignancies, although overexpression of the bcl-2 protein or other members of the anti-apoptotic bcl-2 family has been demonstrated in 80 to 100% of myeloma patient specimens and cell lines examined *(104–107)*. Bcl-2 is a 25-kDa protein that has been proposed to function as an ion gate within the mitochondrial membrane. Overexpression of *bcl-2* allows it to form stable homodimers in the mitochondrial membrane and, thus, prevent the release of cytochrome *c* and inhibit the terminal steps of the apoptotic cascade. Additionally, high levels of bcl-2 protein lead to the formation of heterodimers with pro-apoptotic members of the bcl-2 family, including bax and bad, thereby blocking their apoptotic activity. Inhibition of *bcl-2* expression has been shown to increase the ratio of pro-apoptotic to anti-apoptotic factors, thereby facilitating apoptosis. Strategies designed to inhibit the expression of anti-apoptotic proteins include the inhibition of translation by antisense oligonucleotides and the destruction of their mRNA by ribozymes or siRNA.

Antisense oligonucleotides (ODN) are short segments of DNA that are complementary to a target mRNA. ODNs selectively hybridize to their complementary RNA and prevent the translation of target RNA, thereby blocking gene expression. Two mechanisms of action have been described, one in which the complementary ODN physically inhibits the splicing or translational machinery, and the other in which it directs the activity of endogenous RNase-H to degrade the RNA strand in the RNA/DNA duplex *(108,109)*. The majority of antisense drugs currently being investigated in clinical trials function by means of an RNase-H-dependent mechanism, although the precise mechanism by which RNase-H recognizes the RNA/DNA hybrids is not well understood. Targeted sequences must be selected on the basis of the accessibility of the mRNA for heteroduplex formation within the context of the predicted mRNA secondary structure. Additionally, the development of ODN-based therapeutics requires chemical modification of the ODN to prevent its degradation by exonucleases and endonucleases, both during drug delivery and following tumor uptake of the drug. One of the most common modifications used is the substitution of a sulfur atom for oxygen in the phosphate backbone to form a phosphorothioate.

During phase I clinical trials of ODN that targeted the *bcl-2* mRNA in non-Hodgkin's lymphoma, investigators detected one patient with a complete response, two patients with minor responses, nine patients with stable disease, and nine patients with disease progression. No important systemic toxicity was

identified at doses up to 147.2 mg/m^2 daily, and phase II trials have been initiated
(110). The prevalence of *bcl-2* overexpression in MM suggests that *bcl-2* ODNs
may represent a therapeutic strategy for this disease. However, the bcl-2
family members bcl-xl and mcl-1 may be even more relevant as survival factors in multiple myeloma. Their overexpression has been associated with drug-
resistant tumors. A large randomized trial of patients with MM is now being
conducted using anti-sense ODN that targets *bcl-2*.

Preclinical studies have also demonstrated the efficacy of antisense or inhibitory RNA that blocks the expression of MDR1 and reverses the drug-resistant
phenotype *(111–113)*. In studies using cell lines selected for MDR1 expression
through long-term drug exposure, investigators have observed a 65 to 91% reduction in mRNA expression and up to 42% enhancement of drug activity. Animal
models suggest that the primary challenges for the clinical use of RNA inhibition
will be agent stability and delivery to the tumor. However, inhibitory oligonucleotides display minimal toxicity and cross-reactivity and, thus, may be extremely
useful in combination therapy *(114)*.

4.5. Proteasome Inhibitors

One of the most novel molecular pathways to emerge as a target for cancer
therapy is the ubiquitin–proteasome system of protein degradation. The
ubiquitin–proteasome system regulates intracellular protein turnover and is
involved in multiple cellular activities, including gene transcription, signal transduction, cell–cycle progression, and cell survival. Based on these observations,
proteasome inhibitors have been developed as anti-cancer agents *(115,116)*. A
dipeptide boronic acid, Velcade (formerly known as bortezomib/PS-341) has
received FDA approval for the treatment of patients with MM who received at
least two treatments previously and demonstrated disease progression during the
last treatment *(117)*. Velcade forms a covalent bond with the active-site threo-
nine in the core of the 20S proteasome and inhibits chymotrypsin activity of the
proteasome. Its exact mechanism of cytotoxic activity and selectivity for transformed cells is not well understood. Several studies have suggested NF-κB as a
potential Velcade target. Using 8226 myeloma cell lines selected for resistance
to standard chemotherapeutic drugs, *(118–120)* Berenson and associates demonstrated inhibition of NF-κB activity in MM cells and enhanced chemotherapeutic
cytotoxicity when Velcade was combined with PS-341 *(121)*. Additionally,
Cusack and colleagues demonstrated that the combination of PS-341 with CPT-11
(an agent that activates NF-κB) significantly enhances the drug response in
human colorectal cancer cells *(122)*. However, in both studies, the dose of
PS-341 required to inhibit NF-κB activity was far greater than the toxic dose.

In addition to displaying a high degree of tumor specificity, it has been suggested that Velcade targets the microenvironment. Preclinical studies in human
myeloma cells have demonstrated that PS-341 acts directly on the tumor cells as

well as the bone marrow microenvironment *(123)*. Hideshima and colleagues reported that PS-341 inhibits paracrine growth of MM cells by decreasing their ability to adhere to bone marrow stromal cells. This, in turn, reduces tumor necrosis factor (TNF)-α-stimulated NF-κB activation and inhibits the mitogen-activated protein kinase signaling pathway in both myeloma cell lines and in freshly isolated myeloma cells obtained from patient bone marrow aspirates. Similar activity has been reported in MCF-7 breast carcinoma *(116)* and ovarian and prostate carcinomas grown in spheroid culture (a model of solid tumor "multicellular resistance") *(124)*. Using an ovarian cancer multicellular spheroid model, Frankel and colleagues demonstrated greater cytotoxicity in the SKOV3 cell line when grown in spheroid culture than when they were grown in a mono-layer culture. These data support the hypothesis that Velcade molecular targets may be more active in cells following cell–cell or cell–matrix interactions, such as those that would be encountered in the bone marrow microenvironment. In vivo studies using mouse mammary carcinoma and Lewis lung carcinoma demonstrated anti-tumor activity in both primary and metastatic disease *(116)*, again supporting the role of the microenvironment in the activation of molecular targets for proteasome inhibitors.

In phase I clinical trials, Velcade was well tolerated, with the MTD determined at 1 to 2 mg/m². Primary toxicities included low-grade fever and fatigue, non-dose-limiting thrombocytopenia, and low-grade diarrhea—all of which were manageable. The drug was also associated with peripheral neuropathy. More recently, reports from a large phase II trial that enrolled more than 200 patients at nine centers indicated a 35% response rate, including 19 patients (10%) with a complete or near complete response, 7 of whom had an M-protein component that became undetectable (as determined by both electrophoresis and immunofixation) *(125)*. The median overall length of survival was 16 mo, with a median duration of response of 12 mo. The most clinically significant adverse event cited was a cumulative, dose-related peripheral sensory neuropathy, which was reported by 34% of patients, with complete resolution or improvement of neural symptoms during follow-up in some patients. The results of this trial led to the FDA approval in May 2003 *(117)*. Additional phase II studies are planned in Mantle cell lymphoma, indolent non-Hodgkin's lymphoma, chronic myelogenous leukemia, diffuse large B-cell leukemia, and chronic lymphocytic leukemia. The first phase III trial of Velcade in multiple myeloma was anticipated in 2003. This trial included a randomized comparison of Velcade alone vs combination therapy with dexamethasone.

Recent laboratory studies demonstrating that Velcade could readily reverse chemotherapy resistance in highly chemo-resistant myeloma cells *(121)* have led to several clinical trials *(125a,125b)*. The combination of escalating doses of oral melphalan with lower doses of Velcade (0.7 mg/m² on days 1, 4, 8, and 11) was evaluated as part of a 4-wk cycle in relapsed patients with MM *(125a)*.

Responses were observed in all five cohorts, including those patients receiving only 0.02 mg/kg for 4 d.

Importantly, very limited neuropathic effects were observed with this reduced dose intensity of Velcade. Similarly, Orlowski has evaluated a combination of liposomal doxrubicin with standard dose Velcade with responses in ore than half of patients despite half of the patients having been previously exposed to doxirubin *(125b)*.

The drug is also being evaluated with ATO because preclinical studies show synergism with the combination in MM.

5. THE TUMOR MICROENVIRONMENT AS A TARGET FOR NOVEL THERAPY

5.1. Anti-Angiogenesis

Tumor growth in solid tumors is known to depend on angiogenesis *(126)*. Recently, there have been reports that angiogenesis also occurs in hematopoietic malignancies, including MM *(10,11)*. Vacca and colleagues reported that angiogenesis was significantly associated with active myeloma, compared with non-active myeloma or a monoclonal gammopathy of unknown significance (MGUS) *(10)*. Myeloma patients who had the highest proliferative fraction also had the highest bone marrow microvessel area. In a recent report by Bellamy and colleagues at the University of Arizona, vascular endothelial growth factor (VEGF) (an important mediator of angiogenesis) was found to be overexpressed in all human myeloma cell lines studied and in myeloma cells obtained from 12 of 16 patients *(127)*. In contrast, plasma cells obtained from normal subjects expressed little or no VEGF. Folkman and colleagues demonstrated that anti-angiogenesis drugs can induce tumor dormancy *(128)*; when given continuously, they can completely eradicate tumors *(129)*. Targeting the tumor vasculature should produce minimal toxicity and avoid the development of acquired drug resistance. These findings support the possibility that anti-angiogenic drugs may inhibit myeloma growth and progression.

5.1.1. THALIDOMIDE

Thalidomide was originally introduced as a sedative in Europe and Canada in the late 1950s and was widely used for insomnia and nausea during pregnancy. Severe teratogenic effects led to its withdrawal in 1961. Subsequent investigation demonstrated that thalidomide is a potent anti-angiogenic and immunomodulatory agent with anti-cancer activity *(130)*. It was approved for use as an anti-angiogenic agent in the United States in July 1998 under 21 CFR 314.520 Subpart H, which restricts the distribution of drugs with special safety concerns.

Thalidomide has been investigated in a number of cancers, including MM, myelodysplastic syndromes, gliomas, Kaposi's sarcoma, renal cell carcinoma, advanced breast cancer, and colon cancer. The mechanism by which thalidomide inhibits angiogenesis is unclear. Its teratogenicity is believed to be due to intercalation into G-rich promoter regions of DNA and inhibition of growth factor transcription during limb bud outgrowth, which suggests that the regulation of specific gene expression is a potential action *(131,132)*. As an anti-inflammatory agent, thalidomide has been reported to block the production of TNF-α, IL-6, IL-10, and IL-12, while enhancing the production of IL-2, IL-4, and IL-5, and stimulating T-cell cytotoxicity. Nonetheless, thalidomide and thalidomide analogs have been remarkably active as both monotherapy and combination therapy in MM *(133)*.

In 1999, Singhal and colleagues reported a 32% response rate to thalidomide, with 20% of the responders demonstrating at least a 50% reduction in M protein. Drowsiness, constipation, weakness, fatigue, and tingling, numbness, or both sensations in the hands and feet, as well as dizziness and a skin rash were reported as the predominant adverse effects. However, most side effects were grade I or II, and only 10% of patients chose to discontinue the study *(134)*. Additionally, a large trial reported by Barlogie and associates *(135)*, in which 169 patients were enrolled, demonstrated a major and partial response in 30% of patients, with 9% of patients displaying toxicity of a neuropathy grade greater than 3, which improved in most patients with a reduction in dose. The thalidomide dose used in this study was 400 to 800 mg/d administered as a single oral dose. Based on the 6- to 7-h half-life reported for this drug, the Swedish group of Juliusson and colleagues examined the benefit of divided doses, starting at 200 mg/d and escalating to 400, 600, or 800 mg/d *(136)*. In the divided-dose group, 43% of patients achieved a partial response, with the median time to partial response being 31 d compared with 70 and 116 d in the two responding patients who received one dose per day. The findings of a retrospective analysis *(137)* of the cumulative dose effect on progression-free survival and overall survival by Neben and colleagues further supports the use of a dose-intensive treatment schedule at least for the first 3 mo of therapy. However, these findings additionally indicated that dose intensity correlated with the incidence of serious adverse events, e.g., deep vein thrombosis (DVT). Durie and Stepan noted that initial responses tended to occur early and dose escalation significantly increased toxicity. In a trial of the efficacy of lower, less toxic doses, patients experiencing a relapse or progressive myeloma were treated with thalidomide 50 to 400 mg/d. Dose escalation was based on a lack of response following an 8-wk course. The overall response in this trial was 25 to 35% in patients with a relapse and 35 to 45% in front-line therapy—highly comparable to trials described above. All responding patients remained in remission at 6 mo, 67% at 18 mo, and 22% at 2 yr. *(138)*. Interestingly, the two patients who were still in remission at 30 mo had received the lowest dose (50 mg/d). Progressive peripheral neuropathy appeared as a long-term toxicity. Thus, the optimum dose of thalidomide and the factors contributing to response and toxicity remain to be determined *(139)*.

Patients with MM frequently display paraprotein-associated coagulopathies, including both hypercoagulability and anticoagulant syndromes. Recently, several studies have identified an increased risk of thromboembolism in myeloma patients receiving thalidomide, particularly when given with anthracycline or steroid therapy *(140–145)*. In the largest of these studies, Zangari and colleagues reported an incidence of DVT in 14 of 50 patients (28%) randomly assigned to thalidomide, but in only 2 of 50 patients (4%) who did not receive the agent. The mechanism for this phenomenon is unknown in most cases. Thromboses were successfully treated with anticoagulant therapy, and patients were able to continue thalidomide treatment.

The thalidomide analogs known as selective cytokine inhibitory drugs (SelCIDs), which are phosphodiesterase 4 inhibitors, and immunomodulatory drugs (ImiDs) have recently entered phase I and I/II clinical trials. SelCIDs have been well tolerated and have shown reduced toxicity compared with thalidomide. Richardson and colleagues reported a phase I dose-escalation trial of the ImiD CC-5013 (Revlimid) at doses of 5–50 mg/d in 27 patients with relapsed and refractory multiple myeloma *(146)*. Dose escalation identified the MTD as 25 mg/d, with limiting toxicities appearing after 28 d of therapy. The most common serious adverse events included grade 3 thrombocytopenia and grade 3 and grade 4 neutropenia. A clinical response was noted in 17 of 24 evaluable patients (71%), primarily at 25 or 50 mg/d. Currently, a large phase II trial is evaluating CC-5013 at a daily dose of 30 mg in 200 relapsing myeloma patients.

Thalidomide and other ImiDs may be best utilized in combination therapy in patients who do not respond to or experience a relapse while taking thalidomide monotherapy or a standard cytotoxic therapy. Two combinations have been reported—DT-PACE (consisting of dexamethasone, thalidomide, cisplatin, doxorubicin, cyclophosphamide, etoposide) and BLT-D (consisting of clarithromycin, thalidomide, and dexamethasone)—with varied results. Additionally, thalidomide has been reported to overcome resistance of myeloma cells to standard chemotherapy *(147)*, which suggests that it may be highly effective in patients with relapsed or refractory disease.

More recently, thalidomide has been suggested for first-line therapy, either as a single agent or in combination with dexamethasone. There have been two clinical trials of either thalidomide or thalidomide plus dexamethasone in newly diagnosed or previously untreated myeloma patients *(148,149)*. This protocol was proposed as a less toxic alternative to VAD for induction therapy in preparation for autologous stem cell transplant. In 28 patients treated with thalidomide alone, Weber and colleagues reported 10 patients (36%) with disease remission and a median time to remission of 4.2 mo. Combination therapy using thalidomide (100–400 mg/d) plus dexamethasone resulted in a significantly higher response rate (72%; $N = 40$), with 5 patients (16%) achieving a complete remission. Similarly, Rajkumar and colleagues reported 32 of 50 patients (64%) demonstrating a response to thalidomide (200 mg/d)–dexamethasone therapy, with an additional 14 patients (28%) categorized as stable. Dose-limiting toxicities were comparable to those reported when thalidomide is used as salvage therapy in patients with advanced or refractory disease. In both studies, the tumor burden was reduced as effectively as with VAD induction. Unfortunately, the long-term effects of thalidomide on stem cell yield or engraftment are not known. In addition, the duration of response from this combination will not be evaluable because most patients underwent an additional high-dose therapy procedure. Currently, a randomized phase III trial comparing thalidomide with dexamethasone to dexamethase alone in patients newly diagnosed with MM is being conducted. Further studies are warranted to identify the most appropriate time to use this therapy during the course of the disease, as well as the long-term toxicity of thalidomide and thalidomide analogs.

5.2. Attacking Cell-Adhesion-Mediated Drug Resistance (CAM-DR)

It has long been realized that intercellular interactions may contribute to tumor cell survival and progression (150). Within the last 5 yr, it has been appreciated that cell–cell adhesion or adhesion between the extracellular matrix (ECM) components of adjacent cells can regulate apoptosis and cell survival in a wide variety of tumor types (151). Recently, the integrin family of cellular adhesion molecules—a major class of receptors through which cells interact with ECM components—has been implicated as being involved in the pathology of myeloma (11,152,153). Integrins have been shown to participate in intracellular signal transduction pathways that may contribute to tumor cell growth and survival. Experimental evidence suggests that the $\beta1$ integrins and fibronectin play a part in apoptotic suppression and cell survival (154). Damiano and colleagues showed that drug-sensitive 8226 myeloma cells, known to express both VLA-4 ($\alpha4\beta1$) and VLA-5 ($\alpha5\beta1$) integrin fibronectin receptors, are relatively resistant to the apoptotic effects of doxorubicin and melphalan when preadhered to fibronectin, compared with cells exposed to either drug while in suspension (120). The term CAM-DR was used to describe this phenomenon, which has been extended to multiple classes of drugs, including topoisomerase II inhibitors, alkylating agents, microtubule inhibitors, and antimetabolites, as well as ionizing radiation and death receptor ligation (155). Multiple intracellular mechanisms contributing to this anti-apoptotic effect have been identified, including increased levels of the cyclin-dependent kinase inhibitor p27kip^1 (156), reduction in DNA double-stranded breaks (157), altered intracellular localization of apoptotic mediators (158), and induction of anti-apoptotic signal transduction pathways (159). These findings provide evidence that antagonists of VLA-4 and VLA-5 adhesion or intracellular signaling cascades may serve as a means of inducing myeloma cell apoptosis or improving the efficacy of anti-cancer therapy for myeloma (160). Similar studies examining the mechanisms of resistance associated with myeloma cells adhered to bone marrow stromal cells have demonstrated a complex interaction involving both direct cell–cell contact and soluble factors, including IL-6 and TNF-α *(161–163)*. Thus, it has become apparent that successful therapy for myeloma will likely be most efficacious with combination therapies that consider not only the tumor itself, but also the microenvironment.

5.3. Immunotherapy As a Novel Approach to Drug-Resistant Minimal Residual Disease

As mentioned earlier, the acquisition of drug resistance is a major obstacle preventing the cure of myeloma. Immunotherapy may represent a novel approach to the control or eradication of the disease. Preclinical investigations have shown that this form of therapy is most effective in preventing disease progression when the disease is in its earliest stages. For this reason, approaches using immunotherapy are being considered following high-dose chemotherapy, when the patient is most likely to have minimal residual disease. Unfortunately, any myeloma cells that survive dose-intensive chemotherapy are likely to be selected for drug resistance. Thus, although high-dose chemotherapy induces a state of minimal residual disease, it also selects for drug-resistant cell, and raises the need for post-high-dose therapy approaches to be capable of eliminating the drug-resistant population of cells.

This could be achieved if the remaining drug-resistant cells are sensitive to the effector mechanisms used by the immune system. The granzyme B/perforin and APO-1/CD95/fas ligand pathways are considered the two main pathways for mediating the lytic effects of cytotoxic lymphocytes (CTLs). Recent reports have questioned the susceptibility of drug-resistant cells to immune-based effector systems *(164)*. Several tumor cell lines selected for resistance to different chemotherapeutic drugs were also resistant to lymphokine-activated killer (LAK) or natural killer (NK) cells *(165)*. Recent reports have also shown that myeloma cells selected for drug resistance are also resistant to fas-mediated apoptosis *(166)*. In contrast, Scheper and colleagues demonstrated that RPMI 8226 myeloma cells selected for drug resistance to doxorubicin (P-gp-positive) or mitoxantrone (P-gp-negative) remain sensitive to LAK- or NK-cell-mediated lysis *(167)*. Given these findings, it is possible that myeloma cells selected for drug resistance may coselect for resistance to one immune effector system, such as the caspase-dependent pathway utilized by fas-mediated killing, but remain sensitive to a nonapoptosis initiating system, such as the perforin-induced necrosis mediated by CTLs. To investigate this possibility, Shtil and colleagues examined the question of whether the selection for drug resistance mediated by MDR1/ P-gp overexpression affected the susceptibility of myeloma cells to a CTL-based vaccine *(168)*. Using a murine myeloma model, the investigators determined whether CTLs that generated a response to immunization with GM-CSF/ IL-12-transfected myeloma cells were capable of killing isogenic drug-resistant vari-

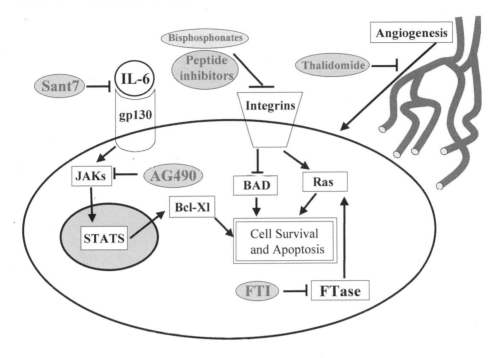

Fig. 2. New therapeutic targets in myeloma. Effective therapy for myeloma will require agents that target both intrinsic and extrinsic factors. Abbreviations: IL-6, interleukin-6; JAK, Janus kinase; STATs, signal transducers and activators of transcription; FTI, farnesyl transferase inhibitor; Ftase, farnesyl transferase.

ants. They found that immunization with either drug-sensitive or drug-resistant cells transfected with GM-CSF/IL-12 caused a highly efficient and prolonged cross-protection of mice challenged with either parental or drug-resistant cells, and that this effect was mediated by granzyme B/perforin-secreting CTLs. Thus, it appears that immunotherapy based on pore-forming CTLs is an attractive option for the treatment of drug-resistant myeloma. Other immunotherapeutic approaches are described in detail elsewhere in this volume.

6. ESSENTIALS FOR DEVELOPING NEW THERAPEUTIC APPROACHES

The treatment of myeloma has not improved substantially over the past three decades, and the mainstay of treatment continues to be based on cytotoxic drugs and glucocorticoids. The use of high-dose chemotherapy with stem cell rescue has improved response duration; however, even with this treatment, most patients experience a relapse with drug-refractory disease. Curative therapy has thus far been elusive. Enhancing the efficacy of currently used drugs by preventing or overcoming drug resistance may improve the frequency of response and response duration, but is also likely result in relapse. To substantially improve the treatment outcome for myeloma patients, a multifaceted approach that capitalizes on newly discovered biological aspects of myeloma is necessary. A wealth of new information is now available regarding the pathogenesis of myeloma, which should be useful in developing new therapeutic targets (Fig. 2). To date, most of these new targets are likely to be effective in preventing disease progression or enhancing the efficacy of more traditional approaches. Therefore, a major challenge to improving treatment outcome is not only discovering new therapeutic targets, but also determining how to integrate these new approaches with treatments that are known to be effective in most patients.

Developing a "total approach" to the treatment of myeloma will likely involve the use of one approach that first reduces tumor burden, followed by a second that eradicates residual disease, and finally a third that minimizes the growth and progression of residual myeloma cells. Additionally, it is likely that combination therapy will be required as demonstrated by the recent preclinical and early clinical results with drugs such as ATO or Velcade when combined with chemotherapy. Because no single "total approach" is likely to be effective for all patients, another challenge will be to identify the patients are suitable for any given approach. Once again, the discovery of the biological aspects of myeloma and consideration of the unique circumstances of each patient will assist the physician in the treatment of patients with myeloma.

REFERENCES

1. Bergsagel DE, Cowan DH, Hasselback R. Plasma cell myeloma: response of melphalan-resistant patients to high-dose intermittent cyclophosphamide. Can Med Assoc J 1972; 107:851–855.
2. Oken MM, Harrington DP, Abramson N, Kyle RA, Knospe W, Glick JH. Comparison of melphalan and prednisone with vincristine, carmustine, melphalan, cyclophosphamide, and prednisone in the treatment of multiple myeloma: results of Eastern Cooperative Oncology Group Study E2479. Cancer 1997; 79(8):1561–1567.
3. Combination chemotherapy versus melphalan plus prednisone as treatment for multiple myeloma: an overview of 6,633 patients from 27 randomized trials. Myeloma Trialists' Collaborative Group. J Clin Oncol 1998; 16:3832–3842.
4. Salmon SE, Haut A, Bonnet JD, et al. Alternating combination chemotherapy and levamisole improves survival in multiple myeloma: a Southwest Oncology Group Study. J Clin Oncol 1983; 1:453–461.
5. Dalton WS. Alternative (non-P-glycoprotein) mechanisms of drug resistance in non-Hodgkin's lymphoma. Hematol Oncol Clin North Am 1997; 11:975–986.
6. Barlogie B, Smith L, Alexanian R. Effective treatment of advanced multiple myeloma refractory to alkylating agents. N Engl J Med 1984; 310:1353–1356.
7. Dalton WS. Mechanisms of drug resistance in hematologic malignancies. Semin Hematol 1997; 34:3–8.
8. Uchiyama H, Barut BA, Mohrbacher AF, Chauhan D, Anderson KC. Adhesion of human myeloma-derived cell lines to bone marrow stromal cells stimulates interleukin-6 secretion. Blood 1993; 82:3712–3720.

9. Damiano JS, Cress AE, Hazlehurst LA, Shtil AA, Dalton WS. Cell adhesion mediated drug resistance (CAM-DR): role of integrins and resistance to apoptosis in human myeloma cell lines. Blood 1999; 93:1658–1667.

10. Vacca A, Di Loreto M, Ribatti D, et al. Bone marrow of patients with active multiple myeloma: angiogenesis and plasma cell adhesion molecules LFA-1, VLA-4, LAM-1, and CD44. Am J Hematol 1995; 50:9-14.

11. Vacca A, Ribatti D, Roncali L, et al. Bone marrow angiogenesis and progression in multiple myeloma. Br J Haematol 1994; 87:503–508.

12. Hannun YA. Apoptosis and the dilemma of cancer chemotherapy. Blood 1997; 89: 1845–1853.

13. Friesen C, Herr I, Krammer PH, Debatin K-M. Involvement of the CD95 (APO-1/fas) receptor/ligand system in drug-induced apoptosis in leukemia cells. Nature Med 1996; 2:574–577.

14. Landowski TH, Qu N, Buyuksal I, Painter JS, Dalton WS. Mutations in the Fas antigen of multiple myeloma patients. Blood 1997; 90:4266–4270.

14a. Yang HH, Ma MH, Vescio RA, Berenson JR. Overcoming drug resistance in multiple myeloma: The emergence of therapeutic approaches to induce apoptosis. J Clin Oncol 2003; 21:22:4239–4247.

15. Harada N, Nagasaki A, Hata H, Matsuzaki H, Matsuno F, Mitsuya H. Down-regulation of CD98 in melphalan-resistant myeloma cells with reduced drug uptake. Acta Haematol 2000; 103:144–151.

16. Wang ZM, Chen ZP, Xu ZY, et al. In vitro evidence for homologous recombinational repair in resistance to melphalan. J Natl Cancer Inst 2001; 93:1473–1478.

17. Spanswick VJ, Craddock C, Sekhar M, et al. Repair of DNA interstrand crosslinks as a mechanism of clinical resistance to melphalan in multiple myeloma. Blood 2002; 100:224–229.

18. Bellamy WT, Dalton WS, Meltzer P, Dorr RT. Role of glutathione and its associated enzymes in multidrug-resistant human myeloma cells. Biochem Pharmacol 1989; 38:787–793.

19. Pegg AE. Mammalian O6-alkylguanine-DNA alkyltransferase: regulation and importance in response to alkylating carcinogenic and therapeutic agents. Cancer Res 1990; 50:6119–6129.

20. Gerson SL, Trey JE, Miller K. Potentiation of nitrosourea cytotoxicity in human leukemic cells by inactivation of O6-alkylguanine-DNA alkyltransferase. Cancer Res 1988; 48: 1521–1527.

21. Shustik C, Dalton WS, Gros P. P-glycoprotein-mediated multidrug resistance in tumor cells: biochemistry, clinical relevance and modulation. Mol Aspects of Med 1995; 16:1–78.

22. Gottesman MM, Pastan I. Biochemistry of multidrug resistance mediated by the multidrug transporter. Ann Rev Biochem 1993; 62:385–427.

23. Dalton WS, Grogan TM, Rybski JA, et al. Immunohistochemical detection and quantitation of P-glycoprotein in multiple drug-resistant human myeloma cells: association with level of drug resistance and drug accumulation. Blood 1989; 73:747–752.

24. Abbaszadegan MR, Cress AE, Futscher BW, Bellamy WT, Dalton WS. Evidence for cytoplasmic P-glycoprotein location associated with increased multidrug resistance and resistance to chemosensitizers. Cancer Research 1996; 56:5435–5442.

25. Salmon SE, Grogan TM, Miller T, Scheper R, Dalton WS. Prediction of doxorubicin resistance in vitro in myeloma, lymphoma, and breast cancer by P-glycoprotein staining. J Natl Cancer Inst 1989; 81:696–701.

26. Sonneveld P, Marie JP, Huisman C, et al. Reversal of multidrug resistance by SDZ PSC 833, combined with VAD (vincristine, doxorubicin, dexamethasone) in refractory multiple myeloma: a phase I study. Leukemia 1996; 10:1741–1750.

26a. Berenson JR, Crowley JJ, Grogan TM, et al. Maintenance therapy with alternate-day prednisone improves survival in multiple myeloma patients. Blood 2002; 99:3163–3168.

27. Thomas H, Coley HM. Overcoming multidrug resistance in cancer: an update on the clinical strategy of inhibiting p-glycoprotein. Cancer Control 2003; 10:159–165.
28. Mistry P, Stewart AJ, Dangerfield W, et al. In vitro and in vivo reversal of P-glycoprotein-mediated multidrug resistance by a novel potent modulator, XR9576. Cancer Res 2001; 61:749–758.
29. Stewart A, Steiner J, Mellows G, Laguda B, Norris D, Bevan P. Phase I trial of XR9576 in healthy volunteers demonstrates modulation of P-glycoprotein in CD56+ lymphocytes after oral and intravenous administration. Clin Cancer Res 2000; 6:4186–4191.
30. Cole SPC, Bhardwaj G, Gerlach JH, et al. Overexpression of a transporter gene in a multidrug-resistant human lung cancer cell line. Science 1992; 258:1650–1654.
31. Doyle LA, Yang W, Abruzzo LV, et al. A multidrug resistance transporter from human MCF-7 breast cancer cells. Proc Natl Acad Sci U S A 1998; 95:15665–15670.
32. Abbaszadegan MR, Futscher BW, Klimecki WT, List A, Dalton WS. Analysis of multidrug resistance-associated protein (MRP) messenger RNA in normal and malignant hematopoietic cells. Cancer Res 1994; 54:4676–4679.
33. Hazlehurst LA, Foley NE, Gleason-Guzman MC, et al. Multiple mechanisms confer drug resistance to mitoxantrone in the human 8226 myeloma cell line. Cancer Res 1999; 59:1021–1028.
34. Ross DD, Yang W, Abruzzo LV, et al. Atypical multidrug resistance: breast cancer resistance protein messenger RNA expression in mitoxantrone-selected cell lines. J Natl Cancer Inst 1999; 91:429–433.
35. Kickhoefer VA, Stephen AG, Harrington L, Robinson MO, Rome LH. Vaults and telomerase share a common subunit, TEP1. J Biol Chem 1999; 274:32712-32717.
36. Raaijmakers HG, Izquierdo MA, Lokhorst HM, et al. Lung-resistance-related protein expression is a negative predictive factor for response to conventional low but not to intensified dose alkylating chemotherapy in multiple myeloma. Blood 1998; 91:1029–1036.
37. Rimsza LM, Campbell K, Dalton WS, Salmon S, Willcox G, Grogan TM. The major vault protein (MVP), a new multidrug resistance associated protein, is frequently expressed in multiple myeloma. Leuk Lymphoma 1999; 34:315–324.
38. Futscher BW, Foley NE, Gleason-Guzman MC, Meltzer PS, Sullivan DM, Dalton WS. Verapamil suppresses the emergence of P-glycoprotein-mediated multi-drug resistance. Int J Cancer 1996; 66:520–525.
39. Valkov NI, Sullivan DM. Drug resistance to DNA topoisomerase I and II inhibitors in human leukemia, lymphoma, and multiple myeloma. Semin Hematol 1997; 34(4 suppl 5):48–62.
40. Kraut EH, Crowley JJ, Wade JL, et al. Evaluation of topotecan in resistant and relapsing multiple myeloma: a Southwest Oncology Group study. J Clin Oncol 1998; 16:589–592.
41. Kraut EH, Ju R, Muller M. The use of topoisomerase I inhibitors in multiple myeloma. Semin Hematol 1998; 35(3 suppl 4):32–38.
42. Waxman S, Anderson KC. History of the development of arsenic derivatives in cancer therapy. Oncologist 2001; 6(suppl 2):3–10.
43. Voorzanger-Rousselot N, Favrot M-C, Blay J-Y. Resistance to cytotoxic chemotherapy induced by CD40 ligand in lymphoma cells. Blood 1998; 92:3381–3387.
43a. Friedman JM, Ma MH, Manyak SJ, et al. Arsenic trioxide causes apoptosis, growth inhibition and increased sensitivity to chemotherapeutic agents in multiple myeloma cells through inhibition of nuclear factor (NF)-κB activity. Proc Am Assoc Cancer Res 2002; Abstract 4585.
44. Zhang W, Ohnishi K, Shigeno K, et al. The induction of apoptosis and cell cycle arrest by arsenic trioxide in lymphoid neoplasms. Leukemia 1998; 12:1383–1391.
45. Jia P, Chen G, Huang X, et al. Arsenic trioxide induces multiple myeloma cell apoptosis via disruption of mitochondrial transmembrane potentials and activation of caspase-3. Chin Med J 2001; 114:19–24.
46. Grad JM, Bahlis NJ, Reis I, Oshiro MM, Dalton WS, Boise LH. Ascorbic acid enhances arsenic trioxide-induced cytotoxicity in multiple myeloma cells. Blood 2001; 98:805–813.

47. Gartenhaus RB, Prachand SN, Paniaqua M, Li Y, Gordon LI. Arsenic trioxide cytotoxicity in steroid and chemotherapy-resistant myeloma cell lines: enhancement of apoptosis by manipulation of cellular redox state. Clin Cancer Res 2002; 8:566–572.

48. Bahlis NJ, McCafferty-Grad J, Jordan-McMurry I, et al. Feasibility and correlates of arsenic trioxide combined with ascorbic acid-mediated depletion of intracellular glutathione for the treatment of relapsed/refractory multiple myeloma. Clin Cancer Res 2002; 8:3658–3668.

48a. Munshi NC, Tricot G, Desikan R, et al. Clinical activity of arsenic trioxide for the treatment of multiple myeloma. Leukemia 2002; 15:1835–1837.

48b. Hussein MA, Paradise C, Carozza R, et al. Arsenic trioxide in patients with relapsed or refractory multiple myeloma: Final report of a phase II clinical study. Blood 2002; 100:Abstract 5138 (ASH 44th Annual Meeting).

48c. Berenson JR, Yang H, Vescio R, et al. Preliminary findings in a phase I/II study of Trisenox dosed twice weekly in patients with advanced multiple myeloma. Blood 2002; 100:Abstract 5140 (ASH 44th Annual Meeting).

48d. JM, Ma MH, Manyak SJ, et al. Arsenic trioxide causes apoptosis, growth inhibition and increased sensitivity to chemotherapeutic agents in multiple myeloma cells through inhibition of nuclear factor (NF)-κB activity. Proc Am Assoc Cancer Res 2002; Abstract 4585.

48e. Ma MH, Yang HH, Parker K, et al. The proteasome inhibitor PS-341 markedly enhances sensitivity of multiple myeloma tumor cells to chemotherapeutic agents. Clin Cancer Res 2003; 9:1136–1144.

49. Sagaster P, Kokoschka EM, Kokron O, Micksche M. Antitumor activity of imexon. J Natl Cancer Inst 1995; 87:935–936.

50. Salmon SE, Hersh EM. Sensitivity of multiple myeloma to imexon in the human tumor cloning assay. J Natl Cancer Inst 1994; 86:228–230.

51. Dvorakova K, Payne CM, Landowski TH, Tome ME, Halperin DS, Dorr RT. Imexon activates an intrinsic apoptosis pathway in RPMI8226 myeloma cells. Anticancer Drugs 2002; 13:1031–1042.

52. Dvorakova K, Waltmire CN, Payne CM, Tome ME, Briehl MM, Dorr RT. Induction of mitochondrial changes in myeloma cells by imexon. Blood 2001; 97:3544–3551.

53. Dvorakova K, Payne CM, Tome ME, et al. Molecular and cellular characterization of imexon-resistant RPMI8226/I myeloma cells. Mol Cancer Ther 2002; 1:185–195.

54. Miller HJ, Leong T, Khandekar JD, Greipp PR, Gertz MA, Kyle RA. Paclitaxel as the initial treatment of multiple myeloma: an Eastern Cooperative Oncology Group Study (E1A93). Am J Clin Oncol 1998; 21:553–556.

55. Dimopoulos MA, Arbuck S, Huber M, et al. Primary therapy of multiple myeloma with paclitaxel (taxol). Ann Oncol 1994; 5:757–759.

56. Marks PA, Richon VM, Kiyokawa H, Rifkind RA. Inducing differentiation of transformed cells with hybrid polar compounds: a cell cycle-dependent process. Proc Natl Acad Sci U S A 1994; 91:10251–10254.

57. Siegel DS, Zhang X, Feinman R, et al. Hexamethylene bisacetamide induces programmed cell death (apoptosis) and down-regulates BCL-2 expression in human myeloma cells. Proc Natl Acad Sci U S A 1998; 95:162–166.

58. Baldassarre G, Barone MV, Belletti B, et al. Key role of the cyclin-dependent kinase inhibitor p27kip1 for embryonal carcinoma cell survival and differentiation. Oncogene 1999; 18:6241–6251.

59. Ibrahim A, Scher N, Williams G, et al. Approval summary for zoledronic acid for treatment of multiple myeloma and cancer bone metastases. Clin Cancer Res 2003; 9:2394–2399.

60. Berenson JR, Lichtenstein A, Porter L, et al. Efficacy of pamidronate in reducing skeletal events in patients with advanced multiple myeloma. Myeloma Aredia Study Group. N Engl J Med 1996; 334:488–493.

61. Aparicio A, Gardner A, Tu Y, Savage A, Berenson J, Lichtenstein A. In vitro cytoreductive effects on multiple myeloma cells induced by bisphosphonates. Leukemia 1998; 12:220–229.
62. Shipman CM, Croucher PI, Russell RG, Helfrich MH, Rogers MJ. The bisphosphonate incadronate (YM175) causes apoptosis of human myeloma cells in vitro by inhibiting the mevalonate pathway. Cancer Res 1998; 58:5294–5297.
63. Passeri G, Girasole G, Manolagas SC, Jilka RL. Endogenous production of tumor necrosis factor by primary cultures of murine calvarial cells: influence on IL-6 production and osteoclast development. Bone Miner 1994; 24:109–126.
64. van der PG, Vloedgraven H, van Beek E, Wee-Pals L, Lowik C, Papapoulos S. Bisphosphonates inhibit the adhesion of breast cancer cells to bone matrices in vitro. J Clin Invest 1996; 98:698–705.
65. Heider U, Langelotz C, Jakob C, et al. Expression of receptor activator of nuclear factor kappaB ligand on bone marrow plasma cells correlates with osteolytic bone disease in patients with multiple myeloma. Clin Cancer Res 2003; 9:1436–1440.
66. Croucher PI, Shipman CM, Van Camp B, Vanderkerken K. Bisphosphonates and osteoprotegerin as inhibitors of myeloma bone disease. Cancer 2003; 97(3 suppl):818–824.
67. Dhodapkar MV, Singh J, Mehta J, et al. Anti-myeloma activity of pamidronate in vivo. Br J Haematol 1998; 103:530–532.
68. Treon SP, Teoh G, Urashima M, et al. Anti-estrogens induce apoptosis of multiple myeloma cells. Blood 1998; 92:1749–1757.
69. Chauhan D, Catley L, Hideshima T, et al. 2-Methoxyestradiol overcomes drug resistance in multiple myeloma cells. Blood 2002; 100:2187–2194.
70. Dingli D, Timm M, Russell SJ, Witzig TE, Rajkumar SV. Promising preclinical activity of 2-methoxyestradiol in multiple myeloma. Clin Cancer Res 2002; 8:3948–3954.
71. Tinley TL, Leal RM, Randall-Hlubek DA, et al. Novel 2-methoxyestradiol analogues with antitumor activity. Cancer Res 2003; 63:1538–1549.
72. Wang LH, Yang XY, Mihalic K, Xiao W, Li D, Farrar WL. Activation of estrogen receptor blocks interleukin-6-inducible cell growth of human multiple myeloma involving molecular cross-talk between estrogen receptor and STAT3 mediated by co-regulator PIAS3. J Biol Chem 2001; 276:31839–31844.
73. Yamamoto T, Matsuda T, Junicho A, Kishi H, Saatcioglu F, Muraguchi A. Cross-talk between signal transducer and activator of transcription 3 and estrogen receptor signaling. FEBS Lett 2000; 486:143–148.
74. Halgren RG, Traynor AE, Pillay S, et al. 8Cl-cAMP cytotoxicity in both steroid sensitive and insensitive multiple myeloma cell lines is mediated by 8Cl-adenosine. Blood 1998; 92:2893–2898.
75. Gandhi V, Ayres M, Halgren RG, Krett NL, Newman RA, Rosen ST. 8-chloro-cAMP and 8-chloro-adenosine act by the same mechanism in multiple myeloma cells. Cancer Res 2001; 61:5474–5479.
76. Portier M, Moles J-P, Mazars G-R, et al. p53 and RAS gene mutations in multiple myeloma. Oncogene 1992; 7:2539–2543.
77. Corradini P, Ladetto M, Inghirami G, Boccadoro M, Pileri A. N- and K-Ras oncogenes in plasma cell dyscrasias. Leuk and Lymph 1994; 15:17–20.
78. Liu P, Leong T, Quam L, et al. Activating mutations of N- and K-ras in multiple myeloma show different clinical associations: analysis of the Eastern Cooperative Oncology Group phase III trial. Blood 1996; 88:2699–2706.
79. Kato K, Cox AD, Hisaka MM, Graham SM, Buss JE, Der CJ. Isoprenoid addition to Ras protein is the critical modification for its membrane association and transforming activity. Proc Natl Acad Sci U S A 1992; 89:6403–6407.
80. Sebti SM, Hamilton AD. Inhibition of Ras prenylation: a novel approach to cancer chemotherapy. Pharmacol Ther 1997; 74:103–114.

81. Bolick SC, Landowski TH, Boulware D, et al. The farnesyl transferase inhibitor, FTI-277, inhibits growth and induces apoptosis in drug-resistant myeloma tumor cells. Leukemia 2003; 17:451–457.
82. Shi Y, Gera J, Hsu JH, Van Ness B, Lichtenstein A. Cytoreductive effects of farnesyl transferase inhibitors on multiple myeloma tumor cells. Mol Cancer Ther 2003; 2:563–572.
83. Alsina M, Fonseca R, Wilson EF, et al. Farnesyl transferase inhibitor Zarnestra is well tolerated, induces stabilization of disease and inhibits farnesylation and oncogenic tumor survival pathways in patients with advanced multiple myeloma. Blood, DOI 2004 Jan 15 (published on-line).
84. Cortes J, Albitar M, Thomas D, et al. Efficacy of the farnesyl transferase inhibitor R115777 in chronic myeloid leukemia and other hematologic malignancies. Blood 2003; 101:1692–1697.
85. Lerner EC, Qian Y, Blaskovich MA, et al. Ras CAAX peptidomimetic FTI-277 selectively blocks oncogenic Ras signaling by inducing cytoplasmic accumulation of inactive Ras-Raf complexes. J Biol Chem 1995; 270:26802–26806.
86. Prendergast GC, Rane N. Farnesyltransferase inhibitors: mechanism and applications. Expert Opin Invest Drugs 2001; 10:2105–2116.
87. Sebti S, Hamilton AD. Inhibitors of prenyl transferases. Curr Opin Oncol 1997; 9:557–561.
87a. Luckman SP, Hughes DE, Coxon FP, Graham R, Russell G, Rogers MJ. Nitrogen-containing bisphosphonates inhibit the mevalonate pathway and prevent post-translational prenylation of GTP-binding proteins, including Ras. J Bone Min Res 1998; 13:4:581–589.
87b. Shipman CM, Croucher PI, Russell RGG, Helfrich MH, Rogers MJ. The bisphosphonate incadronate (YM175) causes apoptosis of human myeloma cells in vitro by inhibiting the mevalonate pathway. Cancer Res 1998; 58:5294–5297.
87c. van de Donk NWCJ, Kamphuis MMJ, van Kessel B, Lokhorst HM, Bloem AC. Inhibition of protein geranylgeranylation induces apoptosis in myeloma plasma cells by reducing Mcl-1 protein levels. Blood 2003; 102:9:3354–3362.
87d. Walmsley MJ, Ooi SKT, Reynolds LF, et al. Cirtical roles for Rac1 and Rac2 GTPases in B cell development and signaling. Science 2003; 302:459–462.
87e. Joyce PL, Cox AD. Rac1 and Rac3 are targets for geranylgeranyltransferase I inhibitor-mediated inhibition of signaling, transformation, and membrane ruffling. Cancer Res 2003; 63:7959–7967.
88. Suematsu S, Matsusaka T, Matsuda T, et al. Generation of plasmacytomas with the chromosomal translocation t(12;15) in interleukin 6 transgenic mice. Proc Natl Acad Sci U S A 1992; 89:232–235.
89. Bataille R, Barlogie B, Lu ZY, et al. Biologic effects of anti-interleukin-6 murine monoclonal antibody in advanced multiple myeloma. Blood 1995; 86:685–691.
90. Lu ZY, Brailly H, Wijdenes J, Bataille R, Rossi JF, Klein B. Measurement of whole body interleukin-6 (IL-6) production: prediction of the efficacy of anti-IL-6 treatments. Blood 1995; 86:3123–3131.
91. Hirata T, Shimazaki C, Sumikuma T, et al. Humanized anti-interleukin-6 receptor monoclonal antibody induced apoptosis of fresh and cloned human myeloma cells in vitro. Leuk Res 2003; 27:343–349.
92. Savino R, Lahm.A., Salvati AL, et al. Generation of interleukin-6 receptor antagonists by molecular-modeling guided mutagenesis of residues important for gp130 activation. EMBO J 1994; 13:1357–1367.
93. Sporeno E, Savino R, Ciapponi L, et al. Human interleukin-6 receptor super-antagonists with high potency and wide spectrum on multiple myeloma cells. Blood 1996; 87:4510–4519.
94. Honemann D, Chatterjee M, Savino R, et al. The IL-6 receptor antagonist SANT-7 overcomes bone marrow stromal cell-mediated drug resistance of multiple myeloma cells. Int J Cancer 2001; 93:674–680.

95. Tassone P, Galea E, Forciniti S, Tagliaferri P, Venuta S. The IL-6 receptor super-antagonist Sant7 enhances antiproliferative and apoptotic effects induced by dexamethasone and zoledronic acid on multiple myeloma cells. Int J Oncol 2002; 21:867–873.

96. Tassone P, Forciniti S, Galea E, et al. Synergistic induction of growth arrest and apoptosis of human myeloma cells by the IL-6 super-antagonist Sant7 and Dexamethasone. Cell Death Differ 2000; 7:327–328.

96a. Lacy MQ, Donovan KA, Heimbach JK, Ahmann GJ, Lust JA. Comparison of interleukin-1β expression by in situ hybridization in monoclonal gammopathy of undetermined significance and multiple myeloma. Blood 1999; 93:1:300–305.

97. Akira S, Nishio Y, Inoue M, et al. Molecular cloning of APRF, a novel IFN-stimulated gene factor 3 p91-related transcription factor involved in the gp130-mediated signaling pathway. Cell 1994; 77:63–71.

98. Darnell JE. STATs and gene regulation. Science 1997; 277:1630–1635.

99. Catlett-Falcone R, Landowski TH, Oshiro MM, et al. Constitutive activation of Stat3 signaling confers resistance to apoptosis in human U266 myeloma cells. Immunity 1999; 10:105–115.

100. Oshiro MM, Landowski TH, Catlett-Falcone R, et al. Inhibition of JAK kinase activity enhances Fas-mediated apoptosis but reduces cytotoxic activity of topoisomerase II inhibitors in U266 myeloma cells. Clin Cancer Res 2001; 7:4262–4271.

101. Hallek M, Bergsagel PL, Anderson KC. Multiple myeloma: increasing evidence for a multistep transformation process. Blood 1998; 91:3–21.

102. Reed JC. Bcl-2 family proteins: regulators of apoptosis and chemoresistance in hematologic malignancies. Semin Hematol 1997; 34(4 suppl 5):9–19.

103. Strasser A, Huang DCS, Vaux DL. The role of the bcl-2/ced-9 gene family in cancer and general implications of defects in cell death control for tumourigenesis and resistance to chemotherapy. Biochim Biophys Acta 1997; 1333:F151–F178.

104. Pettersson M, Jernberg-Wiklund H, Larsson LG, et al. Expression of the bcl-2 gene in human multiple myeloma cell lines and normal plasma cells. Blood 1992; 79:495–502.

105. Harada N, Hata H, Yoshida M, et al. Expression of Bcl-2 family of proteins in fresh myeloma cells. Leukemia 1998;. 12:1817–1820.

106. Hamilton MS, Barker HF, Ball J, Drew M, Abbot SD, Franklin IM. Normal and neoplastic human plasma cells express bcl-2 antigen. Leukemia 1999; 9:768–771.

107. Nishida K, Taniwaki M, Misawa S, Abe T. Nonrandom rearrangement of chromosome 14 at band q32.33 in human lymphoid malignancies with mature B-cell phenotype. Cancer Res 1989; 49:1275–1281.

108. Galderisi U, Cascino A, Giordano A. Antisense oligonucleotides as therapeutic agents. J Cell Physiol 1999; 181:251–257.

109. Tamm I, Dorken B, Hartmann G. Antisense therapy in oncology: new hope for an old idea? Lancet 2001; 358:489–497.

110. Waters JS, Webb A, Cunningham D, et al. Phase I clinical and pharmacokinetic study of bcl-2 antisense oligonucleotide therapy in patients with non-Hodgkin's lymphoma. J Clin Oncol 2000; 18:1812–1823.

111. Ramachandran C, Wellham LL. Effect of MDR1 phosphorothioate antisense oligodeoxynucleotides in multidrug-resistant human tumor cell lines and xenografts. Anticancer Res 2003; 23:2681–2690.

112. Nieth C, Priebsch A, Stege A, Lage H. Modulation of the classical multidrug resistance (MDR) phenotype by RNA interference (RNAi). FEBS Lett 2003; 545:144–150.

113. Wu H, Hait WN, Yang JM. Small interfering RNA-induced suppression of MDR1 (P-glycoprotein) restores sensitivity to multidrug-resistant cancer cells. Cancer Res 2003; 63:1515–1519.

114. Collis SJ, Swartz MJ, Nelson WG, DeWeese TL. Enhanced radiation and chemotherapy-mediated cell killing of human cancer cells by small inhibitory RNA silencing of DNA repair factors. Cancer Res 2003; 63:1550–1554.
115. Adams J. Proteasome inhibition in cancer: development of PS-341. Semin Oncol 2001; 28:613–619.
116. Teicher BA, Ara G, Herbst R, Palombella VJ, Adams J. The proteasome inhibitor PS-341 in cancer therapy. Clin Cancer Res 1999; 5:2638–2645.
117. Adams J, Behnke M, Chen S, et al. Potent and selective inhibitors of the proteasome: dipeptidyl boronic acids. Bioorg Med Chem Lett 1998; 8:333–338.
118. Dalton WS, Durie BGM, Alberts DS, Gerlach JH, Cress AE. Characterization of a new drug resistant human myeloma cell line that expresses P-glycoprotein. Cancer Res 1986; 46:5125–5130.
119. Bellamy WT, Dalton WS, Gleason MC, Grogan TM, Trent JM. Development and characterization of a melphalan resistant human multiple myeloma cell line. Cancer Res 1992; 51:995–1002.
120. Damiano JS, Dalton WS. Integrin-mediated drug resistance in multiple myeloma. Leuk and Lymph 2000; 38:71–81.
121. Berenson JR, Ma HM, Vescio R. The role of nuclear factor-kappaB in the biology and treatment of multiple myeloma. Semin Oncol 2001; 28:626–633.
122. Cusack JC Jr, Liu R, Houston M, et al. Enhanced chemosensitivity to CPT-11 with proteasome inhibitor PS-341: implications for systemic nuclear factor-kappaB inhibition. Cancer Res 2001; 61:3535–3540.
123. Hideshima T, Richardson P, Chauhan D, et al. The proteasome inhibitor PS-341 inhibits growth, induces apoptosis, and overcomes drug resistance in human multiple myeloma cells. Cancer Res 2001; 61:3071–3076.
124. Frankel A, Man S, Elliott PJ, Adams J, Kerbel RS. Lack of multicellular drug resistance observed in human ovarian and prostate carcinoma treated with the proteasome inhibitor PS-341'. Clin Cancer Res 2000; 6:3719–3928.
125. Richardson PG, Barlogie B, Berenson J, et al. A phase 2 study of bortezomib in relapsed, refractory myeloma. N Engl J Med 2003; 348:2609–2617.
125a. van de Donk NWCJ, Kamphuis MMJ, van Kessel B, Lokhorst HM, Bloem AC. Inhibition of protein geranylgeranylation induces apoptosis in myeloma plasma cells by reducing Mcl-1 protein levels. Blood 2003; 102:9:3354–3362.
125b. Shipman CM, Croucher PI, Russell RGG, Helfrich MH, Rogers MJ. The bisphosphonate incadronate (YM175) causes apoptosis of human myeloma cells in vitro by inhibiting the mevalonate pathway. Cancer Res 1998; 58:5294–5297.
126. Folkman J. Angiogenesis in cancer, vascular, rheumatoid and other disease. Nat Med 1995; 1:27–31.
127. Bellamy WT, Richter L, Frutiger Y, Grogan TM. Expression of vascular endothelial growth factor and its receptors in hematopoietic malignancies. Cancer Res 1999; 59:728–733.
128. O'Reilly MS, Holmgren L, Chen C, Folkman J. Angiostatin induces and sustains dormancy of human primary tumors in mice. Nat Med 1996; 2:689–692.
129. O'Reilly MS, Holmgren L, Shing Y, et al. Angiostatin: a circulating endothelial cell inhibitor that suppresses angiogenesis and tumor growth. Cold Spring Harb Symp Quant Biol 1994; 59:471–482.
130. Singhal S, Mehta J. Thalidomide in cancer. Biomed Pharmacother 2002; 56:4–12.
131. Stephens TD, Bunde CJ, Fillmore BJ. Mechanism of action in thalidomide teratogenesis. Biochem Pharmacol 2000; 59:1489–1499.
132. Stephens TD, Fillmore BJ. Hypothesis: thalidomide embryopathy-proposed mechanism of action. Teratology 2000; 61:189–195.
133. Mitsiades N, Mitsiades CS, Poulaki V, et al. Apoptotic signaling induced by immuno-modulatory thalidomide analogs in human multiple myeloma cells: therapeutic implications. Blood 2002; 99:4525–4530.

134. Singhal S, Mehta J, Desikan R, et al. Antitumor activity of thalidomide in refractory multiple myeloma. N Engl J Med 1999; 341:1565–1571.
135. Barlogie B, Desikan R, Eddlemon P, et al. Extended survival in advanced and refractory multiple myeloma after single-agent thalidomide: identification of prognostic factors in a phase 2 study of 169 patients. Blood 2001; 98:492–494.
136. Juliusson G, Celsing F, Turesson I, Lenhoff S, Adriansson M, Malm C. Frequent good partial remissions from thalidomide including best response ever in patients with advanced refractory and relapsed myeloma. Br J Haematol 2000; 109(1):89–96.
137. Neben K, Moehler T, Benner A, et al. Dose-dependent effect of thalidomide on overall survival in relapsed multiple myeloma. Clin Cancer Res 2002; 8:3377–3382.
138. Durie BG. Low-dose thalidomide in myeloma: efficacy and biologic significance. Semin Oncol 2002; 29(6 suppl 17):34–38.
139. Cavenagh JD, Oakervee H. Guideline. Thalidomide in multiple myeloma: current status and future prospects. Br J Haematology 2003; 120:18–26.
140. Zangari M, Anaissie E, Barlogie B, et al. Increased risk of deep-vein thrombosis in patients with multiple myeloma receiving thalidomide and chemotherapy. Blood 2001; 98:1614–1615.
141. Zangari M, Siegel E, Barlogie B, et al. Thrombogenic activity of doxorubicin in myeloma patients receiving thalidomide: implications for therapy. Blood 2002; 100:1168–1171.
142. Camba L, Peccatori J, Pescarollo A, Tresoldi M, Corradini P, Bregni M. Thalidomide and thrombosis in patients with multiple myeloma. Haematologica 2001; 86:1108–1109.
143. Cavo M, Zamagni E, Cellini C, et al. Deep-vein thrombosis in patients with multiple myeloma receiving first-line thalidomide-dexamethasone therapy. Blood 2002; 100:2272–2273.
144. Escudier B, Lassau N, Leborgne S, Angevin E, Laplanche A. Thalidomide and venous thrombosis. Ann Intern Med 2002; 136:711.
145. Osman K, Comenzo R, Rajkumar SV. Deep venous thrombosis and thalidomide therapy for multiple myeloma. N Engl J Med 2001; 344:1951–1952.
146. Richardson PG, Schlossman RL, Weller E, et al. Immunomodulatory drug CC-5013 overcomes drug resistance and is well tolerated in patients with relapsed multiple myeloma. Blood 2002; 100:3063-3067.
147. Hideshima T, Chauhan D, Shima Y, et al. Thalidomide and its analogs overcome drug resistance of human multiple myeloma cells to conventional therapy. Blood 2000; 96:2943–2950.
148. Rajkumar SV, Hayman S, Gertz MA, et al. Combination therapy with thalidomide plus dexamethasone for newly diagnosed myeloma. J Clin Oncol 2002; 20:4319–4323.
149. Weber D, Rankin K, Gavino M, Delasalle K, Alexanian R. Thalidomide alone or with dexamethasone for previously untreated multiple myeloma. J Clin Oncol 2003; 21:16–19.
150. Durand RE, Sutherland RM. Effects of intercellular contact on repair of radiation damage. Exp Cell Res 1972; 71:75–80.
151. Verma S, Zhao LJ, Chinnadurai G. Phosphorylation of the pro-apoptotic protein BIK: mapping of phosphorylation sites and effect on apoptosis. J Biol Chem 2001; 276:4671–4676.
152. Caligaris-Cappio F, Gregoretti MG, Merico F, et al. Bone marrow microenvironment and the progression of multiple myeloma. Leuk Lymphoma 1992; 8:15–22.
153. Shain KH, Landowski TH, Dalton WS. The tumor microenvironment as a determinant of cancer cell survival: a possible mechanism for de novo drug resistance. Curr Opin Oncol 2000; 12:557–563.
154. Clark EA, Brugge JS. Integrins and signal transduction pathways: the road taken. Science 1995; 268:233–239.
155. Hazlehurst LA, Dalton WS. Mechanisms associated with cell adhesion mediated drug resistance (CAM-DR) in hematopoietic malignancies. Cancer Metastasis Rev 2001; 20:43–50.
156. Hazlehurst LA, Damiano JS, Buyuksal I, Pledger WJ, Dalton WS. Adhesion to fibronectin via beta1 integrins regulates p27kip1 levels and contributes to cell adhesion mediated drug resistance (CAM-DR). Oncogene 2000; 19:4319–4327.

157. Hazlehurst LA, Valkov N, Wisner L, et al. Reduction in drug-induced DNA double-strand breaks associated with beta1 integrin-mediated adhesion correlates with drug resistance in U937 cells. Blood 2001; 98:1897–1903.
158. Shain KH, Landowski TH, Dalton WS. Adhesion-mediated intracellular redistribution of c-Fas-associated death domain-like IL-1-converting enzyme-like inhibitory protein-long confers resistance to CD95-induced apoptosis in hematopoietic cancer cell lines. J Immunol 2002; 168:2544–2553.
159. Landowski TH, Olashaw NE, Agrawal D, Dalton WS. Cell adhesion-mediated drug resistance (CAM-DR) is associated with activation of NF-kappa B (RelB/p50) in myeloma cells. Oncogene 2003; 22:2417–2421.
160. Damiano JS. Integrins as novel drug targets for overcoming innate drug resistance. Curr Cancer Drug Targets 2002; 2:37–43.
161. Nefedova Y, Landowski TH, Dalton WS. Bone marrow stromal-derived soluble factors and direct cell contact contribute to de novo drug resistance of myeloma cells by distinct mechanisms. Leukemia 2003; 17:1175–1182.
162. Cheung WC, Van Ness B. The bone marrow stromal microenvironment influences myeloma therapeutic response in vitro. Leukemia 2001; 15:264–271.
163. Chauhan D, Anderson KC. Mechanisms of cell death and survival in multiple myeloma (MM): therapeutic implications. Apoptosis 2003; 8:337–343.
164. Yanovich S, Hall RE, Weinert C. Resistance to natural killer cell-mediated cytolysis by a pleiotropic drug-resistant human erythroleukemia (K562-R) cell line. Cancer Res 1986; 46:4511–4515.
165. Kimmig A, Gekeler V, Neumann M, et al. Susceptibility of multi-drug-resistant human leukemia cell lines to human interleukin-2 activated killer cells. Cancer Res 1990; 50:6793–6799.
166. Landowski TH, Gleason-Guzman MC, Dalton WS. Selection for drug resistance results in resistance to Fas mediated apoptosis. Blood 1997; 89:1180–1187.
167. Scheper RJ, Dalton WS, Grogan TM, et al. Altered expression of P-glycoprotein and cellular adhesion molecules on human multi-drug-resistant tumor cells does not affect their susceptibility to NK- and LAK-mediated cytotoxicity. Int J Cancer 1991; 48:562–567.
168. Shtil AA, Turner JG, Durfee J, Dalton WS, Yu H. Cytokine-based tumor cell vaccine is equally effective against parental and isogenic multidrug-resistant myeloma cells: The role of cytotoxic T lymphocytes. Blood 1999; 93:1831–1837.

Index